WA 220 JAC

J.P. Jackson (Ed.)

A PRACTICAL GUIDE TO MEDICINE AND THE LAW

With a Foreword by The Right Honourable
Kenneth Clarke, QC, MP

Springer-Verlag
London Berlin Heidelberg New York
Paris Tokyo Hong Kong
Barcelona Budapest

J.P. Jackson, MB, FRCS
Emeritus Consultant Surgeon, University of Nottingham, and Emeritus
Consultant Orthopaedic Surgeon, Harlow Wood Orthopaedic Hospital

Saddlers Cottage, The Green, Farnsfield, Newark,
Nottinghamshire, UK

ISBN 3-540-19677-3 Springer-Verlag Berlin Heidelberg New York
ISBN 0-387-19677-3 Springer-Verlag New York Berlin Heidelberg

British Library Cataloguing in Publication Data
A practical guide to medicine and the law.
  I. Jackson, J. P. (John Peter)
  342.441
  ISBN 3-540-19677-3

Library of Congress Cataloging-in-Publication Data
A Practical guide to medicine and the law / J.P. Jackson (ed.).
    p. cm.
  Includes index.
  ISBN 3-540-19677-3 (alk paper). – ISBN 0-387-19677-3 (alk. paper)
  1. Medical jurisprudence. 2. Forensic medicine. I. Jackson, J.P. (John Peter),
  1915- .
  [DNLM: 1. Jurisprudence. 2. Malpractice. W 32.6 P895]
  RA1051,P65 1991
  614' .1–dc20
  DNLM/DLC   91-4879
  for Library of Congress   CIP

© Springer-Verlag London Limited 1991
Printed in Germany

Typeset by Fox Design, Surbiton, Surrey
2128/3830-543210 Printed on acid-free paper

Foreword

From: The Rt. Hon. Kenneth Clarke, QC, MP

HOUSE OF COMMONS
LONDON SW1A 0AA

When I practised at the Bar in the Midlands some years ago, I had quite a large industrial injury and negligence practice. I therefore must have read thousands of medical reports prepared for litigation. I also encountered medical issues in cases quite frequently, and found myself involved in the presentation of the evidence by non-medically qualified advocates to non-medically qualified Judges who had to determine differences of professional opinion between the expert witnesses on each side. When I turned to politics and became a Minister at the Department of Health, I of course experienced, from a different perspective, problems for everyone in the Health Service that arise from the rapid growth of litigation involving medical issues that is now taking place. I am convinced that we are going to see a continuing expansion of these medico-legal problems. There is therefore a growing need for good practical guidance to all who might find themselves involved.

Peter Jackson is a good friend and also a very distinguished orthopaedic surgeon. He has gathered an extremely impressive list of colleagues to produce this new Guide. It is written by consultants and lawyers in a way designed to be of great assistance to those practising Consultants and lawyers who wish to have a useful reference guide. I am also sure that students preparing for both professions will find this an invaluable introduction to the issues that they are bound to encounter in the course of their professional lives when they are advising upon or engaged in potential litigation.

London
January 1991

Preface

Litigation involving doctors has greatly increased during the past decade. This is of two types, the first and perhaps of more immediate interest to doctors arises from negligence claims against them for errors of diagnosis or treatment. The second involves the suing of an employer as the result of alleged negligence involving the health of his employees. Despite the fact that nowadays few doctors can remain aloof from litigation, no appropriate formal teaching is given to most medical students or doctors. Furthermore there is only a limited amount of literature available to which reference may be made. The purpose of this book is to give practical guidance to all who may be involved.

The book is presented in three parts. The first part relates to those problems which may affect the doctor in the examination of patients and the preparation of medical reports. In order not to infringe the rights of the plaintiff, when arranging an appointment or obtaining information from hospital or practitioner's notes, or indeed any other source, knowledge of the problems of confidentiality and consent is required. These aspects do not normally arise in clinical practice and accordingly a chapter has been included on this subject. In addition, the writing of reports is discussed so that the results may give most help to solicitors and the courts.

The second part is devoted to clinical problems. The specialties chosen are those carrying the highest risk of leading to litigation. The authors all have experience in the various medico-legal problems in their subjects, mostly being members of council of the two defence societies. They have been asked to cover the contentious issues that arise most frequently in their specialties. Some of these complaints such as perinatal damage and the viability of the unconscious patient may be primarily related to the negligence of doctors. Other problems such as backache or deafness caused by accidental or industrial negligence are more concerned with damage assessment.

Finally a third part, written by those with legal expertise sets out advice to the doctor on the law, both on the writing of reports, Court attendance and includes a discussion of medical negligence. This will perhaps give some instruction to doctors on the problems that may arise, and occasionally allow them to avoid the dangers of litigation. As a result, earlier and appropriate contact with the medical protection societies may be made.

The hope is that the book will prove useful not only to all students and younger doctors but in addition to some of their older colleagues for reference. The second and largest part should also be of interest to many of the legal profession who, often with limited medical knowledge, have to deal with the conditions discussed. General Practitioners also should find much helpful information in this section. Many of them may well be approached by their patients for advice on whether or not there has been negligence in the handling of their case at the hospital. The advice given, may well determine whether or not there are reasonable grounds for litigation.

Finally, following the reorganisation of the National Health Service, Practitioners may well wish to undertake a number of minor procedures of a surgical nature, which would previously have been referred to hospital. The clinical part gives some guidance in the snags which may be encountered and how to avoid them. There may as a result be an increase in negligence claims. Hopefully much of this will be avoided.

March 1991   J.P. Jackson

Contents

PART II: THE MOST CONTENTIOUS PROBLEMS IN THE
HIGH-RISK SPECIALITIES

4 Anaesthesia

5 General Surgery

13 Paediatrics

14 Psychiatry

Part III: LEGAL ADVICE FOR DOCTORS INVOLVED WITH
MEDICO-LEGAL PROBLEMS

Contributors

Prof. A. R. Aitkenhead, BSc, MD, FFARCS*
Professor of Anaesthesia, Department of Anaesthesia, University
Hospital, Queens Medical Centre, Nottingham NG7 2UH, UK

Mr. K.P. Gibbin, FRCS
Consultant Otolaryngologist, Department of Otolaryngology, B Floor,
West Block, University Hospital, Nottingham NG7 2UH, UK

Dr. R.B. Godwin-Austen, MD, FRCP
Consultant Neurologist, Department of Neurology, C Floor, Queen's
Medical Centre, Nottingham NG7 2UH, UK

Dr. G.L. Harrison, MD, MRCPsych
Consultant Psychiatrist, Academic Department of Psychiatry,
University Hospital, Nottingham NG7 2UH, UK

Prof. D. Hull, BSc, FRCP, DCH*
Professor of Child Health, Department of Child Health, E Floor, East
Block, University Hospital, Nottingham NG7 2UH, UK

Mr. J.P. Jackson, MB, FRCS
Emeritus Orthopaedic Surgeon, Clinical Teacher, University of
Nottingham. Saddlers Cottage, The Green, Farnsfield, Newark, Notts.
NG22 8HF, UK

Mr. N. Keddie, BM, BCh, FRCS, FRCS (Ed)*
Consultant Surgeon, Hon. Clin. Lecturer, Manchester and Newcastle
Universities. White Spar, Bridekirk, Cockermouth, Cumbria CA13
OPE, UK

Prof. B. Knight, MD, MRCP, FRC(Path), DMJ(Path), Barrister*
Professor of Forensic Pathology and Home Office Pathologist, Wales
Institute of Forensic Medicine, University of Wales, College of
Medicine, Royal Infirmary, Cardiff CF2 1SZ, UK

Mr. R. Maxwell, QC,
24 The Ropewalk, Nottingham NG1 5EF, UK

Dr. R.N. Palmer, LLB, MB, MRCS
Secretary, The Medical Protection Society, 50 Hallam Street, London
W1N 6GE, UK

Mr. J. Punt, FRCS
Consultant Neurosurgeon, Department of Neurosurgery, C Floor,
Queen's Medical Centre, Nottingham NG7 2UH, UK

Mr. G.C. Reed, Solicitor
Browne Jacobson, 44 Castle Gate, Nottingham NG1 6EA, UK

Dr. K.V. Sanderson, MB, BS, FRCP, FRACP
Hon. Consulting Dermatologist, St Georges Hospital, The Lizard, 49
Cuckfield Road, Anstey, Sussex RH17 5AG, UK

Mr. J.H.S. Scott, FRCS
Consultant Orthopaedic Surgeon, Murrayfield Hospital, 122
Corstorphine Road, Edinburgh EH12 6UD, UK

Prof. E.M. Symonds, MD, FRCOG*
Professor of Obstetrics, Department of Obstetrics and Gynaecology,
D Floor, East Block, University Hospital, Nottingham NG7 2UH, UK

---

*Member of Council of the Medical Defence Union

PART 1:

**The Writing of Reports and
Related Problems**

CHAPTER 1

The Medico-legal Consultation

J.P. Jackson

Although examination of patients is essentially the same whether they are seen for medico-legal purposes, or have simply come for advice in a normal consultation, there are certain differences in the way that they are referred and seen. This chapter is therefore concerned with the differences between the two so that problems can be avoided.

Arranging to See Patients

Initiation of the process for seeing patients for the purposes of assessment of medico-legal disability should start with a letter asking for an examination and report. This request usually comes from either a solicitor or an insurance company. Most will be from private firms of solicitors but large organisations such as British Telecom or British Coal utilise their own legal departments. Trade unions may also approach the doctor directly and on occasions smaller firms may need a report which they ask for without employing a solicitor. If the doctor is in doubt as to the standing of the organisation or person making the request, it is as well to make further enquiries, if necessary from their Medical Defence Organisation. There are "insurance assessors" of doubtful integrity. At this stage there is no necessity for the general practitioner to be involved as would be the case if it were a normal clinical consultation.

Whatever the initiating body, reports can only be given with the consent of the person to be examined. This may seem self-evident when the patient is specifically sent an appointment for an examination. On most occasions the appointment is sent direct to the patient and the instructing solicitor will usually make clear whether this is to be done, or request an appointment and take the responsibility of informing the plaintiff. If the report is on behalf of the defendant then permission must be sought through the plaintiff's legal representative. When a report is compiled from previous notes, the same necessity for consent applies.

In those cases in which medical negligence is involved, a briefing letter will also be required from a solicitor. In no case is the doctor under any obligation to see and report on any patient. In a negligence case it may be wiser to refuse if the doctor concerned is a colleague or acquaintance.

The details of the case, so far as they are known to the instructing solicitor, should be stated in the initial briefing letter. On occasion, the process will be initiated by a phone call asking whether the doctor is prepared to carry out the examination and, if so, requesting an appointment. Should the initial approach be by phone, the doctor or secretary should ask that a briefing letter, setting out the details as far as possible, should be forwarded. Until an appropriate letter is received, it is unwise to proceed.

There may well be some difference in the amount of information which is given in the briefing letter, depending on whether the doctor is being employed by the plaintiff or the defendant. Solicitors, representing the latter, may be ignorant of a number of the facts. Indeed there may well be a reluctance on behalf of a plaintiff's solicitors to disclose at this stage some of the details of how the actual accident occurred. If the request is on behalf of the plaintiff no further action need be taken. On rare occasions there may be an objection to the defendant's choice of doctor by either the plaintiff or his solicitor. In this event, no further action need be taken. Most defending solicitors are well aware of the necessity for permission for examination and have already obtained this prior to contacting the doctor.

On occasions the plaintiff may not keep the appointment. If the doctor is satisfied that reasonable time has elapsed after the request has been delivered and there is no good cause for non-attendance, the instructing solicitor should be informed. Further instructions may then be given to the doctor, either immediately or at a later date when enquiries have been made, as to whether a second appointment should be given. In the event that there is no good reason for non-attendance, a modified charge should be made for waste of the doctor's time.

Accompanying Persons

Relatives

In most cases the relationship is close, being either husband or wife. There should be no objection to their presence during either the interview or the clinical examination, provided that the plaintiff requests it. Not all patients may wish to have their spouse present, and in consequence it is wise to obtain permission before admitting them. There should be no difficulty in doing this without causing offence.

If the plaintiff is under age (less than sixteen) a parent or authorised guardian must be present, otherwise the appointment should be cancelled. The reason for cancellation should be explained and the plaintiff told that in all probability a further attendance will be necessary. The patient is told to return at a later date, accompanied by a suitable person. Problems in connection with this are most usual in those who are nearly sixteen, and they often feel rather irritated by this request. Nonetheless there is unlikely to be any difficulty, once it is explained that the examination is purely for legal purposes.

Interpreters

Prior to the appointment the doctor may have been warned that an interpreter will be accompanying the plaintiff. On many occasions the plaintiff appears with a friend or relation who has come for this purpose without prior notice. Unfortunately not all interpreters are of a quality that can be considered reliable. Indeed on occasions the plaintiff may appear to speak and understand English better than the interpreter. The doctor may then have to decide whether or not the facilities are adequate, since it is vital that the plaintiff understands the questions that are put. Furthermore the clinician must comprehend the replies. If not, there should be no hesitation in cancelling the visit and arranging a further attendance with a more suitable person. If during the taking of the history it is apparent that there is a language difficulty, the plaintiff should be asked to return at a later date when arrangements have been made for an interpreter. In a mixed society this is not at all uncommon.

It is essential of course that satisfactory screening facilities for disrobing are available if the interpreter is of the opposite sex. Problems may arise, if the patient has difficulty in co-operating with the physical examination due to lack of understanding. With a little care and patience this can usually be overcome.

Friends

The accompanying person may be simply a friend. Provided the plaintiff wishes them to be present, there would appear to be no reason against it. Where the friend is of the opposite sex, and unrelated in any way, their presence is largely dependent on the views of the examining doctor. If in doubt, it is probably wiser to request that they remain in the waiting room.

Solicitors

Rarely, there is a request for the patient's solicitor to be present. Once more, there seems no reason to refuse admission though it might be wise to inform the briefing solicitor if the examination is being carried out for the opposite side.

It should be made clear from the outset to all accompanying persons that no interruptions should be allowed, unless asked for by the examining doctor. In the case of a minor, help from the parent or guardian may be very necessary should the plaintiff be too young to give an adequate history. If, in the opinion of the doctor the plaintiff is of an age to speak for him or herself, then they should be encouraged to do so, as far as possible, even if further help is subsequently required. In any event, at the end of the history taking, it is wise to ask the relative or friend (if an interested party) whether they wish to add anything. Whatever they do say, should be noted, but it is not necessary to include it in the subsequent report unless it is informative.

Most doctors will be well aware of the necessity for chaperones when seeing patients of the opposite sex. They will, however, have managed perfectly well without them in most cases in their normal clinical practice, since it is not always convenient or possible to have one present. Medico-legal work does however produce rather more patients with a functional or hysterical component and it is wise to have someone at hand who can act in this capacity if necessary. During the taking of the history, the attitude of the plaintiff, which can at times be very aggressive, may suggest that it would be sensible to have the support of a chaperone during the clinical examination. Unfortunately it is often only with hindsight that the doctor may feel that it would have been wiser to have had a third person present, if only as a witness.

The presence of a third person should be recorded in the notes and subsequently in the report. At the start of the interview the author has found it advisable to explain to the relative or friend that the purpose of the examination is medico-legal and they should not speak unless requested. Despite this warning, on occasions, there may be constant interruptions which may make it difficult to obtain a fair view of the plaintiff's history. If they do not cease, the person should be asked to leave the room. In the author's experience this is a very unusual occurrence.

The Consultation

Prior to the start of the history taking, details of the patient, including name, address and date of birth, should be checked. An explanation of the reason for the consultation should be given, stating that it is on behalf of the solicitors or insurance company who have sent the briefing letter. With some plaintiffs, who are perhaps a little confused as to whether the examination is on their behalf or the defendants, it is as well to make this point clear. The author also explains to the plaintiff that this is a medico-legal examination and that this differs in some respects from a normal clinical consultation.

It should be added that the report has been requested by, and is private to, the briefing solicitors. Occasionally patients are a little upset by this and it may help to tell them that a copy may be made available to them in due course through their own solicitors. If the examination has been requested by their own legal advisors, then there can be no harm in any discussion unless the doctor feels that the claim is ill-advised and likely to fail, when it is better to include this in a covering note with the report. The solicitor can then judge for himself how best to advise his client. The possibility of a further opinion from another doctor may be considered, which may be more favourable to his client. If during the examination, some condition is discovered that the examiner feels should be treated urgently, possibly even life-threatening, then the correct course is to advise the patient to contact his own practitioner. A letter can be sent to the plaintiff's doctor explaining the situation. If it is considered urgent enough, contact by phone should be made. Any comments to the plaintiff, if it is found that there is something which has been overlooked by the patient's medical advisors, should be made with discretion. Also nothing should be said which reflects on their treatment.

The History

As in clinical medicine a good history is essential. Details may be even more important in medico-legal work, since often they may indicate whether a negligence claim against either an employer or doctor will succeed. Moreover the mechanism of the "accident" may well help in an assessment of the injuries suffered by the plaintiff and their subsequent course. In a few cases, however, some solicitors advise their clients not to discuss the history of the accident with the doctor, particularly if the examination is on behalf of the defendants. Presumably it is thought that they might prejudice their case, the more so if the account differs from that given in the statement of claim. Unfortunately this may in some cases make it more difficult to give a balanced opinion on the causation of the plaintiff's condition. There is nothing to be gained by arguing with the plaintiff, who is only carrying out instructions from his advising solicitor. The fact that these details have not been disclosed should be noted and recorded in the subsequent report. Should the case eventually go to court, more often than not the judge may well comment unfavourably on this point, and the author has been in court when damages have been reduced for this reason.

Often, the first time that the plaintiff is seen by the examining doctor may be a very long time after the precipitating accident, even some years, and in consequence the memory may be clouded. Although a good description should be obtained if possible, it is neither wise nor necessary to cross-examine the plaintiff at great length. A description may already have been given to the solicitor at a much earlier date and badgering the plaintiff is likely to produce resentment which in the long run may result in a less satisfactory report. It should also be remembered that the plaintiff is almost certainly rather nervous and, if being examined on behalf of the defendants, possibly a little hostile. In those accidents which involve intra-cranial damage the patient's recollection may well be blurred. Establishing the length of pre-accident amnesia can be difficult and the answers may vary from time to time.

A number of the questions may often appear irrelevant to the plaintiff, particularly relating to the past history. The information, although unrelated to the condition under discussion, may be of importance to the patient's ability to work. For instance, although the complaint may be of backache, work may be impossible because of hypertension or deafness. Plaintiffs may on occasion be unwilling to answer any questions relating to other problems and the doctor can only explain their relevance and hope that a reply will be forthcoming. On one consultation the author had a patient who refused even to state his complaints, he said that that was for the examining doctor to find out! Fortunately such patients are rare.

Enquiry should be made into the injuries or disabilities suffered by the plaintiff. Not infrequently claims may be made of symptoms which are subsequently shown to be unfounded or unrelated to the accident in question. Nonetheless these claims should be recorded since they may make it clear why the claim, particularly in negligence cases, has been brought. Unfortunately, although not qualified to do so, persons other than the doctor may already have proffered much advise and information. Thus, a nurse may incorrectly inform a patient that a fracture has occurred. Indeed junior doctors, who have an unenviable responsibility in Casualty Departments, may also be guilty of incorrect reading of radiographs, either declaring them normal or misinterpreting artefacts as fractures. The patient may be left with the impression that the injury is more serious than is the case. Convincing a plaintiff that there was no fracture may be difficult or even impossible at a date considerably removed from the initial injury. There is nothing to be gained by arguing and this is information which should be confined to the report. Disputes of this sort about the diagnosis can easily lead to medico-legal problems. The examining doctor has the aid of hindsight, not only assisted by the passage of time but also not infrequently by the hospital notes.

The history of any operations or other major treatment needs to be enquired into, though often patients can mislead the examining doctor since they are often unclear as to what operation was carried out and the reasons for it. Clearly these are facts which can later be checked from the notes, but it is important to have the patient's viewpoint. A careful record of the subsequent management of the case should be made. There are often discrepancies between the version given by the plaintiff and that written in the notes. The date of return to work must be requested. Not infrequently there will be a significant difference between the date of a patient's discharge from hospital as fit for work and their eventual signing off by the general practitioner. The latter is often exposed to pressure from the patient; a situation which is not found in hospital practice. Consequently the date of discharge from hospital is in most cases a better guide to the state of the patient's health, although, of course, there may be other factors preventing an early return to work of which the hospital consultant is unaware. For example, the plaintiff who has been discharged from the hospital with a fracture may be suffering from raised blood pressure; there may be in addition some domestic problem which the practitioner needs to take into account.

Past History

Careful enquiry must be made into any previous illnesses or accidents since these may well affect the damages that are awarded. There may be continuing problems which render the plaintiff more vulnerable to further episodes, such as previous back trouble. There may indeed have already been a change of occupation, prior to the incident under discussion, as a result of some previous illness or accident.

Social History

Some knowledge of the plaintiff's background will make it easier to assess the effect of a disability on capacity for work. It is also necessary to enquire into the family status for the same reason. Is the plaintiff married and is their spouse working? Are there any children and of what age? Any sporting and leisure activities are important, since the opinion should extend to the effect that disability may have on them.

Occupation

Enquiry into this aspect must be in some depth since the award of damages will largely turn on the plaintiff's ability to return to work or to a suitable alternative. The type of work will need to be considered in relation to the disability. Is it sedentary? Does it involve any lifting and if so with what frequency and how heavy are the loads? Is there any help? Is there any stair or ladder work? Enquiry as to whether the plaintiff feels equal to the work should be made. The doctor may not always be in agreement with the plaintiff on this point!

Examination

This must of necessity begin as soon as the plaintiff enters the room. A proportion of patients will tend to exaggerate their complaints. This may be due to a quite human desire to make sure that the doctor understands their disability, but unfortunately a small proportion are influenced by the fact that money is involved. True malingering is fortunately rarely encountered (see Chap. 12). In legal practice, however, financial gain undoubtedly affects the presentation of many patients. This may take the form of conscious exaggeration so that relatively minor complaints are made to appear more severe. Only rarely are the plaintiff's claims totally baseless. Since a majority of complaints are subjective, it may be difficult at first sight to evaluate their genuineness. For this reason all the activities that the plaintiff carries out when not actually submitting to formal examination are important. How does the plaintiff walk as he enters the room? How does he sit? How does he undress and dress? All the movements that are carried out in the consulting room need to be assessed. Patients who sit quite comfortably leaning forwards may a few minutes later when lying on a couch, actively resist hip flexion of more than twenty or thirty degrees. Even this amount may be accompanied by groans and grimacing. Apart from assessing rather more critically the total presentation of the plaintiff, there is really no difference from a normal clinical examination. Some clues as to the genuineness of a plaintiff may be gained indirectly from the state of the musculature, the presence of callousing of the hands in a patient who denies having done any labouring for the past few years. The callousing of the feet may indicate considerable activity in someone who states that they have only walked short distances of no more than a few hundred yards in the past year or so.

There are a number of ways in which a patient may be shown to be exaggerating their difficulties. A plaintiff may be unwilling to demonstrate full neck movement but an enquiry whether the scar on the outer side of the arm is due to vaccination may be followed by extreme rotation in a patient who has previously been unable to rotate the neck more than a few degrees. Patients with backache will often complain of pain when the examiner requests rotation of the spine at the same time as the pelvis is rotated manually by the examiner's hands so that in effect no rotation of the lumbar spine is produced. There are in addition other "inappropriate" signs which can be used to distinguish the functional from the physical. Account should be taken of the fact that most patients are nervous and may not therefore react in a normal manner. With experience the doctor is likely to acquire skill in deciding how genuine is the patient's reaction.

The result of the above problems means that more significance must be given to objective evidence than is perhaps usual in normal clinical medicine. Consequently measurement is required so far as is possible in recording all physical signs. Attempts should be made to record as accurately as possible limb measurements, ranges of joint movement and dimensions of any scarring.

Further Investigations

Most cases in whom a report has been requested are not patients of the examining doctor. Requests for further tests should therefore be approached with some caution. In many cases radiographs are required. Whilst theoretically permission should be obtained for these both from the patient and the plaintiff's solicitor, it is rarely that there is any objection to plain films being arranged. In those procedures in which there is an element of intrusion such as a radiculo-gram it would be unwise to proceed. Should they be thought necessary, all that can be done is to make a recommendation in the subsequent report that in the opinion of the examiner the investigation would be of value. Blood tests may be requested from a suitable pathologist but their necessity must be explained to the plaintiff and done with his or her express permission. Before embarking on these investigations it is as well to ask the plaintiff whether they have previously been done. If so, then an attempt must be made to obtain them and only if they are unavailable for some reason should they be arranged with the permission of the patient. For instance the X-ray films could have been lost; a not uncommon event with some filing systems. Photographs will often help to record deformity and scarring. These can be arranged without reference to anyone else, but again the plaintiff's permission is required. If considerable expense is involved the solicitors should be approached first.

Finally, on no account should the findings be discussed with the plaintiff if the report has been requested by the defendants. Whilst patients will frequently ask questions at the end of the examination it is rare for there to be any difficulty once it has been explained that the report has been requested by, and is private to, the defendant's solicitor.

CHAPTER 2

Medico-legal Reports

J.P. Jackson

Much of the advice in this chapter will be common knowledge to most doctors who have had to write reports, but hopefully the information will aid those just embarking on a medical career, and possibly more senior personnel will find something of interest. The purpose of a medico-legal report is to convey to legal advisors the effect that the plaintiff's medical condition has had, and will continue to have, on his or her daily life. While much of the report will consist of a factual account of the physical condition, perhaps the greater and more important part will relate to the opinion of the doctor on the impact of disability on the plaintiff's capacity for work and social and family life. In order that the value of the report may be assessed, it follows that details of the doctor's qualifications and experience should be available to those making the judgement. The opinions expressed by the doctor should be non-partisan. Firms of solicitors engaged in medico-legal work are aware of this and of the necessity to avoid bringing any pressure to bear on the doctor; in the unlikely event that they do so, it should be ignored. Fortunately, and notwithstanding an increase in litigation in the past few years, the great majority of claims are still settled by direct negotiation and only a very small percentage are contested in court. Those claims that do in fact end in court will be used as a yardstick by which other claims will be settled. It should be remembered that any opinions expressed in a report may have to be justified in the courts.

Information gained during the consultation should have been recorded during the interview and examination. Although it is time consuming, there is much to be said for the initial notes to be handwritten. This allows more time to be taken, and hopefully results in greater accuracy. The greatest criticism of notes in longhand, especially those written by doctors, is that they are illegible. Except for those doctors who are consistently unable to decipher their own writing, however, this should be the normal method. Only rarely are the notes read by a third person but on infrequent occasions the judge may wish to see them in court. The practice of seeing a patient and subsequently dictating a report without any written notes is to be deprecated as it is in this way vital points may be overlooked.

Before writing the report, particularly if it is to be dictated, as most are, a short time spent in noting the salient points in longhand is worthwhile. This practice will ensure that the major points are not missed; something that is all too easy to do, particularly if the doctor is not practised in dictation.

Furthermore, there is much to be said for dictating the report as soon as possible after examining the plaintiff. If this is done the same day, it is much easier to colour the report with the overriding impressions of the examination whilst they are still fresh in the memory.

Obtaining Additional Information

The plaintiff's contribution may be supplemented from various sources: hospital notes, practitioner's notes, various accounts from the Departments of Health and Social Security and from the plaintiff's workplace. Note should be made of the date on which these records are obtained. The availability of this information should be recorded in the report so that anyone reading it will be able to judge the authenticity of the record. Frequently these records will be available to the doctor at the time of the consultation. More often they may not be obtained until a later date, often considerably later.

There are a number of problems in gaining access to the various sources of information. Firstly, it will be necessary to obtain the patient's permission even if acting on behalf of the plaintiff. This can be conveniently done by use of a suitable form, such as that illustrated in Fig.2.1. Secondly, some practitioners, when requested, will only send the notes relating to the accident in question. Much of the previous history may be of importance to the investigation, either of other diseases or indeed in direct relation to the condition under discussion. For example, a plaintiff who is suing for compensation for a back injury may neglect to inform the examiner that he has had previous attacks, despite a leading question. This may of course be either deliberate or purely a lapse of memory. Absence from work may be assumed by the examiner to be a result of the back problem under review, whereas it could well be due, say, to hypertension as recorded in the practitioner's notes.

Some family doctors, not unreasonably, are reluctant to commit their notes to the mail since few, if any, keep a copy. If this is so, they can usually be persuaded to send a photocopy. Perhaps the spread of computers will help in this respect, though one can imagine some of the disasters that may occur with this aid. Occasionally there may be some reluctance until it is made clear that any costs will be met.

Request for notes and radiographs

I give my consent for Mr. Smith, orthopaedic surgeon, of [address] to have access to my hospital notes and radiographs and or General Practitioner's records for medico-legal purposes.

I confirm that it is not my intention to take legal action against the Health Authority or any of its employees.

Fig. 2.1. Standard consent form for obtaining a plaintiff's notes. (The second paragraph may be omitted, but some authorities require its inclusion before the hospital notes will be released.)

Hospital notes are the property of the Health Service and, as such, permission to see them must be sought from the appropriate authority. Some hospitals make a charge for this service, but this is not uniform. Although the notes have been written or dictated by a hospital doctor, in most cases there is a blanket agreement to release them without permission being sought from the appropriate consultant. Notes made privately are obtained by direct request to the doctor concerned. Most hospitals require written assurance that no action is contemplated against the Health Authority. In cases of negligence some hospitals can be extremely reluctant to part with the notes, though it is difficult to see what purpose this serves. Indeed, the only effect may be to suggest that there is something to hide.

Should there be difficulty in obtaining the notes even with the plaintiff's permission, then the matter should be referred back to the briefing solicitor. On rare occasions it may be necessary to obtain a court order for their release. The dates on which any notes are requested, when they are received and when returned should all be noted. An added precaution is to return them "recorded delivery".

Compiling the Report

The First Page

Most reports are written on headed notepaper and in consequence certain facts are apparent. The name of the author, his or her qualifications, address and telephone number should appear across the top of the page. In addition, for the purpose of the report, the specialty of the doctor should be stated, though this can be left to the end and typed in under the signature, with the relevant qualifications. The person or firm to whom the document is being sent should be stated. The date of the accident, the date of examination and the date of the report should all be given. The details of the plaintiff should appear. These will include the date of birth (age may also be given but is not so helpful), the marital state and occupation. The presence of any third parties at the consultation should be noted, stating the reason for their attendance.

The Accident

Details of the accident or precipitating incident should be given as related by the plaintiff. If there was a history of unconsciousness, this will not be possible and the facts as given in the briefing letter or from a third person such as a relative or friend should be stated. In any event the writer should make clear the origin of the facts. Following the initial history, there should be a description of any emergency treatment. Any attempt made by the plaintiff to obtain further help and advice, particularly medical, should be noted and any other action by the plaintiff. In a motor accident, for instance, it would be helpful to know that the plaintiff was fit enough to exchange insurance details. In a small minority of cases the plaintiff will have stated that his or her solicitor has advised against giving any history of the accident. This fact should be recorded. In many cases lack of information will make it more difficult to give an opinion.

Following the immediate care, an account of the subsequent course of any injuries and their treatment should be outlined. Was the patient taken by ambulance to hospital or did they go in someone's car? Were they seen in the Casualty Department or was it necessary to admit them? In many cases no medical treatment was given or sought and possibly advice was not given until some days or weeks had passed. All these facts will help in giving an overall impression of the severity of the accident. Where the accident occurred at the plaintiff's workplace, it will help to know whether the accident was recorded in the works accident book. If the plaintiff was admitted to hospital, the history must then continue, to cover any further treatment such as intensive care, operations, physiotherapy, etc. Any complications, such as a deep vein thrombosis or urinary infection should be recorded. The complications may be considered as a result of the accident and therefore part of the total assessment. Their course and treatment should be briefly set down. The length of stay in hospital and subsequent attendance as an out-patient needs to be recorded. Much of this information will be given by the plaintiff, but there may well be poor recollection of events, particularly since the examination may be taking place months or even years after the precipitating event. Subsequently, many of the facts may be amplified and checked by reference to the hospital and practitioner's notes. These aids may of course be available to the examiner at the time of the dictation of the report. The source should be recorded.

Present Complaints

The present complaints should be set down as given by the plaintiff, as nearly as possible in the same words. Some plaintiffs are very longwinded and some editing may be possible, but caution should be exercised so that no significant complaint is missed or incorrectly recorded. Many patients will include complaints that the examiner feels are unrelated to the accident in question but which should nonetheless be included. The examiner can comment on their relationship to the accident in the later opinion section of the report. Exaggeration of symptoms is a fairly common human trait and allowance may need to be made for this. It is not uncommon to have a patient complain that they were in "agony", when they were able to move quite easily, or that their swollen ankle "was as big as a football", when clearly this would have resulted in skin rupture. These expressions are not necessarily evidence of malingering but may only be hyperbole to convince the examiner that their symptoms were of significance. The exact words should be recorded, though suitable comment may be made in the Opinion.

Past History

All the previous medical history needs to be included, even if some of it might be thought irrelevant. Often vital facts are suppressed by a plaintiff. This may be pure forgetfulness but it is difficult to believe that a patient complaining of backache after an accident has forgotten that they had seen their practitioner for low back pain on numerous occasions over the preceding several years. These facts can be established later by a review of the general practitioner's notes. Occasionally when confronted by this evidence at a later examination the plaintiff may claim that they did not understand the question or that the previous complaint related to a different type of pain. Difficulties may arise because of apprehension, particularly where there are language problems, and allowance may have to be made for these factors.

The Examination

As in any notetaking a general description of the patient should be given. In general, the subsequent remarks will relate largely to the system examined by the specialist who is preparing the report.

So far as is possible all relevant information should be included. Inclusion of such evident problems as a generalised skin rash, deafness or pregnancy would not be inappropriate in an orthopaedic report. Indeed, these might be of some immediate significance in a patient with backache. Whilst they may be included, their description may be superficial. If it is felt that these other symptoms are material but not within the scope of the examining doctor, a recommendation should be given that the plaintiff should be examined by the appropriate specialist.

Negative findings may be just as important as positive signs. All "inappropriate" information should be recorded. For instance, a plaintiff may appear to have difficulty in bending, but minutes later may have no difficulty in bending down to do up shoelaces. Pseudo-rotation of the spine, carried out by the doctor rotating the pelvis at the same time as the lumbar spine, may surprisingly cause just as much complaint from the plaintiff. These investigations are peculiar to each specialty, and are perhaps more necessary to medico-legal examinations when there is a greater need to differentiate functional problems or even frank malingering.

Technical terms should be avoided wherever possible since the report will be read by lay persons, though mostly with experience in reading medical reports. Most solicitors and barristers will find no difficulty in coping with such words as femur and it is not necessary to resort to terms such as thigh bone. On the other hand, villo-nodular synovitis might cause some difficulty and if such a diagnosis is used, it should be qualified by a description. Most medical reports are understood by an intelligent lay person provided common sense is used in their composition.

The Opinion

Based on the examination a diagnosis should be made if possible. This, just as in clinical work, may be difficult, if not impossible. The reasons for arriving at a specific diagnosis should be given. If this is not possible, then the various diagnoses should be considered in turn, with the evidence for and against. The examiner may then continue to discuss whether or not there is any functional overlay or indeed evidence of malingering. This latter may either be partial or complete. Total malingering is fairly rare and its detection will in all probability rest on evidence obtained away from the clinical examination. With the increase in litigation in the past few years employment of enquiry agents has increased. The introduction of the video-camera has made recording the plaintiff's activities much easier. The examining doctor may be asked to comment on these films, particularly in the light of the medical report. On the other hand, a number of plaintiffs may well exaggerate their symptoms in order to increase any financial gain. Whilst there may be inappropriate signs elicited during the examination, it should be borne in mind that most patients are apprehensive and furthermore there is a natural tendency for patients to make the most of their complaints.

Should the examiner feel quite genuinely that there is an element of malingering then there is no reason not to say that this is a possibility. At the same time, reasons should be stated as to the evidence for this diagnosis. A psychiatric opinion may help in this context and the opinion should be expressed that it should be sought. In most cases, however, the evidence of a private enquiry agent will probably be needed to obtain confirmation. There may also be evidence from other witnesses confirming dishonesty on the part of the plaintiff. In the normal course of events this information will not be available to the doctor when the report is composed.

In many cases there may be difficulty in coming to any diagnosis. There is every possibility that at this stage the plaintiff's notes, X-ray films and other investigations may not be available to the examiner. If so, then it is in order to complete the report but state that various tests are not available. Unfortunately if a decision is taken to await their arrival, this may often occasion considerable delay. If it is possible to complete a report that is likely to be of immediate help to the solicitors or insurance company, then this should be done, enclosing a note that a supplementary report will be forwarded at a later date when further material becomes available. As mentioned above, it may be possible to initiate various X-rays and tests but these cannot be requested by a reporting doctor if they are of an intrusive nature, unless they are already under treatment by the examiner. On occasion, it may be necessary to suggest that further examination should be carried out at a later date when it is hoped that further development will allow a diagnosis to be made.

Having as far as possible come to a diagnosis, attention should be turned to assessment of the plaintiff's physical capacity. This will necessitate a view on how far the plaintiff can walk, run or perform such tasks as going up and down ladders, carrying loads or undertaking repetitive movements such as bending. Some actions which are perhaps peculiar to the plaintiff's job can be considered under the heading of employment.

Finally in this section, suggestions as to any further treatment can be made if it is thought that these could be helpful. In general, these should not be discussed with the plaintiff although exceptionally they may be put to the plaintiff in order to see how he or she reacts. Would the plaintiff consider a further operative procedure? Has cosmetic surgery been discussed? Care and sensitivity must be shown in making any remark which might upset the plaintiff. On the rare occasion when the examiner thinks that something has not been appreciated by the plaintiff's doctor or particularly if it is thought there is a life-threatening condition, it is wiser to contact the plaintiff's practitioner preferably by phone. The necessity for this type of intervention is happily rare.

Although all doctors may have considerable skill and experience in assessing the psychological aspect of the patient, there is every reason to suggest a further opinion if there is doubt as to how much the plaintiff is affected in this way.

Occupation

This section of the report is concerned with whether the plaintiff is fit to do his or her job. If so, then comment should follow as to when the plaintiff was fit to do this. Clearly before this opinion can be given, knowledge of the type of work carried out by the plaintiff must be obtained. This will need more than just a label, such as lorry driver or factory worker. Enquiry must be made about the detail of the work. Does the work entail lifting and, if so, how much? How heavy are the objects lifted and what is the frequency of lifting? Can the worker sit or must he or she stand or walk all the time? What distances does the driver have to travel? How heavy is the lorry? Does the job include loading? It is only with a knowledge in depth that the examiner can answer the question of whether the plaintiff can reasonably expect to return to work. If the plaintiff is not able to do the work, is there any suitable light work available? Alternatively if the work is too strenuous, what sort of occupation or type of work would be suitable? In many cases particularly with unskilled workers it may only be possible to indicate that a job not involving heavy lifting or repetitive bending is necessary, with perhaps the added proviso that the plaintiff can sit part of the time or even may need an occupation that is almost completely sedentary.

Sport and Social Activity

In most cases comments in this category can be relatively short. Some plaintiffs, however, may have a considerable amount of activity under this heading. They may, for instance, take part in regular team games, possibly professionally. A number of persons may in addition to their normal work have a part-time job, perhaps as a musician for example. This all needs to be mentioned since it may well affect their compensation.

The special needs of a plaintiff may be noted under this heading. Those plaintiffs with continuing disability may require support such as home help, mobility allowance and other aids. Alterations to the home may be necessary or perhaps the provision of an automatic car to enable the plaintiff to continue in work.

Prognosis

If the plaintiff has already reached an end point this needs to be stated. In many plaintiffs there is every possibility that there may be continuing improvement. If so, how long is it estimated it will be before a stable position is reached? Are there likely to be any complications that might arise in the future? If there are, how will it affect the plaintiff and perhaps more importantly, how will it affect the ability to work? So far as possible, an estimate should be given as to when a complication might occur and what is the likelihood of its occurrence, i.e.

osteoarthritis is likely to occur in 15 to 20 years in some 20 per cent of cases of this nature. This knowledge may in many cases require reference to someone else's work. The reference should be cited.

Finally, it may not be possible to give a very dogmatic report if the plaintiff is still some way from an end point and it is impossible to state with any certainty that, for instance, the fracture will unite or the infection be controlled. In cases such as this, it is reasonable to suggest that another report in 6 or 12 months or whatever length of time seems appropriate might yield a great deal more information.

CHAPTER 3

Consent and Confidentiality

R.N. Palmer

Consent

An unlawful touching of someone may be an assault. An assault can be a crime or a civil offence or both. Most doctor/patient consultations involve some physical contact, if only the taking of a pulse. To avoid legal proceedings, therefore, the patient's consent should be obtained before any examination, procedure or treatment. This chapter of advice attempts to summarise relevant law in England and Wales. The applicable statutory provisions in Scotland and in Northern Ireland vary but the general underlying principles are similar.

The legal principles set out in this chapter apply equally to issues about AIDS and HIV testing and also to consent for minor surgery undertaken by general medical practitioners.

General Principles

There is more to consent than getting a patient's signature on a consent form. In seeking consent the doctor is required to provide sufficient details and information about what is proposed to enable the patient to form a proper decision. Misinformed consent or consent given without proper understanding of what is involved is of little legal value: whilst it might protect against allegations of assault or battery, it would not afford a defence against allegations of inadequate counselling or failure to warn.

The extent of the explanation which the doctor should give when seeking consent will depend on many factors and may pose considerable problems, calling for fine clinical judgement. Factors to be taken into account include the patient's age and maturity, physical and mental state, intellectual capacity, and the reason for the procedure, operation or treatment. For example, a routine

This chapter was originally produced as a booklet prepared for members of The Medical Protection Society by R.N. Palmer, LL.B., M.B., B.S., Barrister, Secretary and Medical Director. Permission for its incorporation in this book has been given by Dr. Palmer and The Medical Protection Society.

cosmetic procedure may need to be discussed far more extensively than an emergency operation for a life-threatening condition in an ill patient. The explanation which the doctor gives will also depend upon the questions the patient asks, some patients requiring to know far more than others about side-effects, complications, etc. A careful and truthful answer must be given to a particular patient's request for information.

There is no requirement in English law that every possible complication and side-effect should be explained to the patient. Recent court cases, however, show a trend by judges to require more detailed explanations to be given than those of a few years ago. Obviously a balance must be struck between telling a patient enough to enable him or her to give a real consent and yet not so much as to frighten them needlessly from agreeing to treatment which is demonstrably essential to his or her well-being. Achieving that balance can be very difficult, even for a practitioner of many years' experience.

In one case (*Sidaway* v. *Governors of Bethlem Royal Hospital and another* [1985] AC 871) decided by the House of Lords in 1985, it was affirmed that a decision about what degree of disclosure of risk is best calculated to assist a particular patient to make a rational choice as to whether or not to undergo a particular treatment must primarily be a matter of clinical judgement. However, if there is a conflict of medical evidence as to whether a responsible body of medical opinion approves of non-disclosure of risk in a particular case, the trial judge would have to resolve that conflict. The doctor must decide what information should be given to the patient and in what terms that information should be couched; but the doctor's discretion is always subject to challenge and to scrutiny by the courts.

Age of Consent

In English law, any person of sound mind who has attained the age of sixteen years may give legally valid consent to surgical, medical or dental treatment or procedures (Section 8, Family Law Reform Act 1969). What has been less clear is whether a person under the age of sixteen can give consent. The Act does not say that he or she may not. In a case which reached the House of Lords in 1984 (*Gillick* v. *West Norfolk and Wisbech Area Health Authority and the Department of Health and Social Security* [1984] AC 112) it was held that, save where statute otherwise provides, a minor's capacity to make his or her own decision depends upon the minor having sufficient understanding and intelligence to make the decision, and is not to be determined by reference to any judicially fixed age-limit. The House of Lords held that, as a matter of law, the parental right to determine whether or not a child below the age of sixteen will have medical treatment terminates if and when the child achieves a sufficient understanding and intelligence to enable him or her to understand fully what is proposed.

The House of Lords held that it will be a question of fact whether a child seeking advice has sufficient understanding of what is involved to give consent valid in law. Until the child achieves the capacity to consent, the parental right to make the decision continues save only in exceptional circumstances.

The application of these legal principles to contraceptive advice is discussed below in the sections on Sterilisation and Contraception. The House of Lords has upheld the opinion, held by many legal authorities for many years, that a minor who is capable of appreciating fully the nature and consequences of a particular operation or of a particular treatment can give an effective consent thereto and in such cases the consent of the parent or guardian is unnecessary. However, where the minor is without that capacity any apparent consent by him or her will be of no legal validity, the sole right to consent being vested in the parent or guardian.

Intimate Samples

Section 62 of the Police and Criminal Evidence Act 1984 gives certain powers to take an intimate sample (i.e. of blood, semen or any other tissue, fluid, urine, saliva or pubic hair or a swab from a body orifice) from a person in police detention if appropriate consent is given in writing.

For the purposes of intimate samples the relevant age of consent (section 65) is seventeen years. For those aged between fourteen and seventeen years the consent of the patient and of the parent or guardian is necessary. For those who have not attained the age of fourteen years the consent only of the parent or guardian is statutorily required.

An intimate sample other than a sample of urine or saliva may be taken from a person by a registered medical practitioner only [section 62(9)].

Implied and Express Consent

Legally valid consent may be express or implied. In many consultations and procedures the patient rarely agrees explicitly but will, instead, give an implied consent, e.g. the patient will undress and lie on the examination couch when the doctor indicates a wish to conduct an examination or the patient may roll up a sleeve and offer an arm when the doctor indicates a wish to measure the blood pressure or take a blood sample.

Express consent, of course, is given when a patient states agreement in clear terms, orally or in writing, to a request.

Oral and Written Consent

A perfectly valid consent may be given orally and there is no absolute need for it to be in writing. However, written consent is sometimes preferable since it provides documentary evidence of the agreement. The problem is a practical one: disputes over consent may arise months or years after the event, by which time memories of an oral consent are unreliable. A witness to an oral consent may be dead or untraceable by the time an allegation of assault is made. Thus, for purely evidential reasons, it is wiser to obtain a signed consent form, duly witnessed.

There is no "magic", legal or otherwise, in a consent form. It is simply a piece of documentary evidence of the fact that a consent was sought and obtained. It is the reality of consent which is important. A consent form signed without knowledge about and/or understanding of the procedure to be performed is valueless.

It would be unrealistic to insist upon a written request for all examinations and procedures and common sense is required in deciding when the consent should be evidenced in writing. It is not the intention here to set out rigid guidelines about the need for written consent but, as a general rule, a consent form should be completed for any procedure involving a general anaesthetic (which includes most operations) and for many procedures involving invasive techniques such as endoscopies, biopsies and angiography. It would also be sensible to seek written consent in the case of those whom the practitioner regards as "difficult" patients.

Obtaining Consent

However consent is obtained, whether express or implied, oral or written, the paramount consideration is that care should be taken to explain the intention, nature and purpose of what is proposed so that the patient truly comprehends that for which his or her agreement is sought. Time so spent is time well spent for the avoidance of future medico-legal complications. In many cases obtaining consent is really too important to be delegated to junior staff or others since it often calls for careful clinical judgement and explanation. For example, junior staff may be unaware of the technical details, risks and complications in more specialised surgical procedures, and consent is best obtained by the specialist.

It is necessary to obtain appropriate consent. Consent to "sterilisation" is not a licence to perform a bilateral salpingectomy, for example, and where two or more procedures are planned it is necessary to have consent for each. Sometimes the procedure which was envisaged is amended and the original description of it is crossed through and the amended procedure added to the consent form without the form being re-signed by the patient. If a change is made to a planned procedure it must be explained to the patient and a new form should be completed, signed and witnessed.

Emergencies and Consent

In the case of a genuine emergency the practitioner may safely proceed to do what is reasonably necessary to save life or prevent a deterioration in the patient's health without formal consent. Medical and not legal considerations are of greater importance in life-threatening situations and the courts are most unlikely to censure a practitioner for proceeding to provide essential treatment in an emergency.

However, the doctor should do only that which is immediately necessary for the patient's well-being. If, during an emergency procedure, some coincidental and non-urgent problem is encountered it should not be dealt with until later, after consent has been obtained.

The guiding principle is to act in good faith and in the immediate best interests of the patient's health and safety. If there is any doubt there should be no hesitation in seeking the advice and opinion of one or more colleagues.

If the emergency arises in an unconscious patient the practitioner should, if time permits, endeavour to obtain the assent of the next-of-kin, but if urgent treatment or investigation is essential the doctor should have no hesitation in proceeding to do what is necessary. The next-of-kin's consent is not legally necessary; nor will it justify the treatment of an unconscious patient unless otherwise justified because the situation is one of urgent necessity.

The Mental Health Act 1983 and Consent to Treatment

New, statutory law governing consent for some treatments for mental disorder was introduced by Part IV of the Mental Health Act 1983 and by the Mental Health (Hospital, Guardianship and Consent to Treatment) Regulations 1983. The Mental Health Act 1983 applies to England and Wales only. Different statutory provisions apply in Northern Ireland and Scotland has a different Mental Health Act.

Section 57 applies to all patients, formal or informal, in respect of any surgical operation for destroying brain tissue, or the functioning of brain tissue, and in respect of the surgical implantation of hormones to reduce male sexual drive. Any such treatment requires:

1. The consent of the patient; and
2. certificates from one approved, independent doctor and two lay persons (as defined in the Act) that the patient is capable of giving an informed consent and has given it; and
3. the approved, independent doctor has certified that the treatment should be given, having consulted two other persons who have been professionally concerned with the patient's medical treatment.

Section 58 applies to compulsorily detained patients only, in respect of specified treatments defined in the Act and Regulations (currently ECT and some medicines). Such treatments may not be given unless:

1. The patient has consented to the treatment and either the responsible medical officer or an approved, independent doctor has certified that the patient has given an informed consent; or
2. an independent, approved doctor has certified that the patient is incapable of giving an informed consent, or has not consented to the treatment, but that the treatment should be given.

Consent forms. Special, statutory forms of consent are required for treatments covered by sections 57 and 58 of the Act. Form 37 is required for section 57 treatments and forms 38 and 39 for section 58 treatments. The forms are set out in the 1983 Regulations (S.I. 1983 No. 893). Copies of the forms are available from health authorities.

Emergencies. Section 62 of the Mental Health Act 1983 makes exceptions to the applicability of sections 57 and 58 in certain cases of urgent and essential treatment.

Other treatment for mental disorder in patients liable to be detained under the Act. Section 63 provides that the consent of a patient to whom Part IV of the Act applies (i.e. with some exceptions, patients liable to be detained), is not required for any treatment for his or her mental disorder not covered by sections 57 or 58 if it is given by or under the direction of the responsible medical officer.

Other mentally disordered or mentally impaired or psychopathic patients.
The statutory provisions referred to above do not apply to many of the more
routine aspects of treating and caring for the mentally ill and handicapped,
particularly those who are voluntary patients. Apart from the new, statutory
provisions summarised above, the common law of consent continues to apply,
as before. Valid consent to any treatment whether for a physical or mental
disorder can only be given by a patient who is mentally ill or impaired [as
defined in the Mental Health Act 1983, section 1(2)] if the matter is within his or
her understanding.

Not all patients suffering from mental disorder or impairment or psychopathic disorder are incapable of giving personal consent to such treatment.
Therefore the foregoing general considerations of the law of consent apply to
them as to other patients.

For those adult patients who, through mental illness or impairment, lack the
necessary understanding to give a personal consent to treatment for physical
disorders (or for mental illness where this is not covered by the Act) there is a
legal difficulty. Old common law powers dating back for centuries have been
replaced by statutory powers. As a result of changes in the law in 1983, no
parent, guardian, responsible medical officer nor even the judges of the Supreme
Court have power to consent on behalf of mentally disordered persons over the
age of eighteen who, for whatever reason, are incapable of providing a valid
personal consent.

In the case of *In Re F* ([1989] 2 WLR 1025; [1989] 2 All ER 545), which concerned the proposed sterilisation of a severely mentally handicapped adult, the
House of Lords gave some legal guidance concerning the more general question
of treating such persons. If such a patient is incapable of giving a valid personal
consent – and is likely to remain so throughout any relevant time – a doctor will
not be acting unlawfully in giving treatment or care which he believes the
patient needs, provided it is in the patient's best interests to receive the
treatment or care. The doctor should determine what is in the patient's best
interests by coming to a decision in accordance with standards acceptable to a
responsible body of professional opinion.

While the doctor is unlikely to have great difficulty in deciding what is in the
patient's best interests in the case of routine medical treatment, the approval for
the proposed course of action should be sought from the guardian, responsible
medical officer or relatives as a matter of good practice. A second medical
opinion as to the necessity of the treatment may also be desirable, particularly
where the proposed treatment could have serious consequences for the patient.

While the doctor may feel able to determine the patient's best interests in
most cases, there may be others involving difficult emotional, social or moral
issues, such as sterilisation (see below), where the doctor may wish to seek the
protection of the court by applying for a declaration before proceeding with
treatment.

The advice on emergencies and consent given above applies to these patients
as well as to other patients. In a genuine emergency, treatment which is demonstrably necessary may be given in the absence of the patient's or guardian's
consent. However, a second medical opinion may be a wise precaution if time
permits. This advice applies not only to mental health emergencies but to other
co-existing or supervening medical or surgical emergencies arising in a patient
who is mentally disordered or impaired.

Sterilisation: Medical and Social Grounds

Adults

Where an operation is proposed which, coincidentally, will affect reproductive capacity (e.g. hysterectomy or orchidectomy) the patient should be told of the fact. The patient's consent alone is all that the law requires; there is no obligation to obtain the consent of the spouse.

The same is true of a sterilising operation for medical reasons, but it has for long been good medical practice, with the patient's consent, also to seek the agreement of the spouse. This practice is one which is encouraged in the interests of the doctor/patient relationship.

In the case of sterilisation on social grounds, again, only the patient's consent is required by law. The consent of the spouse or consort is not obligatory but it has long been good medical practice to seek to obtain the assent of the latter as well as that of the patient. Where the parties are unmarried or separated and the assent of the other partner cannot or should not be sought, then the practitioner may safely proceed on the strength of the patient's consent alone.

Where the spouse's or consort's consent is sought but is specifically refused, doctors are reminded that their duty is to the patient only and not to any third party. Since the law does not require the spouse's consent, the doctor may proceed on the patient's consent, albeit with due regard for the effects this might have upon the union between the parties.

In all cases of sterilisation great care should be taken to ensure that no guarantee of success is conveyed to the patient when the procedure is explained and consent obtained. In "social" sterilisations the consequences of failure are of such importance to the patient and give rise to so much costly litigation that it is now the Medical Protection Society's advice that, unless there are sound clinical reasons to the contrary, patients should be warned of the risks of early and late failure of sterilising procedures. The Medical Protection Society now recommends a special form for consent to sterilising operations (Fig. 3.1).

Minors (aged under sixteen years)

Where a sterilisation is an inevitable consequence of treatment for a disease there is no particular problem: the consent of the patient (or, where there is lack of understanding, the parent or guardian) is sufficient, having given the usual explanations. So far as sterilisation of minors for "social" reasons is concerned there is legal authority that this could be unlawful where it is found not to be in the child's best interests. In the case of Re D (a minor) [1976] 1 All ER 326 the judge ruled that a proposed sterilisation on an eleven-year-old girl with Sotos syndrome was neither medically indicated nor necessary and that it would not be in the child's best interests for it to be performed. It has since been said in the House of Lords in the cases of In Re B (a minor) [1987] 2 All ER 206 and Re F [1989] 2 All ER 545 that no sterilisation should be performed on a minor without the approval of the wardship court. It would be necessary to make a minor who is not already one a ward of court for this purpose. These judgements apply to other non-therapeutic procedures on minors which are irreversible and not incontrovertibly in the child's best interests. The fact that

---

STERILISATION: CONSENT OF PATIENT

I ....[name]

of ....[address]

hereby consent to undergo the operation of ....

the nature and purpose of which have been explained to me by

Dr/Mr. ....

I have been told that the intention of the operation is to render me sterile and incapable of further parenthood. I understand that there is a possibility that I may not become or remain sterile.

I also consent to the administration of a general, local or other anaesthetic.

No assurance has been given to me that the operation will be performed by any particular surgeon.

Signature..   Date..
                               (Patient)

I confirm that I have explained to the patient the nature and purpose of this operation.

Signature..   Date..
                     (Medical practitioner)

Fig. 3.1. Form recommended by the Medical Protection Society for consent of a patient to a sterilising operation.

the parent(s) purport to give consent does not necessarily make such a procedure lawful. The principles apply, for example, to issues of abortion and to the donation of tissue for transplantation.

Mentally Impaired Patients

A series of cases, culminating in a judgement of the House of Lords in the case of *Re F* [1989] 2 All ER 545, have been brought concerning the legality of performing sterilisation operations on mentally handicapped women who were physically well, but to whom pregnancy would be seriously contraindicated on psychiatric grounds. As a result there is now greater clarity in an area where doctors will be particularly anxious to understand their legal duties. The law may be summarised as follows:

In the case of a minor (i.e. a person under eighteen years of age) whether or not capable of understanding the nature and consequences of the proposed procedure, no sterilisation which is not the inevitable consequence of treatment for organic disease should be performed without the patient having been made a ward of court and the consent of the court obtained.

In the case of an adult, he or she may, in spite of mental impairment, be able to give valid consent (see previous sections on Obtaining Consent and the Mental Health Act 1983). If so, having taken care to be satisfied that the patient is so capable, the doctor may proceed as in respect of a patient not suffering from a mental handicap.

If the adult patient is incapable of giving valid consent personally, no other person or body, parent, guardian, medical officer or even a court, has the power to give valid consent on behalf of the patient. In such a case it is lawful to perform a sterilisation if it is in the patient's best interests to undergo such a procedure.

In such circumstances the test of whether a doctor is acting in the patient's best interest is whether the doctor's action is in accordance with a responsible body of medical opinion in the relevant specialty.

Because sterilisation is perceived to have moral, social and emotional connotations, and is a procedure which might in some circumstances leave the doctor open to the accusation that the procedure had been performed for the benefit of a carer or relation rather than that of the patient, it is highly desirable for the doctor or responsible health authority to apply to the court for a declaration that the proposed procedure would be lawful and in the patient's best interests, even though such an application is not strictly necessary as a matter of law.

Thus, although the legal position differs in respect of mentally impaired minors and adults, it will be seen that in both cases some form of application should be made to the court before the doctor can perform a sterilisation procedure safely. Before such an application is made it is necessary to ensure that there is evidence to put before the court that the various relevant issues have been considered carefully by those responsible for the care of the patient and that the procedure would be in the patient's best interests.

Consent to Abortion and Contraception

The pregnant mother's consent alone is relevant in the case of abortion under the Abortion Act 1967. The putative father has no legal say in the matter, whether or not he is married to the mother, as was made clear in the cases of *Paton* v. *Trustees of BPAS* [1978] 2 All ER 987 and *C* v. *S* [1987] 1 All ER 1230. However, this is not to discourage the sound medical practice of discussing a proposed abortion with the father (provided that the mother agrees).

Similar considerations apply to contraception as to abortion. For adults there is no legal requirement to seek the consent of the spouse/consort. Many practitioners prefer to ask for the consent of both parties before fitting an intra-uterine contraceptive device and, whilst there is no legal requirement to do so, it is sound medical practice.

Girls under 16 Years of Age

The general principles of the law concerning the age of consent are set out above (see section on Age of Consent). In applying the legal principles to contraceptive and abortion advice and treatment it was stated by Lord Scarman in the *Gillick* case in the House of Lords that it has to be borne in mind that there is much that has to be understood by a girl under the age of sixteen if she is to have legal capacity to consent to such treatment. It is not enough that she should understand the nature of the advice which is being given; she must also have a sufficient maturity to understand what is involved. There are moral and family questions, especially her relationship with her parents; long-term problems associated with the emotional impact of pregnancy and its termination; and there are risks to health of sexual intercourse at her age, risks which contraception may diminish but cannot eliminate. It follows that a doctor will have to be satisfied that the patient is able to appraise these factors before the doctor can proceed safely upon the basis that the patient has at law, capacity to consent to contraceptive treatment. Ordinarily, the proper course for the doctor is first to seek to persuade the girl to bring her parents into consultation, and, if she refuses, not to prescribe contraceptive treatment unless the doctor is satisfied that the patient's circumstances are such that the treatment may proceed without parental knowledge and consent.

Lord Scarman acknowledged that a criticism of this view of the law is that it will result in uncertainty and leave the law in the hands of the doctors. Lord Scarman commented that uncertainty is the price which has to be paid to keep the law in line with social experience, which is that many girls are fully able to make a sensible decision about many matters before they reach the age of sixteen years. This view of the law places great responsibilities upon the medical profession and it is pointed out that abuse of the power to prescribe contraceptive treatment for girls under the age of sixteen would render a doctor liable to severe professional penalty.

Somewhat more detailed guidance was given in the House of Lords by Lord Fraser of Tullybelton who said that the doctor will be justified in proceeding without the parents' consent or even knowledge provided the doctor is satisfied:

That the girl (although under sixteen years of age) will understand the advice

That he cannot persuade her to inform her parents or to allow him to inform her parents that she is seeking contraceptive advice

That she is very likely to begin or to continue having sexual intercourse with or without contraceptive treatment

That, unless she receives contraceptive advice or treatment, her physical or mental health, or both, are likely to suffer

That her best interests require the doctor to give her contraceptive advice and/or treatment without parental consent.

Lord Fraser commented that this result ought not be regarded as a licence for doctors to disregard the wishes of parents on the matter whenever they find it convenient to do so.

Consent and Research, Clinical Trials

Non-therapeutic procedures, research and trials pose very special problems over consent. The problems are much easier for adults than for minors, the mentally ill or subnormal. Guidance on research involving patients was published by the

Royal College of Physicians of London in January 1990 (*Research involving patients,* The Royal College of Physicians of London, 1990) and includes a section on consent. It is important that patients should know that they are taking part in research. In general, research involving a patient should only be carried out with that patient's consent although there are a few exceptions to this general rule (ibid. section 7.7). Research involving patients should be subject to independent ethical review and it must be made clear to patients that participation in research is entirely voluntary and they may decline to participate without giving a reason, without prejudice to their future care. Patients should also be assured that they may withdraw from research, without the need to give a reason, at any time.

Research on healthy volunteers poses special problems over consent. The problems are more easily resolved for adults than for minors, the mentally ill or mentally impaired. Guidance on research on healthy volunteers was published by the Royal College of Physicians of London in 1986. Members who intend to conduct research on healthy volunteers are advised to obtain a copy of this report.

Adults

A special consent form should be drawn up, with expert advice, tailored to the particular features and requirements of the procedure or research. Very great care is needed in explaining the nature, purpose and effects to the subjects if the practitioner is to avoid accusations of duress, coercion, etc. Indeed it may be wise for consent to be obtained by someone wholly independent of the research. The doctors involved with the research may think it wise to tap several sources for advice, including colleagues, ethics committees, research bodies, royal colleges and professional associations. Since the topic is so specialised and individual, further general advice is not likely to be helpful.

Minors, the Mentally Ill or Subnormal

Even greater problems are posed for such subjects. Legal opinion is divided about whether or not a parent or guardian can give a lawful consent for a non-therapeutic procedure or for research and there are few legal cases on the subject in English law. However, the case of *Re D* (see above: Sterilisation of Minors) is some authority for the proposition that non-therapeutic procedures on minors may be unlawful if they are irreversible and of no direct benefit to the subject.

The Medical Protection Society is always pleased to offer advice to members on individual problems or cases.

Consent and Jehovah's Witnesses

Problems of consent can arise for the doctor faced with a patient, usually a Jehovah's Witness, who refuses to receive blood when, in the doctor's opinion, it is necessary. However, the above principles and the law on consent would be meaningless if the doctor could force blood into an unwilling patient. Competent adults are entitled to refuse treatment.

For the *adult* Jehovah's Witness a doctor must first decide whether he or she is willing to treat the patient at all in circumstances where a blood transfusion may be necessary. If the doctor is not prepared to allow the patient to die as a result of his or her religious convictions then it might be better not to accept the patient for treatment. If the doctor is willing to undertake treatment then the nature of the illness and the need for possible blood transfusion should be explained to the patient in the presence of a witness who should be warned, in clear terms, of the possible consequences of refusal.

If, despite an unambiguous warning, the patient adheres to his or her refusal to receive blood, he or she should be asked to sign a written declaration of refusal. Alternatively, oral refusal should be recorded by the doctor in the notes and countersigned by the witness.

There is no doubt that Jehovah's Witnesses appreciate the difficulties for doctors of their religious convictions and they published a pamphlet setting out their position in 1977 which they distributed to members of the medical profession, (*Jehovah's Witnesses and the Question of Blood*. Watchtower Bible and Tract Society of Pennsylvania, USA, 1977). This stated that Jehovah's Witnesses are ready and willing to bear responsibility for their refusal to accept blood and to sign legal waivers which relieve medical staff from any concern about legal actions. Similar categorical assurances were repeated in their 1990 pamphlet "How can blood save your life?".

For the *children* of Jehovah's Witnesses, however, the position is not so simple. No signed waiver can protect the doctor from criminal proceedings, and the Children and Young Persons Act 1933 makes it a criminal offence for anyone over sixteen who has the custody, charge or care of a child under sixteen wilfully to ill-treat, neglect or abandon that child or to expose him to unnecessary suffering or injury to health. Should the child die as a result of ill treatment or neglect, the facts could give rise to a charge of manslaughter.

Some years ago it was common practice for the hospital or health authority to apply to magistrates for the child to be taken into care when blood transfusion was deemed necessary but parental consent was refused. These care proceedings are seldom needed. Rather it should be for the doctor in charge of the care of the child-patient to do what is genuinely believed to be best for the child. These decisions are not easy and should not be left to junior medical staff. Whilst the doctor concerned will hesitate before overriding the wishes of the parents, ultimately a decision will have to be made on the basis that it is the child and not the parent who is the patient. In reaching a decision the doctor will need to have due regard to all the circumstances relevant to the individual case, and to consider possible alternatives to transfusion of blood or its products. The doctor may also wish to consult with medical and nursing colleagues and perhaps others. Consultation with the appropriate medical defence society may give some help and support. If the doctor decides to proceed with a transfusion he or she should of course document the decision, the reasons for it, and the fact that one or more colleagues concur.

Consent and Radioisotopes

In general, the use of radioisotopes for diagnostic purposes does not come within the definition of a hazardous procedure and the minimal radioactivity requires no special consideration concerning the advice and information to be provided to patients. The use of radioisotopes for diagnostic purposes requires that an appropriate explanation be given to patients: the principles involved are the same as for any other radiodiagnostic procedure. It is important that an adequate note is made of the advice and information provided to the patient. A written consent form is not mandatory.

If a radiotherapeutic procedure is to be used which involves the implantation of a radioactive source which could become detached from the patient, and thus present a hazard to the general public, this fact should be clearly explained to the patient and an appropriate entry made in the clinical records. It may be prudent to ask the patient to sign a consent form in respect of such therapeutic procedures, or when radioisotopes are used for treatment, for example, radio-iodine for thyrotoxicosis.

Consent Forms

For many years the Medical Protection Society has advocated the use of a single consent form for all therapeutic and investigative purposes. Others have advocated the use of different forms for different purposes, but the Society considers that a single consent form will suffice and that a variety of different forms is unnecessarily confusing and may lead to the 'wrong' form being completed (Fig. 3.2).

Over the many years during which the Society has advocated the use of one form no legal problems have been encountered as a result. However, in the light of experience of litigation arising from sterilising operations performed on essentially social grounds, the Society now advocates the use of a special form of consent for such procedures (see Fig. 3.1).

As explained earlier, there is no legal or other "magic" in the form. The signed consent is no more than a piece of written evidence, duly witnessed, that a proper explanation was given and a valid consent obtained. The most important piece of the stethoscope is the part which fits between the earpieces - the most important part of the consent is the explanation and preamble to the signature.

Clinical Trials

For research and clinical trials the Society advise that a special consent form should be drawn up to cover the specific circumstances of each.

Consent to Post-mortem Examination and to Removal of Human Tissue

There is still some doubt in law as to who - if anyone - is the lawful owner of a dead body. Some have argued that no-one can claim to own a corpse and that, at best, the issue is one of possession rather than ownership.

In the case of coroners' post-mortem examinations there is no problem over consent: the coroner's order is a complete authority to the pathologist to perform the post-mortem examination.

STANDARD CONSENT FORM

I ....[name]

of ....[address]

* hereby consent to undergo

or

* hereby consent to..undergoing
                                    (name of patient)

the operation/treatment of ....

the nature and purpose of which have been explained to me by

Dr/Mr...

I also consent to such further or alternative operative measures or treatment as
may be found necessary during the course of the operation or treatment and to
the administration of general or other anaesthetics for any of these purposes.
No assurance has been given to me that the operation/treatment will be
performed or administered by any particular practitioner.

Signature .... Date ....
                        (Patient/parent/guardian*)

I confirm that I have explained the nature and purpose of this
operation/treatment to the person(s), who signed the above form of consent.

Signature .... Date ....
                        (Medical practitioner)

* Delete whichever is applicable

Fig. 3.2. A standard consent form.

In the case of hospital post-mortem examinations performed for the purpose of establishing the cause of death or of investigating the existence or nature of abnormal conditions, section 2 of the Human Tissue Act 1961 clears up any doubt about their lawfulness. However, the Human Tissue Act 1961 does require that, before a "hospital" post-mortem examination is performed, and before tissue is removed from a body after death, the authority must be obtained of "the person lawfully in possession of the body". It is the health authority or board of governors who are *prima facie* in lawful possession at the moment of death and remain so until a near relative or executor comes forward to claim the body, and the health authority or board of governors will delegate one or more persons to give authority on their behalf. In the case of a private institution or a Services hospital the person lawfully in possession would be the manager and commanding officer respectively.

Any clinician wishing to remove human tissue under section 1 of the Act must seek the authority of the person approved to give such authority by those

POST-MORTEM DECLARATION FORM

I do not object to a post-mortem examination being carried out on the

body of ....

and I am not aware that he/she had expressed objection or that another
relative objects.

I understand that this examination is carried out:

(a) to verify the cause of death and to study the effects of treatment which may
     involve the retention of tissue for laboratory study;

(b) to remove amounts of tissue for the treatment of other patients and for
     medical education and research.

Signed...   Date......................................

Relationship to deceased ....

Witnessed by ....

Notes on completion of this form

1. The signature of a relative of the deceased should be witnessed by the
   member of staff administering the form.
2. A relative of the deceased should not be invited to sign this form if the
   hospital itself is aware of objections on the part of other relatives.
3. Should a relative agree to paragraph (a) but not to paragraph (b) appropriate
   deletions may be made to the form.

Fig. 3.3. The post-mortem declaration form. Crown copyright: reproduced from Appendix 2
HC(77)28 with the permission of the Controller of Her Majesty's Stationery Office.

lawfully in possession of the body and must ensure that the necessary proce-
dural steps are taken before granting authority, e.g. the existence of a signed
consent or a kidney donor card. Non-compliance with the provisions of the
1961 Act may lead to proceedings in the courts.

Where the patient did not sign a consent or kidney donor card before death
the person lawfully in possession of the body may only authorise the removal of
tissue if, having made such reasonable enquiry as is practicable, he or she has
no reason to believe that the donor would have objected or that the surviving
spouse or relative objects. Specific consent is not necessary, only a lack of
objection.

Where there is any reason to believe that the coroner may require an inquest
or a post-mortem examination to be held, authority to remove tissue may not be
given nor may tissue be removed without the consent of the coroner.

Because of the increasing demand for human tissue for diagnosis, treatment
and research it is often convenient to remove it during the course of routine

SURGICAL IMPLANTS (FOR USE IN ORTHOPAEDIC, CARDIAC AND OTHER DEPARTMENTS WHERE IMPLANTS ARE USED)

....Hospital

Consent for Operation   Unit No. ....

I , ... of ....

.... hereby consent to

* [the submission of my *   (child ....

(ward..........................to]

undergo the operation of ....

the nature and purpose of which have been explained to me by

Dr/Mr * ....

I also consent to such further or alternative operative measures as may be found necessary during the course of the above-mentioned operation and to the administration of general, local or other anaesthetics for any of these purposes.

I acknowledge and agree that any implant supplied to and implanted in me as part of this operation or the further or alternative operative measures mentioned above, is supplied and implanted subject to the condition that if at any time it is removed by or on behalf of a health authority:

(a) for the purpose of replacement, or
(b) where a replacement is not required, to enable it to be examined, or
(c) where in the case of a cardiac pacemaker paragraph (a) or (b) does not
      apply, after my death the ownership of the implant will vest in that health
      authority.

No assurance has been given to me that the operation will be performed by any particular practitioner.

Signed.. Date...
            (Patient/Parent/Guardian)*

I confirm that I have explained the nature and purpose of this operation to the patient/parent/guardian*.

Signed.. Date...
            (Medical/Dental* Practitioner)

Any deletions, insertions or amendments to the form are to be made before the explanation is given and the form submitted for signature.

This form is not suitable for consent to procedures such as electroplexy, sterilisation or vasectomy.

* Delete as necessary.

Fig. 3.4. Consent form for use in orthopaedic, cardiac and other specialised departments where surgical implants are used. Crown copyright: reproduced from HN(83)6 with the permission of the Controller of Her Majesty's Stationery Office.

"hospital" post-mortem examinations. The Human Tissue Act does not require a written agreement to a post-mortem examination or to the removal of tissue but the Medical Protection Society considers it desirable that a written declaration should be made and, for this purpose, recommends to members completion of the post-mortem declaration form set out as Appendix 2 to the Department of Health and Social Security Circular HC(77)28 (Fig. 3.3).

Surgical Implants

Any device or prosthesis implanted surgically and intended to remain within a patient's body becomes, in English law, the property of the person in whom it has been implanted. Following a patient's death such implants form part of the estate unless there is specific provision to the contrary.

If the practitioner or health authority desires the right to retain an implant, removed for examination or replacement, a special form is recommended. The form is set out as an annex to Health Notice HN(83)6 published by the (then) Department of Health and Social Security and is reproduced here as Fig. 3.4.. This form, intended for use in orthopaedic, cardiac and other specialised departments where implants are used, serves two purposes: (i) a form of consent to operation and (ii) a vesting of rights of ownership of the implant in the health authority.

Confidentiality

Perhaps the most fundamental of the principles of medical ethics is that all which passes between patient and doctor in the course of a professional relationship is secret. This principle can sometimes bring the doctor into conflict with others, notably the police and lawyers.

In some countries the law positively obliges the medical practitioner to maintain confidentiality, with criminal sanctions for a breach. In English law there is no general statutory duty of confidentiality, although some people argue that there should be, and that there should be some uniformity in the law within the member states of the European Community. Most lawyers agree that, in English law, confidentiality is an implied term of the contract between a doctor and his patient and that unauthorised disclosure of professional secrets would be a breach of the contract, giving grounds for civil proceedings. Although English courts have, in recent years, considered cases involving issues of confidentiality as between doctors and patients and others, confidentiality remains essentially an ethical as much as a legal principle in the UK. Issues of confidentiality may be complex with scope for differences of opinion arising from conflicts of competing interests.

Venereal Disease

One of the few statutory rules on confidentiality in English law is to be found in the National Health Service (Venereal Diseases) Regulations (SI 1974 No. 29,

Her Majesty's Stationery Office). These require every health authority to take all necessary steps to secure that any information capable of identifying an individual, which is obtained by health authority officers with respect to persons examined or treated for any sexually transmitted disease, shall not be disclosed except to another doctor, or someone employed under his direction, in connection with the treatment or prevention of the spread of such diseases. (See also the section on AIDS below).

The General Rule and Exceptions

The General Rule

This is set out in the UK General Medical Council's publication *Professional Conduct and Discipline: Fitness to Practise* (GMC, 1990). Subject to certain exceptions it is a doctor's duty to observe strictly the rule of professional secrecy by refraining from disclosing voluntarily to any third party information which has been learned directly or indirectly in his or her professional capacity as a registered medical practitioner. The patient's death does not absolve the doctor from the duty to maintain secrecy (see the section on Death and Confidentiality below).

Exceptions

A number of exceptions exist to the general rule of confidentiality. However, whatever the circumstances, a doctor must always be prepared to justify any disclosure of confidential information.

Consent. The secrets are those of the patient, not the doctor, and therefore the doctor is perfectly entitled – perhaps under a duty – to disclose information if asked to do so by the patient or the patient's legal adviser.

Colleagues. Information about a patient may be shared with other registered medical practitioners who assist with clinical management. Information may also be shared, to the extent that the doctor deems necessary, with other professional persons who are properly concerned with the patient's health (e.g. dentists, nurses, professions supplementary to medicine. See also the section on Non-medical Staff below). It is the doctor's duty to ensure that those with whom information is shared appreciate the rule of professional secrecy.

Statutory Duty. There are many legal rules and regulations which positively require the doctor to pass on certain information about his or her patients. Examples include:

Notifications of infectious diseases

Notifications under the provisions of the Factories Act and of the Control of Substances Hazardous to Health (COSHH) Regulations

Notifications under the provisions of the Abortion Act 1967 (as amended)

Notifications of drug addicts under the provisions of the Misuse of Drugs Act 1971

Notifications of births and deaths

Duty to give information which may lead to the identification of a driver (section 168, the Road Traffic Act 1972; *Hunter* v *Mann* (1974).

For a complete list of diseases etc. see the Medical Protection Society's leaflet "Statutory Notifications").

Information to Relatives. Traditionally, the doctor has been willing to discuss a patient's illnesses with relatives to a lesser or greater extent, though some circumspection is called for if complaints are to be avoided. Where it is undesirable on medical grounds to seek the patient's consent the doctor may give information, in confidence, to a relative or other appropriate person.

Third Parties. If, in the doctor's opinion, disclosure of information to a third party other than a relative would be in the best interests of a patient, it is the doctor's duty to make every reasonable effort to persuade the patient to allow the information to be disclosed. If, none the less, the patient refuses to allow this, only in exceptional circumstances should the doctor feel entitled to disregard or override the refusal.

Research. It is ethical to disclose information for the purpose of a proper medical research project which has been approved by a recognised ethics committee.

The Public Interest. This is perhaps the most contentious exception to the general rule where the doctor learns information about a serious matter in the course of his or her professional dealings with a patient or colleague. The doctor is not merely a "healthcare professional" but also a citizen of the country in which he or she practises. There will sometimes be circumstances which give rise to a conflict for the doctor as to whether the greater duty is to the patient or to the public, and there is seldom an easy answer to the dilemma. What seems a problem to one doctor will not be a problem to another. The doctor faced with a dilemma should take advice and consult with colleagues. The Medical Protection Society will be very pleased to advise members. Ultimately, however, the individual practitioner alone must resolve the dilemma and act according to a combination of what is believed to be the patient's best interests and the dictates of the practitioner's conscience.

A Court Order. Despite a widely held belief to the contrary, confidential medical information is not privileged from disclosure. This contrasts sharply with the privileges accorded to the barrister and solicitor; any information passed to them by a client in the course of a professional relationship cannot be the subject of an order for disclosure. If, in the course of legal proceedings, a court requires knowledge about a patient's medical details, an order can be made which compels the doctor to reveal the details - or face proceedings for contempt of court. A verbal or written request from a lawyer or court official is not sufficient: the doctor should divulge no secrets about a patient unless directed to do so by the judge or other presiding officer of a court, or upon receipt of a formal, sealed court order. If in doubt the doctor should seek advice; if necessary, an adjournment may be sought to permit advice to be obtained.

Some Practical Problems

In the Medical Protection Society's experience practical difficulties over confidentiality tend to arise from requests for medical reports, usually by the police, solicitors or insurance companies.

Where the police seek information about a patient the doctor is perhaps wise, in most routine circumstances, to ask the police to provide the patient's informed agreement to pass on the information. Occasionally the police will not wish to do this for fear of impeding their inquiries or warning off the suspect and, in these circumstances, often concerning serious crime, the doctor is faced with deciding between professional duty to the patient and public duty as a citizen. A general rule of wide application is that matters are very seldom so urgent that a doctor cannot reasonably ask the police for time to consider their request and to take advice.

Where a solicitor seeks information the doctor should take care to check for whom he acts and for what he asks. If he specifies that he acts for Mr. AB and seeks information only about Mr. AB the doctor may safely prepare a report since the professional relationship between solicitor and client is such that no further formalities are indicated or necessary. Any improper approach from a solicitor would be a matter for investigation by the Law Society.

However, the doctor should confine the report entirely to information about Mr. AB and should not pass on details about Mrs AB, Mr. CD or anyone else. Failure to respect this elementary point has led to complaints being made against doctors, sometimes to the General Medical Council.

Furthermore, if the solicitor specifies that he acts for Mr. AB but asks for details about Mr. and Mrs. AB, the doctor should respond by saying that he is unable to supply details about Mrs. AB unless either the solicitor acts also for her or the solicitor supplies the doctor with her own consent. This sort of trap for the unwary tends to arise in the course of separation or divorce proceedings, or disputes over the custody of children. The doctor who inadvertently passes on to, say, the husband's solicitors details about the wife may soon find that he incurs the wrath of the latter or her solicitor, and may become the subject of a formal complaint.

The same general principles apply to anyone (e.g. insurance companies, housing departments, social work departments, etc.) seeking information about a patient: they should provide the patient's specific agreement to the disclosure of the information to them by the doctor.

Death and Confidentiality

Where information is sought by a third party about a dead patient the appropriate consent to be given is that of all the personal representatives of the estate of the deceased, i.e. his executors or, if none, those who take out letters of administration.

Not infrequently, a life insurance office or agent will write to a doctor for information before agreeing to pay out on a life policy, especially if it was taken out not long before the death. The doctor is wise not to release any details until the office or agent has provided the consent of the personal representatives.

Confidentiality and Non-medical Staff

If the ethical principle is to mean anything it is clearly important that all members of the healthcare team should honour it. Nurses, like doctors, are reared on the principle, but other members of the team may not be. Medical practitioners should ensure that all members of staff with whom they associate, be they receptionists, secretaries, porters, practice managers, technicians or whomever, are fully aware, and constantly mindful, of the duty to respect the patients' secrets. Casenotes should be kept securely, and access to them should be controlled most strictly. It is the clinician in charge of the care of the patient who is ethically responsible for the confidentiality of medical records, and this should not be overlooked even though the responsibility may, for example, be delegated to medical records officers.

Other members of the team may feel that they have loyalties different from those of the doctor. Social workers, for example, may consider that their duty is to the community which has given them the task of providing services. Some caution may therefore be called for from the doctor who is asked to participate in case conferences which are also attended by the police and/or social workers.

Fitness to Drive

The duty to notify the licensing authorities about medical conditions which affect the ability to drive rests with the patient. If a doctor has reason to believe that an epileptic patient is continuing unlawfully to drive a motor vehicle the Medical Protection Society suggests that in the first instance he or she should give a firm warning to the patient to stop driving and should record this warning in writing, either by making an entry in the notes or by writing to the patient and keeping a copy of the letter. The patient may also be warned that, if he or she continues to drive, the doctor may have no alternative but to report the matter to the licensing authority. If, despite the warning, the doctor has good evidence that the patient is continuing to drive it may be ethical to report the facts to the Driver and Vehicle Licensing Authority. For borderline or problematic cases the Authority has a medical department with which a practitioner may discuss a case. Similar principles apply to other conditions affecting fitness to drive (e.g. diseases, disabilities, drug or alcohol abuse, etc.).

Non-accidental Injury to a Child

Where a practitioner has reasonable grounds to suspect child abuse, his or her paramount duty and responsibility is to the child-patient and there need be no fear of taking such action as is deemed to be most appropriate medically. It is perfectly legitimate to supply reasonable information to the children's department of the local authority or to the National Society for the Prevention of Cruelty to Children.

The Occupational Health Physician

Special problems of confidentiality may arise for a medical practitioner having divided loyalties, as in occupational health practice. This is particularly true where a general practitioner may be asked, as an occupational health adviser, to see his or her "own" patient. The doctor should ensure that any employee who is seen in that capacity understands the reason for the consultation and the duties which the doctor may have to the employer, such as certifying fitness to perform in a job. A confusion of roles in the mind of an employee, patient or doctor may lead to problems in general at the workplace and, in particular, when a request is made for access to medical records.

Non-clinical and Administrative Medical Officers

The duty of confidentiality applies not only to doctors who have received information in a clinical relationship with a patient but also to doctors who receive information indirectly, in the course of administrative or non-clinical duties, e.g. with health authorities, commercial firms, insurance companies, local authorities, pharmaceutical industry, journalism or authorship.

AIDS: HIV Status

Neither AIDS nor positive HIV status are statutorily notifiable conditions. Thus the ordinary principles of law and ethics apply to information about patients with AIDS or about HIV status. Particular care is necessary over confidentiality in view of the profound social consequences for the patient, e.g. over personal relationships, housing, employment and life insurance.

In the case of *X* v. *Y* [1988] 2 All ER 648 the High Court ruled that the public interest in maintaining confidentiality about the identity of actual or potential AIDS sufferers outweighed the public interest in the freedom of the press. Hospital employees are under a duty not to disclose the identity of AIDS victims and this duty will be enforced by the courts. The judgement confirmed that confidentiality is of paramount importance to AIDS patients, including doctors suffering from the disease. If confidentiality is breached, or if patients have grounds for believing it may be or has been breached, patients will be reluctant to come forward for and to continue with treatment and counselling. The case gives clear legal authority in support of the preservation of confidentiality in the public interest.

Audit

In 1990 the Standing Medical Advisory Committee for the Secretaries of State for Health and for Wales produced a report entitled "The Quality of Medical Care" which dealt with audit and related matters (HMSO, 1990). This report recognised that "confidentiality is essential" and recommended that the documentation in audit meetings be provided in such a form that the general conclusions of audit meetings and recommended action are recorded "while the cases used in discussion are not in any way identifiable".

The report recognised that in medical audit a patient's medical records would be open to scrutiny by doctors other than the doctors responsible for the patient's clinical care but that this sharing of information was legitimate because all doctors share the same ethical principles. However audit sessions should be organised so as to avoid referring to patients by name or revealing information by which patients may be identified. The report states "it is possible to conduct medical audit without using patients' names".

PART 2:

The Most Contentious Problems in the High-Risk Specialties

CHAPTER 4

Anaesthesia

A.R. Aitkenhead

Anaesthesia represents a high insurance risk for the medical profession primarily for two reasons. Anaesthetists manipulate the physiology of the cardiovascular and respiratory systems and administer potentially lethal drugs which are not primarily therapeutic; consequently, when a serious accident occurs, it may result in hypoxaemia or ischaemia within seconds or minutes, culminating in death or permanent neurological damage. In addition, because the majority of patients are healthy, even minor morbidity attributed to anaesthesia or the anaesthetist may be regarded as unacceptable to the patient, even though more serious forms of morbidity which are perceived as an inevitable complication of surgery may be tolerated without complaint.

For the overwhelming majority of patients anaesthesia is uneventful. However, both surgery and anaesthesia carry a finite risk. Mortality is related usually to the extent of surgery and the pre-operative condition of the patient (Table 4.1). However, deaths occur as a consequence of anaesthesia alone, and some of these are avoidable. Lunn and Mushin [34] estimated that the risk of death attributable to anaesthesia alone was approximately 1 in 10 000. In a later study of approximately 500 000 operations [15], the overall death rate after anaesthesia and surgery was 0.7%. Anaesthesia alone was responsible for only three deaths (an incidence of approximately 1 in 160 000 operations), but *contributed* to 14% of all deaths; in almost one-fifth of these deaths, avoidable errors occurred. Factors which contributed to death in these cases are listed in Table 4.2.

Table 4.1. The ASA (American Society of Anesthesiologists) physical status scale, and associated mortality [57]

Grade	Description	Mortality rate (%)
I	A normally healthy individual	0.1
II	A patient with mild systemic disease	0.2
III	A patient with severe systemic disease that is not incapacitating	1.8
IV	A patient with incapacitating systemic disease that is a constant threat to life	7.8
V	A moribund patient who is not expected to survive for 24 hours with or without operation	9.4

Table 4.2. Factors involved in deaths attributable in part to anaesthesia, in decreasing order of frequency [15]

Failure to apply knowledge
Lack of care
Failure of organisation
Lack of experience
Lack of knowledge
Drug effect
Failure of equipment
Fatigue

Table 4.3. Causes of anaesthetic-related death or cerebral damage in 750 cases reported to the Medical Defence Union between 1970 and 1982 [56]

Mainly misadventure		Mainly error	
Coexisting disease	14%	Faulty technique	43%
Unknown	6%	Failure of post-operative care	9%
Drug sensitivity	5%	Drug overdosage	5%
Hypotension/blood loss	4%	Inadequate pre-operative assessment	3%
Halothane-associated hepatic failure	3%	Drug error	1%
Hyperpyrexia	2%	Anaesthetist's failure	1%
Embolism	2%		

The incidence of morbidity related to anaesthesia is more difficult to assess. The causes of major morbidity (causing permanent disability) are, not surprisingly, often similar to those associated with mortality. Table 4.3 lists the causes of death or cerebral damage reported to the Medical Defence Union between 1970 and 1982 [56]; the majority were associated with errors. Table 4.4 shows the detailed causes of the incidents which resulted from errors. Recently, death attributable to negligence by anaesthetists has resulted in convictions for manslaughter [13] as well as civil litigation. Less serious incidents may also result in distress or physical injury, and may be followed by

Table 4.4. Causes of anaesthetic-related death or cerebral damage reported to the Medical Defence Union between 1970 and 1982 in 326 cases thought to be the result of errors in technique [56]

Cause	% of total
Errors associated with tracheal intubation	31
Misuse of apparatus	23
Inhalation of gastric contents	14
Errors associated with induced hypotension	8
Hypoxia	4
Obstructed airway	4
Accidental pneumothorax/haemopericardium	4
Errors associated with extradural analgesia	3
Use of nitrous oxide instead of oxygen	2
Use of carbon dioxide instead of oxygen	2
Errors associated with Bier's block	2
Underventilation	1
Use of halothane with adrenaline	1
Mismatched blood transfusion	<1
Vasovagal attack	<1

Table 4.5. Untoward anaesthetic-related events (other than death or cerebral damage) in 1501 cases reported to the Medical Defence union between 1970 and 1982 [56]

Event	% of total
Damage to teeth	52
Peripheral nerve damage	9
Extradural foreign bodies (e.g. needles, catheter tips)	7
Superficial thrombophlebitis and minor injuries (e.g. abrasions)	7
Awareness	7
Spinal cord damage	4
Pneumothoraces	3
Extravasation of injected drugs	2
Lacerations, falls from table	2
Impaired renal function (mismatched blood transfusion)	1
Burns	1
Others	5

claims for compensation. The most common events reported to the Medical Defence Union between 1970 and 1982 are shown in Table 4.5.

This chapter will deal with three categories of incident which result relatively frequently in litigation. All three categories have attracted considerable public attention. In each category, the maxim *res ipsa loquitur* is often relied upon by the plaintiff. However, in many instances this may be inappropriate, as injury may occur despite the highest standards of care.

Cerebral Damage

Damage to the central nervous system during anaesthesia and in the post-operative period may result in death, a variable degree of disability, or complete recovery. Causes related to anaesthesia itself, or to administration of drugs in the post-operative period, are associated almost exclusively with arterial hypoxaemia or cerebral ischaemia. In addition, cerebral damage may occur as a result of treatment in the intensive therapy unit; in most cases, the causes are similar to those of brain damage during anaesthesia.

Hypoxaemia

This is the commonest reason for cerebral damage during anaesthesia and the post-operative period. It may arise from failure to deliver an adequate inspired oxygen concentration, an abnormality of the lungs which impairs oxygenation of pulmonary capillary blood, or a failure of ventilation.

Inspired Oxygen Concentration

Oxygen Supply. During anaesthesia, oxygen is supplied from either a pipeline system or oxygen cylinders, regulated by a needle valve, and the flow rate measured by a rotameter tube [58]. Occasionally, errors have occurred in the connections of pipelines at source, and nitrous oxide has been delivered through the oxygen pipeline. There have been instances in which the nitrous oxide pipeline bas been connected to the oxygen inlet of the anaesthetic machine and vice versa [12].

Faulty air/oxygen mixers may allow contamination of one pipeline gas with the contents of the other. This may cause air to leak into the oxygen pipeline, reducing the oxygen concentration with the potential for delivery of a dangerously low inspired oxygen concentration when the "oxygen" is mixed with nitrous oxide [53].

The anaesthetist may fail to notice that an oxygen cylinder is empty or that the pipeline supply is not connected to the anaesthetic machine. All modern anaesthetic machines incorporate an alarm to indicate a failure of oxygen supply, but these may develop faults; in addition, some machines without such alarms are still in use.

Rotameter bobbins may give erroneous readings if the rotameter tube becomes contaminated with dirt, if static electricity collects on the glass walls, if a rotameter tube breaks, if the O-ring seal is faulty or if there is a leak from components of the rotameter block [16, 24]; delivery of a hypoxic gas mixture may result. Other gases, for example carbon dioxide, may be delivered in the gas mixture in error.

Breathing Systems. A hypoxic gas mixture may be delivered when a circle system (a rebreathing system with carbon dioxide absorber) is supplied with low flow rates of oxygen and nitrous oxide. An appropriately low flow rate of anaesthetic gases to other breathing systems, a leak within the breathing system at its connection with the anaesthetic machine, or a leak within the back bar of the anaesthetic machine may cause rebreathing of gases and inhalation of a progressively hypoxic gas mixture.

Inadequate Ventilation

Inadequate ventilation, or total failure of ventilation, results in a decrease in alveolar and arterial oxygen tension and an increase in carbon dioxide tension (Fig. 4.1); the absolute value of oxygen tension depends principally on the alveolar minute ventilation and the inspired oxygen concentration. Hypoxaemia occurs more rapidly if the functional residual capacity (FRC) is low (e.g. pregnant or obese patients). Total failure of ventilation in a normal patient who has been breathing 33% oxygen (the normal inspired concentration during anaesthesia) results in significant arterial hypoxaemia (arterial Po_2 <50 mmHg) in about 5 minutes, but this occurs in less than 2 minutes in a patient breathing air (e.g. immediately after induction of anaesthesia) and in 1–1.5 minutes, and sometimes less, in a patient with reduced FRC or pulmonary disease.

Pharmacological Depression. Hypoventilation, or apnoea, may be caused by a relative overdose of anaesthetic or opioid drugs in the spontaneously breathing patient during anaesthesia, or in the immediate post-operative period. In the later post-operative period, opioid analgesics given to treat wound pain may cause ventilatory depression and hypoxaemia, especially in elderly patients or if a continuous infusion of an opioid is employed, as cumulation may take place [40]. Respiratory arrest may be of relatively rapid onset. Intrathecal or epidural administration of opioids is often more effective than conventional systemic

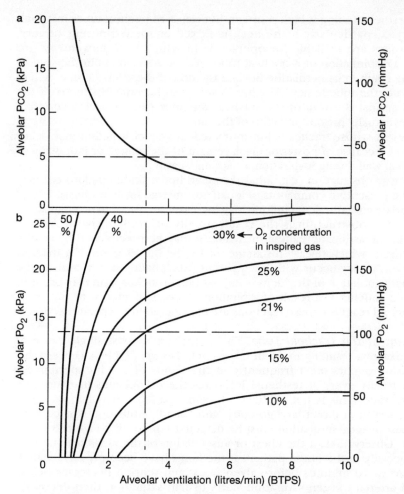

Fig. 4.1. Gas exchange during hypoventilation. **a.** The hyperbolic relationship between alveolar carbon dioxide tension and alveolar ventilation; **b.** the relationship between alveolar oxygen tension and alveolar ventilation for different levels of inspired oxygen concentration. Reproduced, with permission, from Nunn [41]

administration, but there is a documented risk of sudden depression of ventilation many hours after the last administration of analgesic [6].

Residual neuromuscular blockade may cause hypoventilation, or occasionally complete paralysis and apnoea, in the post-operative period, particularly if renal function is impaired (e.g. neonates, the very old, or patients with severe renal disease).

Hypoventilation or apnoea may occur occasionally in association with the injection of local anaesthetic drugs for subarachnoid (spinal) or extradural (epidural) anaesthesia.

Airways Obstruction. The passage of oxygen to the lungs may be obstructed at a number of locations. Anaesthetic breathing systems and connecting tubes may become kinked, or obstructed by a foreign body or manufacturing fault.

Most anaesthetic tubing is kink-resistant, but standard tracheal tubes may kink in the pharynx, particularly if the neck is flexed or rotated during surgery; reinforced tubes are available for operations in which such movements are predictable. Over-inflation of a tracheal tube cuff, or a weakness in the wall of the cuff, may result in its herniation beyond the end of the tracheal tube, where it may obstruct the tube lumen. The lumen may also become obstructed if the bevel abuts against the wall of the trachea; this may cause a ball-valve effect which will eventually prevent inflation of the lungs.

In the patient whose trachea is not intubated, airway obstruction may occur in the pharynx because of posterior displacement of the tongue or indrawing of the pharyngeal wall during inspiration, or laryngospasm.

Upper airway obstruction (e.g. inhaled foreign body, acute epiglottitis) may be one of the presenting complaints of a patient undergoing anaesthesia. Use of an inappropriate anaesthetic technique may increase the risk of hypoxaemia.

Lower airway obstruction is the result usually of bronchospasm. This is commoner in the asthmatic patient, in whom it may be precipitated by administration of drugs which release histamine, or by the introduction of a tracheal tube. However, it may occur with no apparent precipitating factor, and can be so severe that ventilation of the lungs is impossible. Bronchospasm may occur in non-asthmatic patients as a result of aspiration of gastric contents, or as part of an anaphylactoid reaction; these reactions are considered in a separate section.

Misplacement of the Tracheal Tube. This is the commonest single cause of serious hypoxaemia resulting in death or cerebral damage (Table 4.4). Oesophageal intubation occurs most frequently in the hands of the inexperienced. However, virtually every anaesthetist intubates the oesophagus inadvertently from time to time. This is not negligent. In some patients, it is impossible to visualise the larynx at direct laryngoscopy, and "blind" intubation is necessary. However, oesophageal intubation must be detected rapidly, although this is not always easy. Observation of the chest or auscultation of the lungs may be misleading, especially in the obese patient. If the lungs have been pre-oxygenated, it may be up to 10 minutes before alveolar oxygen tension decreases below normal and arterial oxygen saturation starts to fall; saturation then decreases very rapidly.

Disconnection or Ventilator Failure. Most mechanical ventilators are robust and reliable, but occasionally they malfunction and fail to deliver gas to the patient. More commonly, a disconnection occurs either in the hoses connecting the inspiratory or expiratory port to the Y-piece, or between the Y-piece and the tracheal tube. A loose connection may cause gas to leak from the system, resulting in hypoventilation. However, the positive pressure in the system is likely to cause a loose joint to become completely disconnected, resulting in total failure of ventilation.

Other Causes. Ventilation may be impaired by increased diaphragmatic pressure during spontaneous ventilation, particularly if the abdomen is distended (e.g. during laparoscopy) or if the patient is placed in a steep head-down position. Occasionally, ventilation may be inadequate because of the presence of air or fluid in the pleural cavity. A pre-existing pneumothorax may become larger and develop into a tension pneumothorax because of diffusion of nitrous oxide into the cavity. More commonly, pneumothorax is the result of pulmonary trauma, either because of pulmonary disease (e.g. bullae), rib fractures, cannulation of a neck vein or the use of high inflation pressures. High pressures are often required to inflate the lungs of patients with adult respiratory distress syndrome, and positive end-expiratory pressure may be necessary to attain adequate oxygenation of the blood; these may cause a tension pneumothorax during anaesthesia or in the intensive therapy unit. However, on some occasions, inappropriately high inflation pressures are used in patients with normal lungs, usually because of misuse of ventilators or gas injectors. A progressively increasing hydrothorax may be the result of a misplaced central venous catheter; a large haemothorax may develop in patients who have sustained trauma to the thoracic cage.

The development of a large bronchopleural fistula may result in loss through the chest drain of virtually all of the tidal volume in a patient receiving positive pressure ventilation. This is most likely to occur in patients with chronic pulmonary disease, after pulmonary surgery, or as the result of trauma.

Pulmonary Disease

Patients with pulmonary disease may become hypoxaemic during anaesthesia unless a high inspired oxygen concentration is provided. During one-lung anaesthesia (a technique used for pulmonary and oesophageal surgery), arterial oxygen saturation is often subnormal even when 100% oxygen is administered. However, this is anticipated by the anaesthetist, and appropriate steps are taken to monitor and treat excessive decreases in oxygen saturation. It is possible for the bronchial portion of the double-lumen tube to occlude one or more lobes of the ventilated lung [49], resulting in severe hypoxaemia.

Pulmonary oedema may develop during or after anaesthesia. The commonest cause is cardiac disease, but excessive fluid administration may result in accumulation of fluid in the alveoli, and occasionally acute upper airway obstruction (e.g. laryngospasm) may result in pulmonary oedema because of the hydrostatic gradient generated across the pulmonary capillary membrane by the highly negative intra-alveolar pressures which occur when the patient attempts to breathe.

Failure of Oxygen Delivery

Reduced Tissue Blood Flow

This may result from impairment of cardiac output or extreme hypotension for some other reason. Severe anaphylactic reactions to drugs administered during anaesthesia may cause cardiovascular complications; this subject is discussed in a separate section.

Cardiac Contractility. Many anaesthetic agents decrease cardiac contractility in a dose-related manner. This may result in a critical reduction of cardiac output if excessive concentrations particularly of inhaled anaesthetics are given, or if the patient has received other drugs (e.g. beta-blockers) with a negative inotropic effect. Inadvertent intravascular injection of local anaesthetics may reduce contractility, as does high (mid-thoracic or above) spinal or epidural anaesthesia. Patients with pre-existing cardiac disease may be more sensitive to the negative inotropic effects of anaesthetic drugs. Patients with ischaemic heart disease may suffer a reduction of cardiac contractility in the presence of otherwise innocuous degrees of hypoxaemia, tachycardia, hypertension or hypotension.

Cardiac Arrhythmias. Cardiac output may be reduced by atrial or ventricular arrhythmias. However, these rarely result in serious hypotension unless a severe tachycardia or severe bradycardia is present. Arrhythmias may be precipitated by volatile anaesthetic agents or by exogenous adrenaline (administered usually by the surgeon), especially in the presence of halothane, and are commoner in patients taking drugs which affect cardiac excitability or conduction. Hypoxaemia also predisposes to abnormal cardiac rhythm or conduction, as do electrolyte abnormalities.

Cardiac Arrest. Cardiac arrest during anaesthesia is very unusual in the absence of a non-anaesthetic cause (e.g. profound hypovolaemia). Asystole may occur as a result of vagal stimulation, preceded usually by sinus bradycardia. It is also the usual terminal event in severe hypoxaemia. Ventricular fibrillation is less common, but may occur after the administration of adrenaline in a patient receiving halothane, in association with hypoxaemia or because of acute myocardial ischaemia or infarction. Cardiac arrest may also result from intravascular injection of local anaesthetics, particularly bupivacaine, either inadvertently or in association with Bier's block if the tourniquet is applied inadequately or released prematurely or if the drug is injected rapidly into a large vein. Electrolyte abnormalities, especially related to potassium, may precipitate cardiac arrest; abnormalities of serum potassium concentration may be exaggerated by acid-base changes induced by hypercapnia or hypocapnia.

Electromechanical dissociation may precede asystole in patients with severe hypovolaemia, pneumothorax or prolonged hypoxaemia.

Hypotension. Almost all anaesthetic drugs produce some hypotension, by reducing cardiac output, promoting vasodilatation, or both. Hypotension is more marked in the absence of surgical stimulation (e.g. between induction of anaesthesia and the start of surgery) and in the presence of relative hypovolaemia (e.g. after haemorrhage or in the dehydrated patient). However, the presence of low blood pressure is not linked automatically to reduced tissue perfusion or oxygenation, provided that cardiac output is maintained. In the presence of a normal microcirculation, autoregulation maintains flow despite moderate decreases in arterial pressure. Normally, cerebral autoregulation occurs down to a mean arterial pressure of 60 mmHg; below that value, cerebral blood flow decreases progressively. However, the threshold is increased in chronically hypertensive patients, and flow may be pressure-dependent in patients with atherosclerosis of cerebral arteries; care must be exercised in these groups of patients to prevent profound hypotension.

Tissue flow is reduced to a greater degree when hypotension is associated with reduced cardiac output and accompanied by vasoconstriction [2]. Excessive hyperventilation causes profound hypocapnia, which also results in vasoconstriction [8], and may impair tissue perfusion further in the hypotensive patient.

Inadvertent hypotension during anaesthesia may be the result of a relative overdose of general anaesthetic agents, high spinal or epidural anaesthesia or inadequate replacement of blood and plasma losses. For some types of surgery, hypotension is induced deliberately to reduce surgical blood loss; hypotensive techniques are used particularly for middle ear, pelvic and plastic operations. Anaesthetists vary in their enthusiasm for deliberate hypotension, and there have been cases of cerebral damage, myocardial infarction and death attributable to its use. There is no sudden "cut-off" value of blood pressure below which serious complications occur predictably. However, there does appear to be an increased risk of complications if deliberate hypotension is used; the incidence of non-fatal complications has been estimated as 2.5% [32]. A large proportion of these complications can be prevented if deliberate hypotension is avoided in patients with pre-existing hypertension, cerebrovascular or ischaemic heart disease, hypovolaemia or anaemia. Hypotensive techniques associated with myocardial depression (by administration of high concentrations of volatile anaesthetic agents or beta-blockers) are associated with more complications than those that employ vasodilatation. The complication rate is also increased if mean arterial blood pressure is reduced to less than 70 mmHg, or if the anaesthetist is inexperienced. However, there may be some surgical procedures in which the risk of excessive blood loss warrants the use of lower values of blood pressure in otherwise healthy young patients and there is evidence that an adequate cerebral blood flow can be maintained in such patients at systolic blood pressures of 60 mmHg or slightly less [32].

Anaemia

Tissue oxygenation may be impaired despite a normal arterial oxygen saturation if the total amount of oxygen carried by blood is decreased by severe anaemia. The most common cause is massive haemorrhage, with replacement of blood volume by artificial solutions. It is a potential problem in any Jehovah's Witness who undergoes major surgery and refuses permission for blood transfusion.

Embolism

Embolism of air or thrombus may result in cerebral ischaemia. Emboli or air or clot, or reduced cerebral perfusion pressure, may cause focal or global ischaemia after cardiopulmonary bypass [47]; microemboli of platelets, air bubbles or other substances result in a high incidence of minor neurological and psychological sequelae, the majority of which are of little clinical significance and some of which are temporary [14].

Consequences of Cerebral Hypoxia or Ischaemia

The effects of these two insults are not identical. In the presence of an intact cardiovascular system, the brain is able to adjust for temporary episodes of even severe hypoxaemia by a compensatory increase in cerebral blood flow, thereby minimising the reduction in oxygen delivery. If arterial Po_2 decreases to less than 50 mmHg without circulatory arrest, there are increases in intracellular and extracellular brain lactate concentrations. More profound hypoxaemia results in a decrease in intracerebral phosphocreatine concentrations. However, even very severe hypoxaemia is not associated with a significant decrease in adenosine triphosphate (ATP) concentrations because of a rapid compensatory vasodilatation, a resultant increase in blood flow (in excess of four times normal) and a sixfold increase in glucose metabolism [30, 48]. As long as increased cerebral blood flow is maintained, hypoxaemia must be very severe to threaten neuronal survival, although cerebral function may be impaired during the episode of hypoxia. However, prolonged moderate or severe hypoxaemia also affects the heart. There is an initial increase in heart rate and stroke volume as a result of sympathetic nervous system stimulation, but bradycardia or other arrhythmias, followed by cardiac arrest, supervene and permanent cerebral changes ensue. Hypoxic cerebral damage may be followed by initial recovery but subsequent development of a "delayed postanoxic encephalopathy" [42]. This is a specific syndrome which causes irritability, apathy and confusion and changes in gait, and is associated with histological changes in white matter and sometimes in the basal ganglia; there is no evidence that more generalised neuronal damage occurs after a period of normal cerebral function. In severe hypoxaemia with circulatory inadequacy, the sequelae are similar to those caused by primary cerebral ischaemia.

Global ischaemia, as occurs in severe hypotension or cardiac arrest, results much more rapidly in neuronal damage. Brief episodes of ischaemia are often followed by complete recovery. However, as the duration of ischaemia increases, progressively more permanent damage occurs. Resulting lesions are more likely to affect grey matter than white matter, and are frequently bilateral and symmetrical; they may be confined to the parietal and occipital areas of the cerebral hemispheres, but in most cases involve both the supratentorial and infratentorial compartments [23]. Fits may develop during or shortly after the ischaemic episode. A wide range of residual deficits may result, ranging from mild psychological symptoms or personality changes to a vegetative state or brain death. Cortical blindness is not uncommon. Outcome is influenced by the duration and extent of ischaemia and by age. Paradoxically, incomplete ischaemia (e.g. severe hypotension) may result in a worse outcome than a similar period of complete ischaemia; this is thought to be the result of continued delivery of glucose with an inadequate supply of oxygen in incomplete ischaemia, which causes increased lactate production and a lower intracellular pH.

Patients with cerebrovascular disease may develop localised neurological lesions attributable to ischaemic damage in the area of impaired perfusion.

Attempts at reducing the neurological sequelae of hypoxaemia or ischaemia have been disappointing [5]. No specific treatment has been shown to ameliorate the condition in man. However, it is likely that prompt restoration of the circulation reduces secondary ischaemic damage caused by the reperfusion syndrome [43] and moderate hyperventilation may be of theoretical benefit if there are signs of cerebral oedema. There is no clinical evidence that the use of routine artificial ventilation after cardiac arrest influences neurological outcome. Steroids are of no benefit.

Prevention

The risk of hypoxaemia caused by an inadequate supply of oxygen can be minimised by regular servicing of anaesthetic apparatus by qualified engineers, and by a thorough pre-operative equipment check by the anaesthetist before every operating list. The Association of Anaesthetists of Great Britain and Ireland has recently published an appropriate check drill [4].

The importance of training and education of anaesthetists has been recognised as an important method of preventing accidents. Most developed countries now require specialist anaesthetists to undergo training in recognised centres which are inspected regularly to ensure that standards are maintained. Continuing education of specialist anaesthetists is encouraged, and in some countries is compulsory. Simulators have been developed which can mimic disasters and which enable anaesthetists to rehearse diagnosis and treatment of critical incidents [22]. Critical incident analysis has been introduced in a number of centres. Audit methods are being used increasingly to identify the reasons for anaesthetic mishaps and to educate anaesthetists about the causes. Design of new anaesthetic machines incorporates additional safety devices to reduce the risk of delivery of hypoxic or inappropriate gas mixtures [51].

However, the most important advance in the prevention of cerebral damage and anaesthetic-related deaths has been the implementation of minimum monitoring standards.

Intra-operative Monitoring

Anaesthetic associations and societies in virtually all developed countries have issued recommendations about monitoring. In some states in the USA and in Australia, specific items of monitoring equipment are mandatory.

The most important monitor is the anaesthetist, who must remain present, and vigilant, throughout every anaesthetic [3]. However, it is now recognised that the anaesthetist's clinical skills should be supplemented by instrumental monitoring, which provides information which cannot be acquired, or can be obtained only unreliably, by clinical observation.

Inspired Oxygen Concentration. Measurement of inspired oxygen concentration at the gas outlet of the anaesthetic machine or (particularly when a circle breathing system is used) in the inspiratory limb of the breathing system provides protection against delivery of a hypoxic gas mixture for any of the causes outlined above.This is not a substitute for a pre-operative equipment check.

Ventilation and Oxygenation. The use of a ventilator pressure alarm provides warning of partial or total disconnection (the pressure in the breathing system fails to reach a preset minimum pressure) or airway obstruction (the pressure exceeds a preset maximum). These devices must be adjusted to provide appropriate preset minimum and maximum pressures for each patient to ensure accurate detection of abnormalities. There should also be visual displays of airway pressure and expired tidal volume to provide confirmation that ventilation is satisfactory.

Pulse oximetry, although recommended as desirable only in the UK, has become mandatory in many countries. This device estimates arterial oxygen saturation non-invasively, and provides a continuous display of both saturation and pulse rate. It can detect a small decrease in oxygen saturation which is imperceptible clinically, and is much more reliable than the human eye in detecting serious oxygen desaturation, particularly in anaemic patients or those with pigmented skin. However, it may provide a relatively late warning of decreased oxygen supply or pulmonary dysfunction; arterial oxygen tension may already have decreased significantly before oxygen saturation starts to fall. In addition, pulse oximeters often fail to provide a reliable signal in the presence of vasoconstriction, and are subject to interference from diathermy. Nevertheless, they provide valuable information about the state of oxygen supply, pulmonary function and circulation and represent a major advance in the prevention of hypoxic damage.

Capnography (the measurement of carbon dioxide concentration in the respired gases) has been available for some years to provide an index of arterial carbon dioxide concentration, but is now recognised as a very important form of monitoring in the prevention of accidents. A normal capnogram is obtained only if the tracheal tube has passed through the larynx (although the trace may be normal if the tube lies in a main bronchus), and the device therefore provides immediate assistance in diagnosing oesophageal intubation.[1] Although there may be a gradient between arterial and end-tidal carbon dioxide tensions in some circumstances, the capnogram is useful in monitoring the effectiveness of ventilation. In addition, measurement of the inspired carbon dioxide concentration ensures that the anaesthetist can detect inappropriate rebreathing or inadvertent administration of carbon dioxide in the inspired gas mixture.

Cardiovascular Monitoring. The electrocardiogram (ECG) is essential for diagnosis of rhythm or conduction abnormalities in the heart, and also provides evidence of myocardial ischaemia. Its use is regarded as mandatory in all anaesthetised patients. Measurement of blood pressure must be performed intermittently in all patients, and should be undertaken continuously (usually by an intra-arterial cannula) in the presence of cardiac disease or in circumstances when sudden changes or extreme values may be anticipated (e.g. major surgery, deliberate hypotensive techniques). In the absence of continuous blood pressure monitoring, the anaesthetist must have some other indication of a continuous circulation; at present, the pulse oximeter is the most commonly used technique.

Miscellaneous. Hypothermia or hyperthermia may affect oxygenation of the blood, and the facility to measure core temperature must be available in all operating theatres, although its routine use is unnecessary. Monitoring of neuromuscular function is desirable in the paralysed patient, particularly if an infusion of muscle relaxant is employed or if renal insufficiency is present. Measurement of inspired and end-tidal concentrations of nitrous oxide and volatile anaesthetic agents is of value in ensuring that appropriate concentrations are being delivered to the patient, particularly when a circle breathing

---

[1] Only one other device, based on the the inability to aspirate air from the oesophagus [62], is effective in detecting oesophageal intubation.

system is used. If there is a predictable risk of impairment of the cerebral circulation (e.g. carotid artery surgery, cardiac surgery), monitoring of the integrated electroencephalogram signal may be of value. Biochemical and haematological monitoring are indicated during major and prolonged surgery, or in the presence of pre-operative abnormalities.

Monitoring in the Post-operative Period

In most instances, clinical monitoring in the recovery room is sufficient, but each patient requires the dedicated attention of one trained nurse until consciousness has been restored and cardiovascular and respiratory stability have been achieved. After major surgery, and in the compromised patient, instrumental monitoring of the cardiovascular system is usually necessary and it may be appropriate to nurse the patient for 24–48 hours in a high dependency unit; if none is available, then intensive nursing care, with close medical supervision, is required on the surgical ward. If there is instability of one of the major physiological systems, or if ventilatory or cardiovascular support is required, then the patient should be transferred to an intensive therapy unit, where monitoring standards usually equal or exceed those in the operating theatre. There is some controversy about the monitoring requirements of patients who receive post-operative analgesia by continuous infusion (intravenous or subcutaneous), or by epidural or spinal administration, of opioids. These techniques are associated with a small but significant risk of ventilatory depression or arrest, and it is the author's view that these patients should not be nursed in a general ward unless an apnoea alarm is used; it is preferable for such patients to be under close nursing supervision in a high dependency or intensive care area.

Records

In the event of a hypoxic or ischaemic incident in the peri-operative period, it may be difficult or impossible to exonerate the medical and nursing staff from blame if adequate records of all monitored parameters are not available. During anaesthesia, the anaesthetist must make regular recordings of each parameter, and of all drugs and fluids given. It is essential that the timing of every event is clear. Many monitors can produce a paper record, and these should be attached to the anaesthetic chart; they can provide invaluable assistance not only by demonstrating that adequate monitoring was used, but also by excluding many or all of the potential causes of cerebral damage which may be alleged by plaintiffs or their experts. It is inappropriate to keep a contemporaneous record *during* an emergency caused by hypoxaemia or ischaemia, but the anaesthetist should make a full note as soon as possible after the situation has been controlled. It is also essential that comprehensive records of cardiovascular, respiratory and neurological status are maintained by nurses in the post-operative period; if cerebral damage occurs, it is important to know the time at which it developed and to identify any precipitating factors in order to determine its aetiology.

Conclusion

The majority of cases of cerebral damage associated with anaesthesia and surgery are preventable. It must be recognised, however, that mortality and morbidity may be unpredictable and unpreventable despite the highest standards of medical and nursing care. The most important steps which can be taken to minimise their incidence are pre-operative equipment checks and the use of appropriate monitoring during and after anaesthesia. It has been estimated that serious morbidity or mortality might have been prevented, or at least ameliorated, by the use of pulse oximetry and capnography in between one-third and two-thirds of patients who sued their anaesthetist in the United States [18, 54]. There is also evidence that the number of claims for death or cerebral damage has decreased in the United States since monitoring standards were implemented, although some of this reduction may be attributable to the greater defensibility of claims when monitoring has been used.

Anaphylaxis

Anaphylactic reactions represent an exaggerated response of the body to a foreign protein or other substance to which it has previously been sensitised, and are associated with the release of histamine, serotonin and other vasoactive substances. These reactions may occur with a tiny dose of the drug, are worse after repeated exposure and the symptoms and signs are not related to the pharmacological effect of the drug. The clinical features are listed in Table 4.6. Reactions may present with any one or any combination of these signs. Anaphylactoid reactions are clinically indistinguishable from anaphylactic reactions, but other mechanisms are responsible. Anaphylactic and ana-phylactoid reactions are classed as Type B adverse reactions, and must be distinguished from Type A reactions, which are dose-related and represent an extension of the normal pharmacological response of the drug.

It has been recognised for many years that there is a small but clinically important incidence of anaphylactic and anaphylactoid reactions to drugs given intravenously during anaesthesia. Some anaesthetic drugs were associated with a particularly high risk because of a high incidence of sensitivity to Cremophor, which was used as a solvent; these drugs have now been withdrawn. At present,

Table 4.6. Clinical features of anaphylactic reactions, listed in order of severity

Pruritus
Erythema
Flushing
Urticaria
Nausea, vomiting and diarrhoea
Angioedema
Laryngeal oedema
Bronchospasm
Hypotension
Cardiovascular collapse
Death

about 80% of anaphylactic reactions are related to administration of muscle relaxants (about 50% of these involve suxamethonium) and most of the remainder to the anaesthetic agents thiopentone, etomidate or propofol. Public attention was focused on the subject of anaphylaxis during anaesthesia as the result of a fatal accident enquiry in Aberdeen after the death of a patient who had received suxamethonium [29]. The sheriff had been told by an expert witness that between 5000 and 10 000 "operation-disrupting" adverse reactions to general anaesthetics occur in the UK each year out of 3.5 million operations, and that 500 of these may result in death or permanent brain damage. He was told by the expert witness that tests were available which could warn of the probability of anaphylactic reactions to specific anaesthetic drugs, and he recommended that Health Boards should consider screening patients before elective surgery, particularly if the patient was female, had previously received suxamethonium and/or had shown signs of other allergy. The sheriff's report prompted newspaper articles and radio programmes in which these figures and recommendations were discussed. The expert witness put forward the opinion that 300–500 patients die or suffer brain damage each year in the UK as a result of adverse drug reactions and that pre-operative screening with drug-specific radioallergosorbent tests (RASTS) could substantially reduce the number of anaphylactic reactions; this, it was claimed, would be justified financially by the huge reduction in cost incurred from cancelled operations, intensive care management, and awards paid to patients who had suffered damage. Similar advice is still (August 1990) being offered to patients who have suffered such reactions, and to their relatives, who are told that pre-operative screening with RAST could have prevented the cerebral damage which occurred (B. Fisher, personal communication). Such advice has clear medico-legal implications. Selected Members of Parliament were sent a letter by a public relations firm acting on behalf of the manufacturers of RAST kits strongly advocating the use of RAST for routine screening [19].

Incidence

The incidence of "operation-disrupting" adverse reactions suggested by the expert witness is 1 : 700 to 1 : 1400, and is based entirely on extrapolation from the number of patients investigated at his centre and a completely unvalidated estimate of the ratio of patients referred in relation to the total number who suffer a reaction. The number of deaths claimed to result from adverse drug reactions exceeds the estimated *total* number of deaths attributable to anaesthesia by a factor of more than 10 [15]. In fact, the unit which employs the expert witness had been developed to provide a national advice service, and it is likely that more than 50% of patients who suffered a suspected anaphylactic reaction were referred. The centre dealt with blood samples from about 150 patients each year [59]; some of these patients had suffered a Type A reaction. Anaphylactic reactions during anaesthesia may result also from administration of blood, or plasma substitutes. In Australia, the incidence of severe Type B reactions to anaesthetic and muscle relaxant drugs is approximately 1 in 20 000 [21], and it is estimated that in one large British centre one patient in 14 000 suffers such a reaction (J. McG. Imrie, personal communication). This suggests that the *total* number of severe anaphylactic reactions to anaesthetic and muscle relaxant drugs is around 250 per year; the large majority of these patients make an uneventful recovery [21]. This figure is in keeping with the experience of anaesthetists, who would expect to see such a reaction only once every 5 to 10 years, and with information from the Medical Defence Union (Table 4.3) showing that only 5% of *all* reported cases of death or cerebral damage between 1970 and 1982 (when the Cremophor-containing drugs were still in use) were attributable to drug hypersensitivity. Mortality in patients who develop a severe anaphylactic reaction to an anaesthetic drug is believed to be 4%–6%, although this may be an underestimate because some patients may die without diagnosis or investigation.

Consequently, most authorities are of the opinion that the figures given to the Aberdeen sheriff regarding the incidence of anaphylactic reactions to anaesthetic drugs were a gross exaggeration. Nevertheless, anaesthetists appreciate that all reasonable steps must be taken to prevent anaphylactic reactions and to minimise the number of patients who die or suffer cerebral damage, no matter how small the number. A working party of the Association of Anaesthetists of Great Britain and Ireland (AAGBI) has recently considered the problem of anaphylaxis, its prevention and its treatment [38].

Prevention

Predicting the At-risk Population

The only valid predictor is a history of a previous reaction. A history of allergy, atopy or asthma is commoner in patients who develop an anaphylactic reaction to an anaesthetic drug than in patients who undergo uneventful anaesthesia. However, the majority of people who react do not have an atopic history, and the vast majority of those with such a history have no adverse reaction to anaesthetic drugs [20]. Although anaphylactic reactions appear to be commoner in women who are young to middle-aged than in other patients, the major part of this difference is related to the large number of gynaecological operations performed as a proportion of all surgical procedures. Previous exposure to anaesthetic drugs is a particularly poor predictor of subsequent reactions, especially to muscle relaxants. The large majority of patients who receive multiple anaesthetics suffer no anaphylactic reactions. In contrast, 90% of patients who reacted to suxamethonium in one study had no previous exposure to the drug [26]. Foods and cosmetics may sensitise susceptible individuals to the quaternary ammonium group which is common to all muscle relaxants [10].

Screening

As no high-risk group can be identified (other than those with a history of a previous adverse reaction), screening would be required for all patients presenting for anaesthesia, at least before elective surgery. However, the criteria which have been suggested by Whitby [60] for valid screening procedures cannot be met by any of the available methods. In particular, the reactions are not all mediated by the same mechanism; some are related to specific antibodies, but many are not. In addition, none of the available diagnostic tests has been validated as an effective screening method.

Intradermal testing, using high dilutions of suspect drugs, and prick testing, using the standard formulation, have a low incidence of false-positive and false-negative results when used for diagnosis of the cause of a reaction. They have the advantage that a reaction is not dependent on the presence of drug-specific antibodies, but false-positive results may occur with drugs which release histamine, e.g. atracurium. There is a small risk of an anaphylactic reaction when the test is performed. Neither test has been validated prospectively as a screening method.

The HRL (histamine release from leucocytes) test [9] is possibly reliable in diagnosis, but is elaborate, expensive and time-consuming and has not been validated as a screening method.

Measurement of total IgE concentrations is a poor diagnostic method, and is of no value in screening. The RAST technique measures drug-specific IgE antibody concentrations, and it has been claimed that this test would be useful as a routine screening method [19]. However, there are many reasons why this would be inappropriate:

1. At present, RAST kits are available commercially for only three anaesthetic drugs (thiopentone, suxamethonium and alcuronium); thus, even if the technique was sensitive and specific, reactions to any other drug could not be predicted.

2. Only a proportion of allergic reactions to anaesthetic drugs are mediated by drug-specific IgE antibodies. Thus, even if the test was 100% sensitive for IgE-mediated reactions, there would be a high incidence of false-negative results; results of RAST in non-anaesthetic anaphylactic reactions (mostly penicillin-based) suggest that there is a false-negative rate of about 40%.

3. The test has not been validated as a screening method. However, studies are in progress. Preliminary results (J. McG. Imrie, personal communication) show that the incidences of positive RAST to suxamethonium, thiopentone and alcuronium in randomly selected patients are 0.7%, 2% and 7% respectively. None of these patients demonstrated any adverse reaction to anaesthetic drugs; the only patient who did react had negative RASTs to all three drugs. In a similar study of selected patients (mostly young and female), the incidences of positive RAST to the three agents were 3.4%, 3.9% and 9.7% respectively; none of the patients suffered an adverse reaction. In a population of patients with a history of atopy, the incidences of positive RAST results were 5%, 7% and 17% respectively. Not only do these results demonstrate that RAST is totally unsuitable as a screening technique, but they call into question its validity in diagnosis.

The total cost of RAST for all three anaesthetic drugs, including the time of technicians, is approximately £25. Screening of all patients in the UK before every anaesthetic would cost in excess of £17 million. The use of intradermal or prick testing would probably be more expensive. It has been argued that a high false-positive result is unimportant if patients who would be at risk are identified, and use of the drug avoided. However, this is true only if there is no risk, or at least a lower risk, attached to avoidance of the drug in the patients with a false-positive result, who are denied its benefits. The risk of anaphylactic reactions appears to be greatest with suxamethonium, a short-acting muscle relaxant with a rapid onset of action which is used to facilitate tracheal intubation, particularly in patients with a difficult airway, those who develop airway obstruction and those who are at risk from regurgitation and pulmonary aspiration of gastric acid. The incidence of anaphylactic reactions to suxamethonium is probably about 1 in 35 000 (approximately 40% of all reactions). The provisional results from Aberdeen suggest that 245 of each 35 000 patients tested would have a positive RAST for suxamethonium. Even if RAST detects 60% of truly sensitive patients (and this has not been demonstrated), then for each 175 000 patients tested, three would be saved from an anaphylactic reaction, but 1225 would be put at unnecessary risk of complications associated with airway difficulties or aspiration pneumonitis.

After considering all the currently available evidence, the working party of the AAGBI [38] concluded that there is no support at present for routine screening of patients for specific drug antibodies before anaesthesia, and that claims that any form of screening will predict anaphylaxis are without foundation.

Treatment

A severe anaphylactic drug reaction is a life-threatening emergency. Although anaesthetists are trained to respond to such situations and are experienced in the management of the critically ill patient, it is nevertheless essential that they are familiar with the specific as well as the general management of anaphylaxis. The rarity of anaphylactic reactions makes it important that anaesthetists familiarise themselves with the diagnostic features. It has been recommended [39] that every anaesthetist should know an "anaphylaxis drill" and the AAGBI [38] has published an example (Table 4.7). Anaesthetists should rehearse a simulated anaphylactic drill at regular intervals, and these rehearsals should include members of hospital staff who would be called upon to assist. The decision to proceed with the operation must be determined by the severity and duration of the reaction, the response to treatment and the urgency of the

Table 4.7. Anaphylaxis drill [38]. All doses are for a 70-kg patient. Basic monitoring is assumed

Immediate management

Discontinue administration of suspect drug
Summon help
Discontinue surgery and anaesthesia if feasible
Maintain airway and administer 100% oxygen (consider tracheal intubation and IPPV)
Give i.v. adrenaline, especially if bronchospasm present. 50–100μg (0.5–1.0 ml of 1:10 000).
  Further 1 ml aliquots as necessary for hypotension and bronchospasm. Prolonged therapy
  may be required occasionally.
Start intravascular volume expansion, preferably colloid, 10 ml/kg rapidly
Consider external chest compression, even if ECG shows electrical activity

Secondary management

Adrenaline-resistant bronchospasm: consider salbutamol, terbutaline or aminophylline
Bronchospasm and/or cardiovascular collapse: hydrocortisone or methylprednisolone
Antihistamines: chlorpheniramine
Sodium bicarbonate if acidosis severe after 20 minutes of treatment
Catecholamine infusions if hypotension persists: adrenaline or noradrenaline
Consider possibility of coagulopathy: perform clotting screen
Measure arterial blood gas tensions for oxygenation and acid-base status

procedure. There is no evidence that outcome is influenced by the decision to proceed, but it may be unwise if the patient's condition is unstable.

Diagnosis

Diagnosis and investigation of patients who have suffered an anaphylactic reaction to an anaesthetic drug are extremely important, because the drug responsible must be avoided in future. It is also essential to investigate patients who give a history of a previous anaphylactic reaction, but who have not already been investigated. The first step in diagnosis must be a high index of suspicion by anaesthetists when unexpected reactions occur during anaesthesia, and all suspected systemic allergic phenomena should be investigated. Skin tests are the most readily available and useful diagnostic tests (the prick test is safer than intradermal testing) and should be performed a few weeks after the suspected reaction. Skin testing should be performed with a wide range of anaesthetic drugs, and not only the agents used at the time of the reaction, as there is a high incidence of cross-reactivity and cross-sensitivity, especially in respect of muscle relaxants. It may be appropriate also to undertake RAST, although, as alluded to above, there is doubt about its accuracy. Changes in complement, mediator or immunoglobulin concentrations in serial blood samples taken in the hours after the reaction may help to distinguish immune from non-immune mechanisms, but do not identity the responsible drug.

Reporting

Careful recording of all events at the time of the reaction is crucial. All anaphy-lactic reactions should be reported to the Committee on Safety of Medicines. In addition, the patient must be given advice about future anaesthesia; this is the responsibility of the anaesthetist. A full record of the reaction and the results of investigations must be kept in the case notes, and a copy sent to the patient's general practitioner. The patient must be given a written record of the reaction, including the results of investigations, and must be advised to carry an anaesthetic hazard card or a medic-alert bracelet.

Awareness During Anaesthesia

One of the main problems encountered in defining anaesthesia is that there is no satisfactory definition of the term "consciousness". In relation to anaesthesia, consciousness may be taken to mean the ability of the patient to remember events occurring during anaesthesia, i.e. unconsciousness equates with amnesia. However, in patients who are lightly anaesthetised, a purposeful response to command can be obtained if one arm is protected from the effects of muscle relaxants by inflation of a tourniquet [55]; even though there is no subsequent memory of the command or response, it is difficult to argue with the concept that the ability of a patient to respond directly to command during anaesthesia implies that consciousness is present.

The changes in objective response associated with progressively increasing concentrations of anaesthetic drug in the central nervous system may be

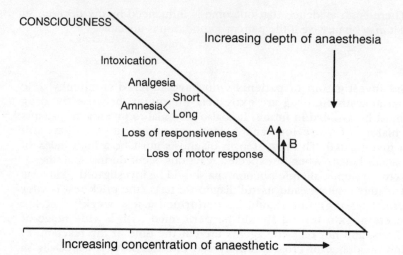

CONSCIOUSNESS

Increasing depth of anaesthesia

Intoxication

Analgesia

Amnesia< Short
          Long

Loss of responsiveness

Loss of motor response

A
B

Increasing concentration of anaesthetic ⟶

Fig. 4.2. Diagrammatic representation of the continuum of anaesthesia, adapted from White [61] with permission. Arrow A represents diagrammatically the response to a surgical stimulus, which tends to produce an effect opposite to that of the anaesthetic agents; arrow B represents the influence of opioids on the response to surgical stimulation. See text for details.

represented by a continuum [61]. As the concentration of drug increases, the patient progresses from full consciousness through a state of intoxication to a "level" at which conscious perception of pain is decreased. There follows a loss of conscious memory of the various sensory modalities. Pain is the first modality to be affected, followed by tactile sensation and subsequently auditory, visual and other senses. At this stage, there may still be responsiveness to stimuli, including the spoken word, but there is no subsequent spontaneous memory of events. Further movement down the continuum results in loss of responsiveness to command and then in loss of motor and autonomic responses to noxious stimuli. Even at this stage of apparently adequate anaesthesia, verbal stimuli may result in alterations of behaviour in the post-operative period, and may be recalled under hypnosis [31, 36]. However, this type of awareness, termed "unconscious perception" is of dubious clinical relevance.

It is important to appreciate that the position on the "continuum" is influenced not only by the concentration of anaesthetic drug but also by the degree of surgical stimulation. Simplistically, it is possible to consider that the effect of noxious stimulation is to promote movement from the continuum in an upward direction (e.g. Arrow A in Fig. 4.2) so that, for a given concentration of anaesthetic in the brain, responses may reappear which had been lost in the absence of stimulation. Thus, to provide adequate anaesthesia, it is necessary to deliver an anaesthetic concentration to the brain which is sufficient to produce amnesia of all sensation in the presence of surgical stimulation, even though this may result in unnecessarily "deep" anaesthesia before surgery starts. Opioid drugs in conventional doses probably have little effect on the position on the continuum, but may reduce the extent of "upward" movement in response to noxious stimuli by reducing the number of impulses which reach the higher centres in the brain (Arrow B in Fig. 4.2).

Spontaneous Recall

Spontaneous recall of intra-operative events, which gives rise to claims of "awareness" during anaesthesia, is confined almost entirely to patients who receive muscle relaxants together with inadequate amounts of anaesthetic drugs, although a few cases have occurred in patients breathing spontaneously a combination of oxygen, nitrous oxide and a volatile anaesthetic agent. Reported incidences of awareness with spontaneous recall vary widely. This is due in part to different methods of detection and to different definitions of "awareness".

It is important to differentiate between true recall of intra-operative events and dreams, hallucinations or illusions. Dreams may occur at any time during the peri-operative period. Their content is not usually related to the operation itself and no specific and verifiable intra-operative events are recalled. There is some evidence that the incidence of dreaming is higher in patients who have received low concentrations of anaesthetic agents. Hallucinations may occur as a side-effect of some drugs which act on the central nervous system. Their content may relate to post-operative events, which may be distorted. Illusions are entirely fictional. Some patients who experience events immediately after operation may attribute their memory to the intra-operative period.

The incidence of spontaneous recall of intra-operative events in patients undergoing non-obstetric procedures has decreased over the last 30 years (Table 4.8). The most recent study [33] suggests that the incidence is about 0.2%. In obstetric practice, the largest study [37] which gave a precise figure suggested that the incidence was about 0.5%, but the incidence has almost certainly decreased since the time of that report and may now be similar to that in general anaesthetic practice. Hearing is the most common sensation to be recalled, as it is the last sense to disappear on losing consciousness. Patients may also recall touch and, if the eyes are not completely closed, vision. Such patients are seldom distressed. Possibly as few as 10% of patients who have spontaneous recall remember pain [17]. These patients are usually distressed, as are those who remember paralysis and an inability to communicate their anxiety to the anaesthetist.

Consequences of Awareness with Recall

Any patient who remembers pain during surgery has undergone an extremely traumatic experience. It is one of the major responsibilities of the anaesthetist to ensure that patients have no memory of intra-operative events, and any failure is

Table 4.8. Summary of incidences of awareness with recall and dreaming in studies using a structured interview 1960–1990

Authors	Date	Awareness (%)	Dreaming (%)	Sample size
Hutchinson [28]	1960	1.2	3.0	656
Harris et al. [27]	1971	1.6	26.0	120
McKenna and Wilton [35]	1973	1.5		200
Wilson et al. [63]	1975	0.8	7.7	490
Liu et al. [33]	1990	0.2	0.9	1000

Table 4.9. Types of operative procedure
associated with cases of awareness with recall
reported to the medical defence organisations
between 1982 and 1986 [25]

Type of procedure	% of cases
General surgery	31
Obstetrics	28
Gynaecology	18
Orthopaedic surgery	11
Miscellaneous[a]	12

[a] Miscellaneous includes dental, ENT and
ophthalmological procedures.

likely to result in a belief that the patient's trust in the anaesthetist has been
betrayed.

Most patients who are distressed report their experience during the first few
post-operative days. Commonly, a relative is told in the first instance, and the
ward nurses may be informed. Until recent years, the relative or the ward nurses
often refused to believe a patient who reported awareness. This resulted often
in the patient failing to report their experience to any medical staff for fear of
being disbelieved and thought mad. Consequently, many anaesthetists remained
ignorant of an experience of awareness by one of their patients. Recent publicity about awareness in the newspapers and television has resulted in wider
knowledge of the condition, and it is likely that this failure of communication
will happen less frequently in future.

The importance of communication relates to the psychological consequences
of recall of intra-operative events if the patient has experienced pain or distress.
A form of traumatic neurosis [11] which includes insomnia, anxiety, irritability,
repetitive nightmares, depression and a preoccupation with death may develop
and there may be a morbid fear of hospitals, doctors and, in particular, of the
need for future surgery. This syndrome may persist for months or years, but is
often ameliorated or cured if the patient is able to discuss their memories
openly, and is assured that the memories are genuine. A similar condition may
develop in patients who have been very lightly anaesthetised, but who do not
recall specific intra-operative events.

For many years up to 1985, there was a small number of claims each year for
compensation on the grounds of alleged awareness. General surgical procedures
accounted for the highest proportion of claims (Table 4.9). In 1985, a patient
who had significant pain and distress during Caesarian section, and who subsequently developed psychological problems, was awarded a sum in excess
of £13 000 amidst a blaze of publicity (*Ackers* v. *Wigan Health Authority* [1]).
Since then, a larger number of patients have attempted to obtain compensation
on the grounds that their anaesthetist acted negligently in providing inadequate
anaesthesia, particularly during Caesarian section; many of these claims have
been successful.

Causes of Awareness with Recall

Spontaneous recall of intra-operative events is, by definition, due to delivery of
inadequate concentrations of anaesthetic agents to the brain for the needs of the

Table 4.10. Causes of awareness with recall reported to the medical defence organisations between 1982 and 1986 [25]

Cause	% of cases
Faulty anaesthetic technique	70
Failure to check equipment	20
Genuine apparatus failure	5
Spurious claims	2.5
Justified risks/unknown cause	2.5

individual patient. The commonest causes in cases reported to the medical defence organisations between 1982 and 1986 [25] are shown in Table 4.10. The specific details discussed in the following paragraphs do not necessarily relate to these cases.

Faulty Anaesthetic Technique. This is the commonest single cause of awareness with recall. A faulty technique is one which could reasonably be predicted to result in recall of intra-operative events, or in which drug doses are not adjusted when clinical signs of inadequate anaesthesia become apparent. In general, the likelihood of awareness is related inversely to the dose or concentration of anaesthetic drug administered (Fig. 4.2). However, high concentrations of most anaesthetic agents result in an increased incidence and severity of side effects, and delayed recovery. Consequently, it became common, particularly in the UK, for anaesthetists to use paralysing doses of a muscle relaxant to prevent movement during surgery (smaller doses are used in some other countries), and to administer anaesthetic agents in concentrations of less than 1 MAC (minimum alveolar concentration which prevents movement in response to surgical stimulation in 50% of individuals).

Inhalational Anaesthetics. The alveolar concentration of inhaled anaesthetic agents required to produce loss of consciousness (i.e. amnesia) (MAC_{awake}) is about 0.6 MAC [50]. However, this is in the absence of surgical stimulation; a higher proportion of MAC is required to ensure amnesia during surgery. In addition, there is individual variability in response; MAC and MAC_{awake} are average values, and the distribution of values among individuals conforms approximately to a normal distribution curve. Thus some patients require significantly higher alveolar concentrations of inhaled anaesthetics than others to ensure loss of consciousness.

Consequently, any technique which results in an alveolar concentration of inhaled anaesthetic which equates to 0.6–0.7 MAC will result predictably in awareness in an unacceptable proportion of patients. The use of unsupplemented nitrous oxide in concentrations of 67%–70% provides about 0.65 MAC, and is unsatisfactory in most circumstances. The addition of opioids may reduce the incidence of awareness slightly, but not significantly. In general, nitrous oxide should always be supplemented with another anaesthetic agent during maintenance of anaesthesia.

The alveolar concentration of an inhalational agent is lower than the delivered concentration and "overpressure" with volatile agents may be required initially to achieve the desired effect. Uptake is more rapid for agents with a low blood/gas solubility coefficient, and this may be of particular importance in preventing awareness during tracheal intubation or at the start of surgery.

The concentration of an inhalational agent delivered to a patient may be considerably less than the concentration set on the flow meters or vaporizer if a circle system with vaporizer outside the circle (VOC) is used, especially with low fresh gas flow rates.

Intravenous Anaesthetics. Anaesthetic drugs administered intravenously are less predictable than inhalational agents. Distribution volumes vary widely between individual patients. While distribution volume has some influence on the rate of uptake of inhalational drugs, its effect is relatively small because increased distribution is to a large extent compensated for by increased uptake from the lungs and the total dose of anaesthetic administered is increased. In contrast, the total dose of an intravenous drug is selected by the anaesthetist, and the blood and brain concentrations are determined, at least in the short term, by redistribution to tissues which receive high blood flow. Awareness may occur during tracheal intubation if a muscle relaxant has been given before clear signs of loss of consciousness have become apparent, or if inhalational anaesthetics are not given between induction and tracheal intubation; this risk is highest if a non-depolarising relaxant has been used. In general, higher doses of anaesthetics are required to ensure lack of awareness in unpremedicated outpatients in comparison to premedicated inpatients.

There may be a higher risk of awareness in the paralysed patient if anaesthesia is maintained by an infusion of an intravenous agent than if inhalational anaesthetics are used. This is true particularly if the lungs are ventilated with oxygen-enriched air (total intravenous anaesthesia) rather than oxygen and nitrous oxide. The minimum infusion rates of intravenous drugs required to produce loss of movement in response to a surgical stimulus vary much more widely among the population than the MAC values for inhalational drugs [45], and the same is almost certainly true for infusion rates required to ensure unconsciousness. The difference between intravenous and inhalational agents in this respect is predominantly because of the relatively unpredictable distribution volumes and rates of drug metabolism of the intravenous drugs. The risk of awareness is even higher if intermittent bolus administration of intravenous agents is used for maintenance.

Obstetric Anaesthesia. The high incidences of recall of intra-operative events which have been reported over the years in obstetric patients who received general anaesthesia are attributable in part to a reluctance to use inhalational agents in adequate concentrations because of fears of inducing depression of the fetus and of increasing haemorrhage from the uterus. There is little evidence that these fears are justified. The dose of intravenous induction agent should not be reduced. If nitrous oxide is used in a concentration of only 50% before delivery, a higher concentration of volatile agent may be required than is necessary to supplement nitrous oxide 67%, and the rate of uptake of the volatile agent is reduced because the influence of the concentration effect is less pronounced. Volatile anaesthetic agents with a low blood/gas solubility coefficient are preferable, because there is usually a very short interval between induction of anaesthesia and the start of surgery. There is normally no good reason to discontinue administration of the volatile agent after delivery of the baby.

Difficult Intubation. It is often desirable to discontinue the administration of nitrous oxide in order to maintain adequate oxygenation if tracheal intubation is difficult. It is essential that anaesthesia is maintained while attempts are made to intubate the trachea, either by administration of adequate concentrations of a volatile agent in oxygen between attempts, or by further doses of an intravenous anaesthetic agent.

Premature Discontinuation of Anaesthesia. A desire to produce inappropriately rapid recovery of consciousness after surgery may lead the anaesthetist to discontinue administration of a volatile anaesthetic agent or intravenous infusion of anaesthetic drug several minutes before the end of the operation, or to switch off the nitrous oxide before reversal of the effects of neuromuscular blockers.

Failure to Understand Apparatus. Air is entrained by some mechanical ventilators if the supply of anaesthetic gases from the anaesthetic machine is less than the total minute volume delivered by the ventilator. Oxygen or air may dilute anaesthetic gases if tubing with an inadequate volume is used to connect a ventilator to a Bain system. Failure to understand the principles of the circle system may result in delivery of inadequate concentrations of anaesthetic gases.

Failure to Check Apparatus. Apparatus must be checked before and during every anaesthetic. Common causes of awareness include failure to ensure that the anaesthetic gases are delivered to a mechanical ventilator of a type which does not depend upon the supply of fresh gas for its power; loose connections in the ventilator tubing or breathing system, which result in loss of fresh gas and rebreathing or entrainment of air; failure to connect the vaporizer into the fresh gas supply at all or at least securely, or to lock the vaporizer on to a Selectatec block; failure to ensure that the vaporizer contains the anaesthetic agent; and failure to notice that a nitrous oxide cylinder has become empty. The emergency oxygen flush may be switched on accidentally, diluting the concentration of anaesthetic gases. An infusion of intravenous agent may become disconnected or leak, or the syringe in the infusion pump may become empty. A number of these events may occur during anaesthesia, even though a pre-anaesthetic check has been undertaken. There may also be misinterpretation of signs of light anaesthesia if ECG monitors and automated blood pressure devices are not checked regularly. Awareness may occur if an inaccurate inspired oxygen monitor or pulse oximeter causes the anaesthetist to increase the inspired concentration of oxygen inappropriately.

Genuine Apparatus Failure

In some circumstances, failure of apparatus could not reasonably have been predicted or detected by the anaesthetist. Flexible hoses connecting the supply of anaesthetic gases to the vaporizer may become perforated, resulting in a reduction in fresh gas flow rate. There may be a loss of fresh gas because of leaks in the back bar of the anaesthetic machine or a damaged flowmeter.

Vaporizers may very occasionally deliver grossly inaccurate concentrations of volatile agent. Infusion pumps may malfunction without sounding an alarm. Ventilators may operate incorrectly despite appropriate external connections.

Spurious Claims

Occasionally, patients complain of awareness without foundation. Others may claim recall of intra-operative events which are found on detailed questioning to be memories of the early post-operative period, or a dream.

Justified Risks

In a very small number of cases, the patient is so seriously ill that there is a genuine risk to life if normally adequate doses or concentrations of anaesthetic drug are administered. The commonest cause is profound hypotension caused by hypovolaemia when only surgery can effect a cure, e.g. ruptured aortic aneurysm, intra-abdominal or intrathoracic haemorrhage caused by trauma.

Prevention of Spontaneous Recall

The large majority of cases of awareness with recall can be prevented by adherence to a small number of principles of clinical practice. All apparatus should be checked before every operating list, and the ventilator, vaporizer and breathing system before every new case. All apparatus must be serviced by qualified personnel at the recommended intervals and full records of servicing kept.

Patients should be resuscitated adequately whenever possible so that concentrations of anaesthetic drugs do not need to be reduced as a result of exaggerated cardiovascular side effects.

An adequate dose of intravenous induction agent should be administered. The "sleep dose" should not be considered as the maximum, especially in young or unpremedicated patients. Consideration should be given to the duration of action of the agent. The induction agent alone should not be relied upon to maintain unconsciousness during tracheal intubation if non-depolarising neuromuscular blockers are used. Anaesthesia must be maintained while waiting for the relaxant to become effective. If intubation is difficult and prolonged, anaesthesia must be maintained either by the use of an inhalational agent with oxygen between attempts, or by supplementary doses of an intravenous drug.

Reliance should not be placed on nitrous oxide-oxygen mixtures alone. A supplementary agent should be used. Volatile agents are probably more predictable than intravenous agents in preventing awareness in the paralysed patient.

Opioids in conventional doses are not effective anaesthetic agents. They form an important part of a balanced anaesthetic technique, but must not be used as an alternative to adequate doses of anaesthetic agents.

Frequent checks of apparatus should be made during anaesthesia to ensure that all connections are intact and that reserves of anaesthetic agents in cylinders, vaporizers or infusion pumps are adequate. The patient's condition must be monitored continuously (see below). The anaesthetist must never leave the patient unattended.

If nitrous oxide is used, its administration should be continued until there is objective evidence of reversal of neuromuscular blockade. If other agents are employed, their anticipated elimination profile should be considered carefully when determining the time at which their administration is discontinued. Volatile agents with a low blood/gas solubility coefficient are eliminated rapidly.

General Monitoring

Monitoring apparatus can be a valuable aid in prevention of awareness in addition to its other functions, provided that the principles of operation are understood and that the measurements are correlated with clinical signs and with information from other equipment. Monitoring of inspired oxygen concentration is a guide to the nitrous oxide concentration when nitrous oxide-oxygen mixtures are administered through non-rebreathing delivery systems. The end-tidal carbon dioxide concentration profile may indicate some types of ventilator malfunction or partial loss of fresh gas flow, as may monitoring of expired tidal and minute volumes. Anaesthetic agent monitors are of great value in ensuring that the anticipated concentrations of agent are being delivered, and in titrating the delivered concentration to achieve the desired end-tidal concentration; they are of particular benefit when circle systems are used with low flow rates of fresh gas.

Monitoring Depth of Anaesthesia

Clearly, the probability of awareness is related to depth of anaesthesia. This can be difficult to assess accurately. In some circumstances, clinical signs of inadequate anaesthesia may be unreliable, and a number of alternative methods of monitoring have been investigated. However, clinical monitoring remains the only routine method of detecting depth of anaesthesia.

Clinical Signs. In the paralysed patient, the only clinical signs of inadequate anaesthesia are those which result from stimulation of the sympathetic nervous system. These may be affected by intercurrent disease or by the actions of other drugs.

The pupil size tends to decrease with increasing depth of anaesthesia, although the degree of constriction varies with different anaesthetic drugs, and the pupil may dilate during very deep anaesthesia. The response to light may be present during inadequate anaesthesia. Opioids constrict the pupil, and anticholinergics dilate it.

Arterial pressure tends to decrease as anaesthesia deepens. Heart rate tends to decrease with increasing depth of anaesthesia. However, other drugs, e.g. muscle relaxants, may influence cardiovascular parameters without altering the conscious level. Anticholinergic drugs may produce an inappropriately high heart rate and beta-blockers may mask tachycardia and hypertension which would otherwise result from inadequate anaesthesia. In addition, haemorrhage, drug reactions, and body fluid abnormalities may affect the interpretation of arterial pressure and heart rate. Peripheral vasoconstriction may be associated with light anaesthesia, but may also be influenced by body temperature and volaemic status.

Sweating and lacrimation may be found during light anaesthesia, but may be present when anaesthesia is adequate. Lacrimation is a more sensitive index of light anaesthesia than sweating. Both may be reduced if anticholinergic drugs have been administered.

Clearly, there may a number of reasons why clinical signs may be unreliable in detecting inadequate anaesthesia in some patients. In addition, patients may awaken, and subsequently recall conversation and touch, but may not be distressed; in the absence of distress or pain, clinical signs would not be expected to change. However, in the large majority of patients who recall pain during the operation, or are distressed by awakening, clear signs of sympathetic nervous system stimulation are found unless relative hypotension exists (as a result of drug administration or hypovolaemia) or significant beta-blockade is present. It is, of course, common for hypertension, tachycardia, sweating and, to a lesser extent, lacrimation to occur in patients who do not subsequently complain of recall of intra-operative events. Nevertheless, the presence of these clinical signs should be taken as a possible indication of inadequate anaesthesia and the doses or concentrations of anaesthetic agents increased, at least temporarily. It may be appropriate for clinical reasons to administer additional doses of opioid or muscle relaxant drugs, but in these circumstances, such agents should be used only as an adjunct to the provision of an effective concentration of anaesthetic drug.

Instrumental Monitoring. Many types of instrumental monitor of depth of anaesthesia have been described, but only the EEG-based methods (spectral edge, median EEG frequency and early cortical auditory evoked response) show any promise in providing possible indices of depth of anaesthesia [44, 46, 52]. These devices are undergoing clinical investigation, but, at the present time, none has been demonstrated to be useful in preventing recall of intra-operative events.

The Anaesthetic Record

Attention has already been drawn to the fact that most cases of awareness are preventable by checks of apparatus, appropriate dosage of drugs and careful monitoring of clinical signs of anaesthesia. However, in some cases, patients may complain of awareness (justifiably or not) when an appropriate technique has been employed and when no clinical signs of inadequate anaesthesia are present. It is very difficult to defend any claim of negligence arising from alleged awareness unless there is a comprehensive anaesthetic record which details the doses, concentrations and timings of all drugs as well as frequent recordings of clinical observations and measurements.

What Should the Patient be Told?

It is important that any patient who has experienced recall of intra-operative events should be identified. Ideally, this would be achieved by regular post-operative visits by all anaesthetists. However, this is not always achieved in practice and it is important that ward nurses and non-anaesthetic medical staff are educated about the subject in order that any complaint is dealt with appropriately. If informed of a patient who complains of awareness, the anaesthetist should interview the patient in the presence of a witness and listen carefully to the complaint. If it is clear that intra-operative awareness has occurred, the anaesthetist should acknowledge the fact that he/she believes the account of events. The anaesthetist should apologise to the patient and explain that awareness can occur without fault during anaesthesia in which muscle relaxants are employed because of the desire to avoid high and potentially toxic concentrations of anaesthetic drugs and because of difficulty in interpreting clinical signs. The patient should be reassured and informed that a note will be made in the hospital record so that other anaesthetists will know of the problem if anaesthesia and surgery are required in future. A full account of the interview should be recorded in the clinical notes. Junior anaesthetists should inform a consultant, who should be present when the patient is counselled.

It is advisable [7] to warn all "high-risk" patients (e.g. the seriously ill, and patients undergoing Caesarian section under general anaesthesia if low concentrations of anaesthetic agents are to be used) of the possibility of awareness during anaesthesia. Many patients are anxious about the possibility of awareness because of recent publicity. In addition, the psychological stress resulting from awareness may be reduced if a warning has been given. However, this should not be used as an excuse to omit the measures outlined above to reduce to a minimum the occurrence of this extremely distressing experience.

References

1. Ackers v Wigan Health Authority (1986), referred to in Current Law, March 1986.
2. Adams AP (1975) Techniques of vascular control for deliberate hypotension during anaesthesia. Br J Anaesth 47: 777-792
3. Adams AP, Baird WLM, Sykes MK et al. (1988) Recommendations for standards of monitoring during anaesthesia and recovery. Association of Anaesthetists of Great Britain and Ireland, London
4. Adams AP, Bickford-Smith PJ, Henville JD et al. (1990) Checklist for anaesthetic machines. Association of Anaesthetists of Great Britain and Ireland, London
5. Aitkenhead AR (1986) Cerebral protection. Br J Hosp Med 35: 290-298
6. Aitkenhead AR (1988) Regional and local anaesthetics and spinal narcotics for postoperative pain management. Curr Opin Anaesthesiol 1: 352-358
7. Aitkenhead AR (1990) Awareness during anaesthesia: what should the patient be told? Anaesthesia 45: 351-352
8. Alexander SC, Smith TC, Strobel G, Stephen GW, Wollman H (1968) Cerebral carbohydrate metabolism of man during respiratory and metabolic alkalosis. J Appl Physiol 24: 66-71
9. Assem ESK (1990) Anaphylactic anaesthetic reactions: the value of paper radioallergosorbent tests for IgE antibodies to muscle relaxants and thiopentone. Anaesthesia 45: 1032-1038
10. Baldo BA, Fisher MM (1983) Substituted ammonium ions as allergenic determinants in drug allergy. Nature 306: 262-264
11. Blacher RS (1975) On awakening paralysed during surgery. JAMA 234: 67-68
12. Bonsu AK, Stead AL (1983) Accidental cross-connexion of oxygen and nitrous oxide in an anaesthetic machine. Anaesthesia 38: 767-769
13. Brahams D (1990) Medicine and the law. Two anaesthetists convicted of manslaughter. Lancet 336: 430-431
14. Brierley JK, French JM, Cartlidge NEF (1991) A comparison of the neurological and neuropsychological sequelae in patients undergoing different types of cardiopulmonary bypass surgery. (In press)

15. Buck H, Devlin HB, Lunn JN (1987) The report of a confidential enquiry into perioperative deaths. Nuffield Provincial Hospitals Trust, London
16. Cole AGH, Thompson JB, Fodor IM, Baker AB, Sear JW (1983) Anaesthetic machine hazard from the Selectatec block. Anaesthesia 38: 175–177
17. Crawford JS (1984) Principles and practice of obstetric anaesthesia. Blackwell Scientific Publications, Oxford, p 297
18. Eichhorn JH (1989) Prevention of intraoperative anesthesia accidents and related severe injury through safety monitoring. Anesthesiology 70: 572–577
19. Faulkner A (1989) Incidence of fatal reactions to commonly used anaesthetic drugs. Letter from Ledger Bennett Public Relations Ltd. to Dame Jill Knight MP, October 26, 1989
20. Fisher MMcD (1990) Medico-legal aspects of anaphylaxis. J Med Defence Union, Spring: 4–5
21. Fisher MMcD, Baldo BA (1984) Anaphylactoid reactions during anaesthesia. Clin Anaesthesiol 2: 677–692
22. Gaba DM, DeAnda A. A comprehensive anesthesia simulation environment: re-creating the operating room for research and training. Anesthesiology 69: 387–394
23. Garcia JH, Conger KA (1981) Ischemic brain injuries: structural and biochemical effects. In: Grenvik A, Safar P (eds) Brain failure and resuscitation. Churchill Livingstone, New York, pp 35–54 (Clinics in critical care medicine, vol 2)
24. Hanning CD, Kruchek D, Chunara A (1987) Preferential oxygen leak – an unusual case. Anaesthesia 42: 1329–1330
25. Hargrove RL (1987) Awareness under anaesthesia. J Med Defence Union, Spring: 9–11
26. Harle DG, Baldo BA, Fisher MM (1984) Detection of IgE antibodies to suxamethonium after anaphylactoid reactions during anaesthesia. Lancet ii: 930–932
27. Harris TJB, Brice DD, Hetherington RR, Utting JE (1971) Dreaming associated with anaesthesia: the influence of morphine premedication and two volatile adjuvants. Br J Anaesth 43: 172–178
28. Hutchinson R (1960) Awareness during surgery. Br J Anaesth 33: 463–469
29. Kelbie D (1989) Sheriff D. Kelbie, Sheriffdom of Grampian, Highlands and Islands Determination given on 9 May 1989 at Aberdeen
30. Kolata GB, Marx JL (1976) Epidemiology of heart diseases: searches for causes. Science 194: 509–511
31. Levinson BW (1965) States of awareness during general anaesthesia. Br J Anaesth 67: 544–546
32. Lindop MJ (1975) Complications and morbidity of controlled hypotension Br J Anaesth 47: 799–803
33. Liu D, Thorp S, Graham S, Aitkenhead AR (1990) Incidence of recall of awareness during anaesthesia for non-obstetric surgery. Br J Anaesth 65: 575–576
34. Lunn JN, Mushin WW (1982) Mortality associated with anaesthesia. Nuffield Provincial Hospitals Trust, London
35. McKenna T, Wilton TNP (1973) Awareness during endotracheal intubation. Anaesthesia 28: 599–602
36. Millar K (1989) Recall, recognition and implicit memory for intra-anaesthetic events. In: Jones JG (ed) Depth of anaesthesia. Baillière Tindall, London, pp 487–510 (Baillière's clinical anaesthesiology: international practice and research, vol 3
37. Moir DD (1976) Obstetric anaesthesia and analgesia. Baillière Tindall, London, p 145
38. Nimmo WS, Aitkenhead AR, Clarke RSJ et al. (1990) Anaphylactic reactions associated with anaesthesia. Association of Anaesthetists of Great Britain and Ireland, London
39. Noble DW, Yap PL (1989) Screening for antibodies to anaesthetics. No case for doing it yet. Br Med J 299: 2
40. Notcutt WG, Morgan RJM (1990) Introducing patient-controlled analgesia for postoperative pain control into a district general hospital. Anaesthesia 45: 406–408
41. Nunn JF (1987) Applied respiratory physiology, 3rd edn. Butterworth, London
42. Plum F, Posner JB (1982) The diagnosis of stupor and coma, 3rd edn. FA Davis Company, Philadelphia
43. Safar P (1981) Resuscitation after brain ischemia. In: Grenvik A, Safar P (eds) Brain failure and resuscitation. Churchill Livingstone, New York, pp 155–184 (Clinics in critical care medicine, vol 2)
44. Schwilden H (1989) Use of the median EEG frequency and pharmacokinetics in determining depth of anaesthesia. In: Jones JG (ed) Depth of anaesthesia. Baillière Tindall, London, pp 603–621 (Baillière's clinical anaesthesiology: international practice and research, vol 3)
45. Sear JW (1983) General kinetic and dynamic principles and their application to continuous infusion anaesthesia. Anaesthesia 38 (Suppl): 10–25
46. Sebel PS (1989) Somatosensory, visual and motor evoked potentials in anaesthetized patients. In:

Jones JG (ed) Depth of anaesthesia. Baillière Tindall, London, pp 587-602 (Baillière's clinical anaesthesiology: international practice and research, vol 3)

47. Shaw PJ, Bates D, Cartlidge NEF et al. (1986) Neurological complications of coronary artery bypass surgery: six-month follow-up study. Br Med J 293: 165-167

48. Siesjo BK, Ljunggren B (1973) Cerebral energy reserves after prolonged hypoxia and ischemia. Arch Neurol 29: 400-407

49. Smith GB, Hirsch NP, Ehrenwerth J (1986) Placement of double-lumen endobronchial tubes: correlation between clinical impressions and bronchoscopic findings. Br J Anaesth 58: 1317-1320

50. Stoelting RK, Longnecker DE, Eger EI (1970) Minimum alveolar concentrations in man on awakening from methoxyflurane, halothane, ether and fluroxene anesthesia: MAC awake. Anesthesiology 33: 5-9

51. Thompson PW (1987) Safer design of anaesthetic equipment. Br J Anaesth 59: 913-921

52. Thornton C, Konieczko K, Jones JG, Jordan C, Doré CJ, Heneghan CPH (1988) Effect of surgical stimulation on the auditory evoked response. Br J Anaesth 56: 372-378

53. Thorp JM, Railton R (1982) Hypoxia due to air in the oxygen pipeline: a case for oxygen monitoring in theatre. Anaesthesia 37: 683-687

54. Tinker JH, Dull DL, Caplan RA, Ward RJ, Cheney FW (1989) Role of monitoring devices in prevention of anesthetic mishaps: a closed claim analysis. Anesthesiology 71: 541-546

55. Tunstall ME (1977) Detecting wakefulness during general anaesthesia for Caesarean section. Br Med J i: 1321

56. Utting JE (1987) Pitfalls in anaesthetic practice. Br J Anaesth 59: 877-890

57. Vacanti D, Van Houten RJ, Hill RC (1970) A statistical analysis of the relationship of physical status to postoperative mortality in 68386 cases. Anesth Anal 49: 564-567

58. Ward CS (1985) The continuous flow anaesthetic machine. In: Ward CS, Anaesthetic equipment, 2nd edn. Baillière Tindall, London, pp 104-121

59. Watkins J (1989) Second report from an anaesthetic advisory service. Anaesthesia 44: 157-159

60. Whitby LG (1974) Screening for disease. Definitions and criteria. Lancet i: 819-822

61. White DC (1987) Anaesthesia: a privation of the senses. An historical introduction and some definitions. In: Rosen M, Lunn JN (eds) Consciousness awareness and pain in general anaesthesia. Butterworth, London, pp 1-9

62. Williams KN, Nunn JF (1989) The oesophageal detector device. A prospective trial on 100 patients. Anaesthesia 44: 412-414

63. Wilson SH, Vaughan RW, Stephen CR (1975) Awareness, dreams and hallucinations associated with general anesthesia. Anesth Analg 54: 609-616

CHAPTER 5

General Surgery

N. Keddie

General surgery is not considered to be a very high risk specialty but the number of claims emanating from it has increased rapidly in recent years. The identity of general surgery is changing and many claims are supported by expert opinions from surgeons who specialise in one part of what was once considered to be a general discipline. They state mostly that a sufficiency of skill is only acquired by those who regularly undertake their particular procedures. This causes difficulty in the defence of the general surgeon concerned if he admits to only performing a certain operation three or four times a year. In the emergency situation general surgeons are expected to tackle all kinds of problems on an occasional basis. The specialisation within general surgery already exists, but is likely to progress further over the next few years with inevitable medico-legal consequences.

What is General Surgery?

In large urban areas such specialties as vascular surgery have already become completely separate, and recently an association was founded for Coloprocto-logical surgeons. Although this diversification is continuing, it might be said that at the present time general surgical practice still encompasses:

Gastroenterology
Vascular surgery
Endocrine surgery
Surgery of the breast
Surgery of the salivary glands
Surgery of the spleen
Surgery of the skin and superficial swellings
Hernia
Head injuries
Sterilisation of male patients
Acute abdomen

This chapter will be considered under these headings, with the exception of head injury. Certain other problems that commonly arise will be mentioned in conclusion.

General Causes for Claims

Inadequate Experience

Claims most commonly follow the results of operations carried out by inexperienced surgeons. When avoidable complications arise defence is impossible. It is not easy to define adequate experience and all surgeons inevitably must go through a learning phase. Experience is required to recognise problems when they arise and to know when help should be sought from a more experienced colleague. The Confidential Enquiry into Peri-operative Deaths (see Bibliography) confirmed that junior and untrained surgeons were responsible for complications and mortality which might well have been avoided had a more senior surgeon been present; a fact which the defence organisations have recognised for many years. Ideally adequate supervision should be provided for surgeons in training at all times, but what is adequate supervision? A number of claims indeed arise from serious complications produced by a junior surgeon when his chief is working in the adjacent theatre. Lack of experience results in a failure to seek help when it is readily available.

Night and Weekend Cover

Another common cause for claims relates to medical cover at night or over weekends when inadequate communication between medical staff occurs. Problems that develop may go unrecognised, leading to avoidable serious morbidity and mortality. When difficulties arise the resident doctor may not appreciate the seriousness of the situation and consequently does not inform the senior doctor sufficiently quickly. Post-operative intra-abdominal bleeding and bacteraemic shock are common examples of causes in this context.

Failure to diagnose the cause of acute abdominal pain is another common problem. It is essential for the on-call staff to visit the patients of the off-duty team each day at the weekend. It is not adequate to rely entirely on the nursing staff to inform them of changes in the patients' condition. It is also vital for the team going off-duty to fully inform the on-duty team about any ill patients. Good clinical records are essential to ensure that a doctor called in an emergency to some unexpected problem knows what has gone before. Holiday times and locum doctors are other potential sources of danger because the normal routines of the surgical unit are not followed in these circumstances.

The Acute Abdomen

Missed Diagnosis

Errors of diagnosis are the commonest cause for claims in this context. These mistakes often involve the general practitioners who are initially called to see the patient, but may also occur in hospital after the patient has been admitted. On occasions, the patient may even be discharged from hospital with an incorrect diagnosis, which leads to claims which are difficult to defend.

Perforation of peptic ulcers is normally very obvious, but in some cases atypical presentations occur, leading to errors in diagnosis. If a proper history has been taken, a thorough examination performed, but an incorrect conclusion has been reached, the claim may be defensible. Sometimes it is impossible to defend a claim because of inadequate records and lack of arrangements to review the patient when a definite diagnosis has not been reached.

Failure to diagnose acute appendicitis is also common. Difficulties may arise due to the anatomical site of the appendix, the extremes of age and the type of appendicitis (catarrhal or obstructive). The problem of gastroenteritis frequently muddles the issue. Acute intestinal obstruction is usually obvious and no difficulty should be experienced in reaching a diagnosis at an early stage. Occasionally, however, some cases are far from typical and even experienced clinicians are well aware of patients in whom the diagnosis has been extremely obscure. It may only be made when the bowel is gangrenous, necessitating a resection. Complications may follow which result in a claim being put forward. Sometimes these claims may be defended on the basis that they are accepted complications of this form of surgery. On other occasions where inadequate care has been provided, a claim can be difficult to defend.

There have been several claims for delay in diagnosis of a ruptured abdominal aortic aneurysm. Often these cases give warning symptoms, such as backache or an episode of acute pain prior to the final rupture. The relatives may allege that the diagnosis should have been made at this stage should the patient die without time for successful treatment to be given.

Ectopic pregnancy can on occasions be very obscure and it is important to bear the diagnosis in mind in young females of childbearing age with lower abdominal symptoms. The menstrual history may not help. Emergency laparoscopy has been helpful in improving the diagnostic accuracy. The availability of rapid pregnancy testing is useful, but may be negative in early cases. The disastrous consequences of sending a young girl out of hospital who has mild iliac fossa discomfort but then ruptures the pregnancy with fatal haemorrhage are obvious.

There are still many claims because of missed torsion of the testicle. The first point to bear in mind is that the early symptoms are in the iliac fossa, not the scrotum and this can cause problems. Acute epididymo-orchitis rarely occurs in young boys. Although rare, torsion must be excluded in all cases of pain and swelling of the testicle. There is only a short time, perhaps 6 hours, in which to act. This is a real emergency of surgery, necessitating the interruption of an ongoing list if no free theatre is available. In addition, it is critically important to fix the other testicle so that it does not twist at a later date.

Post-operative Complications

The Post-operative Acute Abdomen

This is notoriously difficult and may result in a number of claims.

Post-operative Intra-abdominal Bleeding

This usually develops after senior members of the surgical staff have left the hospital and the junior doctor is responsible for the care of the patient. In some cases, it is clear what is happening. The blood pressure falls, the pulse rate rises and it is immediately obvious that there is a serious problem requiring urgent action. In the cases which have been referred to the Medical Defence Union, the blood pressure has been maintained for several hours, although there has been a rise in the pulse rate; then quite suddenly there is a catastrophic fall of blood pressure. Complications, such as spinal artery thrombosis leading to paraplegia and cerebral thrombosis with permanent functional damage may ensue. Acute renal failure may also be a cause of claims for damage. The discharge from a drain is not an accurate guide to the amount of intra-peritoneal haemorrhage.

Post-operative Peritonitis

This does not present the typical features of peritonitis seen in a patient who has not had recent surgery. The usual presentation is rapid, shallow breathing, tachycardia and hypotension and the so-called high-output respiratory failure syndrome due to the elevation of the diaphragm caused by the peritoneal inflammation. An incorrect diagnosis of cardiac failure, myocardial infarction, pulmonary embolism or post-operative pulmonary collapse is frequently made. The pulse rate is often very rapid, the blood pressure low and the blood gases grossly abnormal. The circumstances in which post-operative peritonitis are likely to develop should give a clue to the diagnosis, but there is no simple test that can be done to confirm it. If laparotomy is delayed, fatal complications develop and these have led to claims.

Post-operative Intestinal Obstruction

This can be extremely difficult to diagnose. Once again, the typical features of intestinal obstruction are not obvious because of the resolving paralytic ileus following the laparotomy which merges into the mechanical obstruction. As with post-operative peritonitis the circumstances in which the problem is likely to develop probably give the best clue. Plain abdominal radiographs can be helpful. If closely questioned, the patient usually complains of colicky pain and the typical bowel sounds can be heard occasionally. Radio contrast studies, using water soluble contrast, can be very valuable in determining whether or not there is a mechanical rather than a paralytic obstruction. In general, surgeons rarely regret re-exploring a post-operative abdomen when some catastrophe is suspected. Obviously unnecessary negative explorations are an extra burden for the patient and should be avoided, if possible.

Post-operative Abscesses

The development of modern imaging techniques has certainly improved the diagnosis of post-operative abscesses. Their presence can frequently be confirmed by the radiologist, but sadly, when missed, claims may follow. Defence of the surgeon who has failed to carry out the necessary diagnostic investigations may be difficult.

Successful defence of the management of the acute post-operative abdomen is difficult if the monitoring of patient's progress has been poor. This may be the result of different doctors being involved in the patient's care. The records in these cases are often of poor quality.

Gastroenterology

Many surgeons now carry out their own fibre optic endoscopy. This has led to a massive expansion in the use of endoscopic techniques with resultant increase in negligence claims. Patients do not consider that complications should follow a procedure which they look on as an investigation. The British Society of Digestive Endoscopy has carried out an excellent multicentre prospective study on the complications of endoscopy and these have provided a basis for defending claims in those cases where complications have arisen in the hands of an experienced endoscopist. As stated in the introduction to the chapter, claims against the relatively inexperienced operator may be more difficult to defend. Another area of difficulty is the question as to whether or not warnings about complications should be given and the whole vexed question of informed consent arises. It is certainly not the usual British practice to mention the possibility of a perforation of the gastrointestinal tract as being a significant risk. However, acute pancreatitis should be mentioned as one of the risks during endoscopic retrograde cholangio-pancreatography. This complication may occur however skilful the operator.

Oesophago-gastro-duodenoscopy

The commonest cause for claims following this procedure is a perforation. Claims still arise for perforation using the rigid instrument still used by thoracic surgeons. This account however is confined to the more widely used fibre optic instrument. Perforations can arise in the pharynx during difficult intubation. They are rare in the oesophagus unless associated with interventional procedures, such as dilatation or insertion of tubes into malignant lesions. They rarely occur in the stomach. No cases of perforation in the duodenum have been reported to the Union. There has been a considerable increase in the number of balloon dilatations for functional disorders of the musculature of the oesophagus and a number of claims have arisen after perforation of the oesophagus followed by serious complications. The patient should be warned of this possibility. Whether or not these complications can be defended relates to the promptness of the diagnosis and the adequacy of treatment. Studies by the British Society of

Digestive Endoscopy have shown that perforation is undoubtedly a recognised hazard in a small percentage of cases.

Another source of claims relates to the taking of biopsy material from a number of patients on a large list of upper gastrointestinal endoscopies. The specimens may be labelled wrongly and the dangers that can follow from this are clear. A further source of difficulty may arise from numerous specimens being sent to the laboratory at the same time. They are removed from their pots for staining and examination and during this manoeuvre mistakes can arise. There have been a number of claims when an incorrect diagnosis of carcinoma has been made. The surgeon, as a result, may unwisely proceed to surgical resection, though he may well have been surprised by the result of the biopsy. Patients have developed serious complications or even died following such resections. These claims are indefensible. An unexpected biopsy report should necessitate a repeat endoscopy.

Endoscopic Retrograde Cholangio-pancreatography (ERCP)

Mention has already been made of acute pancreatitis following a diagnostic ERCP. This is well documented and is unavoidable in a small percentage of patients. Fatal cases have led to claims but these have been successfully defended because adequate warnings were given to the patient's relatives. Other claims that have arisen relate to operative interventions associated with ERCP, in particular sphincterotomy, leading to torrential haemorrhage or perforation of the duodenum. Both these hazards are well documented, but the difficulties in defence arise when they have not been recognised and in consequence treated promptly. A gastroenterologist doing ERCP must work very closely with the surgeon so that prompt action can be taken when complications arise.

Colonoscopy

Perforation is a recognised hazard in even the most expert hands. There is a greater risk in bowel which is severely diseased. Perforations can also complicate biopsy or polypectomy. Claims have been defended in those cases in which perforations occurred providing the operator is adequately experienced and has recognised the complication promptly and treated it successfully.

Other claims have arisen when lesions have been missed, in particular carcinomata which came to light many months later. This is a difficult area and defence may not be easy. There is no doubt that colonoscopy is difficult and it is easy to miss small malignant lesions as the instrument slips rapidly through a loop of the colon.

Laparoscopy

This is much more widely practised by gynaecologists than general surgeons in the UK but in future many more general surgeons will be using this technique both for diagnosis and for treatment. The Royal College of Obstetricians and

Gynaecologists have collected detailed information on the complications which may follow this procedure. Most general surgeons are familiar with having to deal with such problems. Injuries are described to the major arteries and veins on the posterior abdominal wall. Bowel injuries occur and are not always immediately obvious. Less commonly, ureteric injuries have been reported to the Medical Defence Union. It would be interesting to see the evolution of laparoscopic surgery which inevitably will give rise to its own selection of claims in the future.

Missed Carcinoma

This is a common cause of claims involving the gastrointestinal tract. Most concern general practitioners, but some involve the surgeon or physician as well. Gastric carcinoma has very mild symptoms in its early stages and these can easily be overlooked even by a caring doctor. Defence is difficult even in those cases where the patient has been seen and a careful history taken. The problem is one of taking a case to court where there is a grieving widow complaining that the doctor failed to diagnose her husband's cancer at the appropriate stage. Pancreatic carcinoma is notoriously difficult to diagnose early, but relatives find this difficult to accept. At the other end of the gastrointestinal tract many cases of missed rectal cancer can cause claims. The doctor may assume the rectal bleeding is from piles, does not carry out a proper examination or refer the patient to the appropriate specialist at an early stage.

Common Bile Duct Injuries

Sadly these continue to occur in significant numbers. Injuries are completely avoidable and totally indefensible. The crucial point is to recognise that the duct has been damaged. Cholangiography used to be recommended as a routine during cholecystectomy, but recently to save cost it has been carried out only in selected cases where common duct stones are thought more likely to be present. The advantage of cholangiography in defining the biliary anatomy is not stressed enough, especially to inexperienced surgeons. When injury occurs it usually presents several days after surgery when jaundice or a biliary fistula is formed. It is important to refer these patients immediately to a surgeon experienced in their management. The individual general surgeon rarely, if ever, has to deal with this problem. He does not have the skill and experience of someone who has made a special study of the condition. He also lacks the necessary backup resources.

Impotence after Rectal Excision

This is recognised as a complication and is well documented in the literature. Patients not unexpectedly sue when it develops. The vexed question of informed consent again arises. Should a warning be given to a man prior to removal of the rectum of the possibility of impotence? The worst situation concerns young men having urgent surgery for inflammatory bowel disease in whom the risk is perhaps greater if the tissue planes behind the rectum are obliterated by fibrous tissue and infection. The operation is difficult and I do not think categorical advice can be given on this point. The author's own view is not to warn the patient.

Incontinence after Anal Procedures

An increasing number of claims have arisen from this source. The most common are related to the use of the cryoprobe to deal with haemorrhoids. The damage arises when the probe has been left in position for longer than the recommended time. This leads to injury of the sphincter. A number of claims have recently been made for sphincter problems following maximal anal dilatation for haemorrhoids. Damage to the anal canal may have been caused by the preoperative enema. This is not recognised at the time and serious septic complications follow, leading to sphincter damage. Each claim has to be considered on its merit as to whether or not it is defensible. The encouraging aspect of these problems is that there are many more methods now available for investigation and for treating patients with incontinence. Thus they are not all necessarily permanently incontinent, as they would have been in the past.

Surgery for Obesity

This is now carried out with increasing frequency. Very obese patients are grave operative risks and claims have arisen for complications of the surgery. It is essential to warn the patient of the risks because they are common and the surgery is being carried out for a non-malignant condition. Patients must only be treated by someone with special experience of this problem in a clinic where they can be thoroughly monitored. Liver failure leading to death has been the commonest cause for claims. Other claims have arisen for fistula formation and difficulties with the wound, including incisional herniae and chronic sinuses.

General Advice

All patients undergoing major gastrointestinal operations should be given prophylactic antibiotics and prophylactic anticoagulants. Claims have arisen from failure to take these precautions.

Vascular Surgery

Varicose Veins

The large number of patients treated for varicose veins has led to numerous claims. Treatment is frequently left to junior surgeons with little experience.

Femoral Vein Damage

The most expensive claims arise from femoral vein injury which remains a common problem. This most often occurs in the hands of a relatively inexperienced surgeon and in any case is never defensible. If the injury is recognised immediately, it is essential that a vascular surgeon is summoned to try and rectify the damage. If a segment of femoral vein has been damaged and a graft is required, it is essential to make a graft of adequate diameter using a cylinder created from an opposite saphenous vein unless the one from the same side is available. Inserting a simple saphenous vein graft is never adequate because of the difference in diameter, though this is often attempted. Another controversial issue concerns whether or not arteriovenous shunt should be established using the external pudendal artery. Judging from cases reported to the Medical Defence Union, this has never appeared to be a successful or useful technique. Most of the patients in whom this is attempted appear to end up with permanent deep venous insufficiency. This results in a substantial settlement as many are young women.

Nerve Damage

Lateral Popliteal Nerve

This nerve is extremely vulnerable at the neck of the fibula and in the popliteal fossa. Numerous claims arise for damage which are all indefensible. The nerve is either cut in error for a vein or stripped out during subcutaneous avulsion of veins. Damage may occur from extravasation of sclerosant or it may be compressed by the bandaging. The latter cases usually recover satisfactorily but the others rarely do so. Immediate suture even using microsurgical methods does not necessarily give good long-term results.

Long Saphenous Nerve

This is in close proximity to the long saphenous vein in the vicinity of the ankle and even if carefully separated from the vein, may be stripped out due to its variable relationship to the vessel. Some surgeons claim damage to the nerve can be avoided by stripping from above downwards. Others restrict stripping to the thigh. It appears that the long saphenous nerve is at risk whatever method of stripping is employed. To avoid injury it is better not to use the stripper, but this is clearly a controversial issue.

Short Saphenous Nerve

Claims for injury to the short saphenous nerve are frequent in surgery carried out for short saphenous incompetence over the popliteal fossa. Local ligations near the course of the saphenous nerve are also a risk.

Wound Problems

Because this surgery is often done for cosmetic reasons, patients claim if the wounds are unsatisfactory, for example, following infection. A number of patients are allergic to catgut, which is frequently used to ligate the veins, and this gives rise to infection. Some patients develop keloid scars for which they may claim.

Injection Therapy

Extravasation of the sclerosant with tissue damage is a hazard. This can result in skin necrosis and subcutaneous tissue loss. An indurated pigmented subcutaneous area which is permanent and unsightly may result. These claims are indefensible as it is such a well-recognised hazard of injection treatment. Difficulties often arise because the procedure is left to a young inexperienced surgeon in less than ideal conditions. There have been a number of claims due to sclerosant entering the posterior tibial artery, leading to tissue loss in the forefoot.

Prophylactic Anticoagulants

Claims have arisen for pulmonary embolism and deep vein thrombosis following varicose vein surgery. It is advisable therefore to give some form of prophylaxis which, although it does not guarantee prevention, does cut down the incidence.

Contraceptive Pill

Operations carried out while the patient is on the pill are controversial. In the past it was considered that this led to a greater risk of deep vein thrombosis. Any patient on the pill was advised to stop it for a minimum of a full month prior to the treatment. In fact, it would normally be recommended that patients with varicose veins are not prescribed the pill. More recent evidence indicates that the risks have been exaggerated. Claims however are still made arising from these risks.

Arterial Injury

Arterial damage may result from penetrating injuries or fractures. The essential point is to be aware of the possibility and to check peripheral pulses in all cases of injury. Paradoxically the serious problems are the result of distal ischaemia rather than local bleeding. There is either failure to appreciate that the distal pulses are absent or the urgency of the situation is not comprehended. Early exploration is essential if the pulses do not recover promptly after manipulation of the fracture or if an arterial injury is suspected. Arteriovenous fistula is a late complication of arterial injury which may be missed.

Compartment Syndrome

This condition results from a rise in compartmental pressure due to oedema or bleeding. The small arterioles are occluded, producing ischaemia primarily affecting nerve tissue. Pulsation in the main vessels may still be felt distal to the obstruction and unless the pressure is relieved by extensive fasciotomies, soft tissue damage may become irreversible. Early diagnosis and treatment are essential.

Arterial Disease

The increasing amount of interventional surgery carried out in patients with mainly degenerative arterial disease has resulted in a rise of the number of claims in this field. Claims for delays in carrying out limb salvage surgery are the commonest The late referral of a patient to a vascular surgeon may lead to the unnecessary loss of a limb or part of a limb due to ischaemia. Difficulty also arises when an abdominal aortic aneurysm is missed or warning symptoms of its rupture are not appreciated. Backache or mild abdominal symptoms are ignored prior to the crisis so that when rupture occurs it may well be fatal. Failure to diagnose diabetes may give rise to problems. The disease may not be recognised when ischaemia of the limb is the presenting feature. Inadequate treatment may be given for septic feet in patients with uncontrolled diabetes and incipient ischaemia. Usually there is a failure to consider the diagnosis and a simple urine test is not carried out.

Arteriography

This is not strictly a surgical procedure. Nevertheless, it gives rise to a considerable number of claims due to inadequate warning of the hazards. The vascular surgeon is called upon to cope with the complications of this investigation. Claims are made due to damage to the artery which is used for access to the arteriogram or for ischaemic complications, such as peripheral embolism or dissection. There is debate as to how much warning should be given to a patient who is about to undergo this procedure.

Angioplasty is also a source of problems. Arterial damage may occur caused by the balloon or peripheral embolism. It is essential that a radiologist and a vascular surgeon work in close conjunction so that any complications that do arise can be promptly handled.

Cervical Sympathectomy

The classical operation for removal of upper sympathetic ganglia carried out through the supra-clavicular fossa is a frequent source of claims. Brachial plexus damage may occur. The anatomy of the plexus is variable and in particular its relationship to the scalene muscles. During exposure of the upper thoracic ganglia through this route damage can occur even in expert hands. There have been claims for other complications, such as Horner's syndrome and pneumothorax which can be defended, but injury to the plexus itself is difficult to defend. If the procedure is carried out through the axillary route these complications can be avoided. An endoscopic method is now in use for carrying out upper thoracic sympathectomy through the rib space.

Endocrine Surgery

Thyroid

Recurrent Laryngeal Nerve Injury

Exposure of the recurrent laryngeal nerves during thyroidectomy minimises the risk of their injury. Even in the most expert hands there is a risk of 1%–2% of nerves being damaged either temporarily or permanently. Should the surgeon be experienced in this operation and has exposed the recurrent laryngeal nerves it is possible to defend claims for injury to one nerve. A pre-operative check of vocal cord function may reveal an unsuspected laryngeal nerve dysfunction. In this case special care will be required to avoid damage to the remaining nerve. Difficulties almost always arise in defence of this complication when the surgeon is an occasional thyroidectomist. A medical report from a surgeon skilled in this operation is likely to support the view that the occasional thyroidectomist should not be carrying out the procedure.

Bilateral Recurrent Laryngeal Nerve Injuries

These cases are generally indefensible. They do not always present in the immediate post-operative period as one might anticipate. They come to light at a later date, the patient having suffered episodes of respiratory infection, bouts of uncontrollable coughing or choking. Voice change may not be very noticeable. A post-operative cord check is essential as delayed palsies of the nerve can occur, not directly due to operative trauma. There is debate as to whether pre-operative warnings of nerve injury should be given. Should every patient be warned of the possibility that their voice may change after thyroidectomy? The risk of this complication is low. In general, British practice has been to warn patients whose voice is critical to their lifestyle but not every patient. This approach has been supported in the courts in similar low risk cases.

Another problem is damage to the external laryngeal nerve. It is not always possible to avoid injury to this structure, though appropriate steps should be taken to prevent it. Most cases of voice change after thyroidectomy are associated with external laryngeal nerve injury rather than recurrent nerve injury.

Other Causes for Claims after Thyroidectomy

The commonest of these relates to haemorrhage. If this is not treated promptly it can lead to respiratory obstruction and hypoxic brain damage. It is vital in a unit where thyroid surgery is carried out that the nursing staff are familiar with the early signs of bleeding in the neck and that the junior medical staff are skilled at passing endotracheal tubes whenever necessary.

Clear instructions must be given that if intubation is unsuccessful the skin clips and sutures in the strap muscles are released in order that the clot can escape to relieve any tracheal pressure.

Other complaints concern the scar. Adequate explanations need to be given pre-operatively about the site and length of the wound. Persons predisposed to keloid formation must be warned of the possibility that this may occur.

A rare cause for claims has been late hypothyroidism. This can be very insidious and for this reason is missed. It may occur many years after the operation has long since been forgotten. It is essential that patients who have had thyroid surgery have their thyroid function checked annually and they should be instructed to attend the general practitioner's surgery for this to be done on discharge from the clinic.

Other Endocrine Problems

Rarely claims have arisen for failure to diagnose the less common endocrine problems. They can on occasions be defended. Sometimes, despite the rarity of the condition, failure to diagnose may not be indefensible, but failure to have the patient seen and investigated by an appropriate specialist cannot be defended. Examples include pheocromocytoma where the blood pressure has not been taken in patients having what in retrospect are clearly typical episodes of intermittent hypertension. A second example is patients having episodes of hypoglycaemia which are labelled as being functional attacks of fainting or fits. In retrospect it may be clear that they were due to hypoglycaemia. The important point is that the doctor should refer the patient for investigation, not that they have failed to make the diagnosis. It is dangerous to label a patient's symptoms as functional without a careful history, full examination and investigation.

Breast

Breast disease is a major source of negligence claims.

Missed Carcinoma

This is undoubtedly the most common problem. A general practitioner may fail to refer a patient with a possible lump in the breast for specialist advice. Alternatively, the surgeon does not consider that biopsy is necessary for a rather vague ill-defined area of thickening which subsequently proves to be a carcinoma. Standard teaching insists that breast lumps must be diagnosed properly. Failure to do so is difficult to defend. Nowadays there are methods readily available for this short of open biopsy, namely, mammography and fine needle aspiration or Trucut biopsy. All these methods have their false positives and false negatives and require expert interpretation.

Breast Screening

This is now practised on a very wide scale and is a major source of claims. Breast screening by mammography is the standard practice. Once more there is the difficulty of the general surgeon who deals with patients with breast disease as against the specialist surgeon running a large breast clinic. What is the standard of care which should be expected for an individual patient? Undoubtedly, it is the standard that can be provided by an expert breast clinic.

Other claims have arisen in cases where a mammogram has been reported as showing the typical appearances of carcinoma. Mastectomy has been performed without confirming that the radiological appearance is in fact due to carcinoma. The pathologist is then unable to find any evidence of malignancy and this inevitably leads to a claim for unnecessary mastectomy. False negatives obviously give rise to claims when a carcinoma comes to light a relatively short time after a mammogram and reassurance of the patient that there was no problem. Because there are problems of interpretation of mammograms such errors can be defended.

Mastectomy

Difficulties arise when a frozen section is reported as showing carcinoma, but subsequent paraffin sections are found to be benign. By this time a mastectomy may have been carried out. Other claims arise for post-operative scarring, severe infection or skin loss. These usually can be defended providing they have been handled in an expert manner by an experienced surgeon. There is no obligation to settle for post-operative complications that are well recognised.

Reconstructive Breast Surgery

This work is technically demanding. Surgery should only be carried out by those surgeons with special training and skill. Should this work be carried out by a plastic surgeon or a general surgeon with a special interest in breast surgery? Claims are often supported by experts from the field of plastic surgery who are critical of general surgeons with breast experience doing reconstructive work that goes wrong. Claims can also follow the implantation of plastic silastic implants. These may be followed by numerous complications that can make the recognition of recurrent disease very difficult.

Salivary Glands

Parotid Surgery

The facial nerve is at risk during the removal of parotid tumours. Patients should be warned of this possibility. In this field also it is essential that surgeons are experienced in carrying out the procedure. Facial nerve injury cannot be defended when it occurs in the hands of an occasional parotidectomist.

Spleen

In recent years it has become increasingly apparent that there is a significant risk of pneumococcal septicaemia after splenectomy. This can be fatal. It has been recognised as a risk in young patients for many years and consequently they were given appropriate prophylaxis when splenectomy was necessary. Now it is essential to give prophylactic treatment prior to and after splenectomy in adults as well. The emphasis is now on the preservation of the spleen if at all possible. Even after injury conservative methods of treatment have been developed. Haemorrhage may be stopped by embolisation of the splenic artery rather than by removal of the spleen.

Other claims have arisen following splenectomy for trauma when fragments of splenic pulp were not replaced in the peritoneal cavity with the possibility of restoring some splenic function. Doubt has been cast on the validity of this method of trying to restore function but there is some evidence that it can be effective and it is simple to do.

Skin and Superficial Swellings

Surgery in this area is frequently carried out by inexperienced surgeons in far from ideal circumstances. The encouragement of general practitioners to carry out minor surgery may well increase the number. There are two areas of skin which are notorious for developing keloid scars. These are over the sternum and the deltoid region. When patients require surgery in these situations they should be warned of the possibility of keloid formation. They may then elect not to have their small lump removed. If it has to be removed because of suspicion as to its nature, the risk of keloid formation has to be accepted.

Neurofibroma

Solid subcutaneous swellings which may lie along the line of the superficial nerve may be neurofibromata. These can be separated from the relevant nerve without much difficulty providing that their nature is appreciated. Claims may arise from permanent damage to the nerve.

Undiagnosed Melanoma

Surgery recommended for removing these tumours is now much less radical than it used to be and there are far fewer claims for inadequate excision. One of the dangers of treating superficial skin lesions in minor operating theatres is that an occasional melanoma will be treated inadequately under local anaesthetic by an inexperienced surgeon. One of the catches is the amelanotic melanoma.

Lymph Node Biopsy

This should never be considered a minor procedure. Access to lymph nodes can present a considerable technical problem. They may lie close to vital structures which can be damaged during their biopsy, particularly when they are adherent or grossly enlarged with distortion of the anatomy. The most common source of this trouble is the lymph node in the posterior triangle close to the spinal accessory nerve. Many claims result from damage to this nerve and they are quite indefensible.

Local Anaesthetic Overdose

This can happen particularly in small patients. If the recommended dose is exceeded, they may develop fits leading to cerebral anoxia and serious complications. It is important therefore when using local anaesthetic to assess the patient's weight so that the maximum safe dose can be calculated. Disasters may follow inadvertent intravenous injection of local anaesthetic.

Inguinal Hernia Repair

This is a common surgical procedure and may be a frequent source of claims. These however form only a small proportion of the operations carried out. Damage to the inguinal nerve can cause a persistent sharp pain in the groin radiating to the scrotum and vicinity of the testicle. It is often impossible to see why this has arisen as all surgeons who have seen the nerve clearly identify it and preserve it. In recurrent hernia it may not be possible however to identify it and in some cases of large herniae the nerve is formally sacrificed without the patient suffering any ill effects. It is difficult therefore to understand why some should suffer such severe discomfort and pain following the operation. Providing the operation has been performed in a proper manner by a surgeon of appropriate experience, the claim is defended.

Another common source of claims is a sinus due to non-absorbable suture material. It is a rare but recognised complication of the use of this material. This claim can be defended.

Testicular Atrophy

There has been an an epidemic of claims in recent years for testicular atrophy following hernia repair. The usual sequence of events is that the patient develops very much more swelling in the scrotum than is usual following a hernia repair. This then slowly resolves. Over a period of 3 or 4 months the testicle atrophies, becomes insensitive or takes up a position high in the scrotum. The cause is not known, though various possibilities have been suggested. Pampiniform plexus thrombosis, arterial damage and haematoma of the inguinal canal have all been put forward as the cause, with suggestions as to their treatment. Thrombosis of the spermatic cord due to excessive dissection has also been suggested. In any case, the patient feels that he has had a common straightforward operation terminating in loss of a testicle. The surgeon, who may well have not deviated in any way from his normal practice, finds explanation difficult. Attempts have been made to defend these claims. As yet, none has been tested in court, but they have been defended.

Vasectomy

This is a frequent source of claims and usually there has been failure in one of the basic recommendations which has led to litigation. It is vital when carrying out a procedure for sterilisation that the patient is fully informed prior to consent. This information must include all the possible complications as the procedure has not been carried out for a disease process, but because of the patient's choice and convenience. It seems that patients are less willing to accept that complications arise following surgery of this kind in contrast to surgery done for an appropriate pathological problem. Consent must include the fact that the procedure may well be irreversible and, if reversed, the success rate is far from 100%. In addition warnings must be given about the possibility of recanalisation with restoration of fertility as a rare consequence. The necessity for post-operative sperm counts must be stressed. Two counts should be done at an interval of a week approximately 12 weeks following the vasectomy. It is essential that the patient waits for the results of these tests prior to assuming that he is sterile. The patient must be informed in writing of the result of such tests. There have been a number of claims in which the patient has alleged that he was given information over the telephone which later proved to be incorrect. The possibility of scrotal swellings and wound infection should also be mentioned.

There is some debate about the value of histology of the vas but obviously it is helpful if this has been obtained as extra support for the view that the procedure was done in a proper manner. The critical point in establishing success or otherwise of the operation is the post-operative sperm tests.

Miscellaneous Problems

Claims arise following pre-operative skin preparation where rashes or blistering develop if the lotion accumulates in a pool beneath the patient. Diathermy problems occur. The booklet published by the defence organisations outlines the ways in which these can be prevented.

Problems due to errors in identification of the patient and the side to be operated upon continue to occur. Swabs and instruments are still occasionally left in the patient. The booklet produced by the medical defence organisations in conjunction with the Royal College of Nursing on Theatre Safeguards fully outlines the steps necessary to prevent these avoidable and indefensible errors.

Further Reading

Specialisation in general surgery
Kings Fund Consensus Statement (1990). Br Med J 300: 1675

Junior doctors' errors
Buck N, Devlin HB, Lunn JN (1987) The confidential enquiry into perioperative deaths. Nuffield Provincial Hospitals Trust , Kings Fund

Acute appendicitis
Thomson HJ, Jones PF (1986) Active observation in acute abdominal pain . Am J Surg 152: 522–525
Malt RA (1986) The perforated appendix . N Engl J Med 315: 1546–1547

Re-operation on post-operative acute abdomen
Kirk RM (1990) Hospital Update 16: 303–310

Endoscopy of the upper gastrointestinal tract
Kirk RM, Stoddard CJ (1986) Complications of surgery of the upper gastrointestinal tract. Baillière Tindall, London, pp 65–91

ERCP
Viceconte G, Viceconte GW, Pietropaulo V, Montori A (1981) Endoscopic sphincterectomy: Indications and results. Br J Surg 68: 376–380

Bile duct injuries
Blumgart LH, Kelley CJ, Benjamin IS (1984) Benign bile duct stricture following cholecystectomy; Critical factors in management. Br J Surg 71: 836

Surgery for obesity
Griffin WO (1979) Gastric bypass for morbid obesity. Surg Clin North Am 59: 1103
Ismail T, Kirby RM, Crowson MC, Baddely RM (1990) Vertical silastic ring gastroplasty: A 6-year experience. Br J Surg 77: 80–82

Prophylactic antibiotics
Keighley MRB (1988) Infection: prophylaxis. Br Med Bull 44: 374–402

Prophylaxis against deep vein thrombosis
Grant PJ, Prentice CRM (1988) Haemorrhage and thrombo-embolic complications associated with surgery. Br Med Bull 44: 453–474

Varicose veins and nerve injury
Holme JB, Skajaa K, Holme K (1990) Incidence of lesions of the saphenous nerve after partial or complete stripping of the saphenous vein. Acta Chir Scand 156: 145–148

Aortic aneurysm
Campbell WB, Collin J, Morris PJ (1986) The mortality of abdominal aortic aneurysm. Ann Coll Surg Engl 68: 275–278

Angioplasty
Lamerton AJ (1986) Percutaneous transluminal angioplasty. Br J Surg 73: 91–97

Recurrent laryngeal nerve injury
Sugrue DD, Drury MI, McEvoy M, Hefferman SJ, O'Malley E (1983) Long-term follow-up of hyperthyroid patients treated by sub-total thyroidectomy. Br J Surg 70: 408–411

External laryngeal nerve injury
Kissin MW, Bradpiece HA, Meikle MS, Auerbach R, Kark AE (1983) Voice changes after thyroid surgery. Br J Surg 70: 306 (Surgical Research Society abstract)

Splenectomy post-operative prophylaxis
Barron PT, Richter M (1990) Immunodeficiency following splenectomy in the early post-immunisation period. Br J Surg 77: 316–319

Autotransplants of spleen
Ludtke FE, Mack SC, Schuff-Werner P, Voth PE (1989) Splenic function after splenectomy for trauma. Acta Chir Scand 155: 533–540

Testicular atrophy after hernia repair
Wantz GE (1989) Ambulatory hernia surgery. Br J Surg 76: 1228–1229

Retained swabs
Rappaport W, Haynes K (1990) The retained surgical sponge following abdominal surgery. Arch Surg 125: 405–409

CHAPTER 6

Dermatology

K.V. Sanderson

The skin is exposed to injury from a variety of sources and some of these injuries may involve negligence. For the purposes of this chapter the most important agents of injury leading to medico-legal claims are employers and the medical profession. Chiropodists, electrologists, hairdressers and beauticians are also at risk through operating on skin and hair. The makers and sellers of cosmetics and other products that may be in close contact with the skin can also be liable. Criminal injury to the skin can be found in the small but important class of abused children.

Three topics have been chosen from the large number possible for consideration in this chapter. Occupational dermatitis will be dealt with in a general way. Some of the common reasons for legal actions being taken against the medical profession in the handling of skin disorders will be considered. Brief mention of the skin signs of child abuse will be made. It has been the writer's aim to present the various aspects in a way that should be comprehensible to those outside dermatology or outside the medical profession.

Whether or not a skin disorder is due to negligence on the part of an employer or the provider of goods or services is frequently the cause of legal argument, in the settling of which the opinion of medical experts may be crucial. It is a specialised field and expertise in the subject is mainly limited to dermatologists. Indeed, aspects such as occupational dermatoses and contact dermatitis require a knowledge of industrial processes, chemistry, toxicology, and cutaneous testing in such detail as to make them almost autonomous subspecialties. The choice of medical expert can thus be most important in the success of a claim. Ideally the expert witness should give unbiased guidance to the lawyers and to the court and not be an advocate for one side or the other. One might hope that the more knowledgeable and experienced the experts are on either side, the more their opinions would approach a consensus.

The Medical Report

Usually, but not always, a medical report is based principally upon an examination of the claimant. Medical reports and sickness certificates may be required at various stages and by different agencies during the course of a case of occupational dermatitis [17]. To get injury benefit under the Prescribed Diseases regulation a worker must show that the disease is a non-infective dermatitis, that his work involves necessary exposure and that the occupation caused the dermatitis.

If the claimant receives Industrial Disablement Benefits he is then likely to claim damages in a civil action against his employer for negligence, especially if he has a trade union to support him. When this happens his solicitors will require an expert report to substantiate his claim and the employer's insurers will require another in an effort to refute it. It is mainly on the facts that these reports contain that the case can either be settled or taken to court.

It cannot be emphasised too strongly that the medical opinion should be based upon a complete and detailed enquiry into the relevant events, an account of their chronology, of the changes seen in the skin and the treatments that have been applied to it, of any constitutional disposition towards skin or other diseases and of any drugs taken.

If the reason for the report has to do with occupational dermatitis a conventional medical history is not sufficient [1, 25]. A brief account of the educational background and occupational history may be helpful in judging whether the claimant is likely to be an intelligent worker capable of avoiding obvious hazards and of likely previous exposures to irritants or sensitising substances. Hobbies and part-time work should also be recorded for the same reason.

A description of the workplace, of the processes on which the claimant is employed, of the protective measures and equipment and the washing facilities provided, and details of other workers who may have been similarly affected are needed as well as the occupational history of the individual. The name of any suspected noxious agent and details of its maker and supplier (for the obtaining of their chemical composition, known hazards and warnings that should have been given to those handling them) should be recorded. If, as often happens, the claimant's account of such details is not precise, a visit to the workplace is by far the most satisfactory way of getting the information. Such a visit is valuable in other ways, and expert guidance on how it should be conducted has been published [4, 25].

Dermatologists, like most specialists, have their own particular descriptive terms and skin diseases have a complex nosology. Practitioners who are not dermatologists need to take care to conform to dermatological usage when these descriptive terms and diagnostic labels are used to record the findings at clinical examination. The whole skin surface should be examined and the morphology, situation and size of all abnormalities described accurately.

Clinical photographs are invaluable in many cases, especially when cosmetic disability is claimed. Photographs are best taken by a medical photographer or at least with a single-lens reflex camera equipped to take close-up views. Amateur snapshots, though better than nothing, are usually lacking in detail and not sharply enough focused. If a photograph cannot be taken a sketch is useful in recording the size, shape and situation of lesions.

Patch testing is an essential way of investigating the precise cause of contact dermatitis due to allergic sensitisation and it is to be recommended in all cases of dermatitis to exclude an unsuspected allergic factor [26]. The procedure is based on the experience of the many workers in the field for some decades and a large body of data has been published [1, 9, 16]. It is a simple procedure in theory but can give very misleading results when performed by the inexperienced [7]. Patch testing will be discussed in more detail in a later section.

When the medical examiner is reporting to the defendant it is necessary to get the consent of the plaintiff and his legal advisers before carrying out patch tests.

Other special investigations are less often required. Fungal infections are proved by examination of scales scraped or hairs pulled from the affected area and a mycological examination should, ideally, be done on all erythemato-squamous lesions seen by a dermatologist. Secondary bacterial infection complicates many cases of dermatitis and needs laboratory confirmation. Impetigo can be distinguished from a cigarette burn, as in a suspected case of child abuse, by microbiological testing of the blister contents or crust. Neoplasms thought to be due to industrial exposure or alleged to have been wrongly managed medically should be examined pathologically to establish a definite diagnosis. The result of all the investigations, whether positive or negative, should be given in the report.

When the report is based on documents only, especially if the documents are the original records that have to be returned, an account of all the relevant details should be given. This may include those from the nursing record in hospital notes, as day-to-day matters are invariably covered more completely by nursing than medical notes. A careful reading of all the records often brings to light significant facts that may have been overlooked by others. If the facts are complicated a summary of the salient features is useful in concentrating attention on what is important.

The final section of the report presents the expert opinion, which should be reasoned from the facts and expressed in terms that are understandable to those without expert knowledge. Diagnosis and causation should be given with an estimate of their probable correctness, an indispensable aspect of cases where there is debate about occupational versus constitutional factors; prognosis is notoriously difficult in occupational dermatitis [15]. Any facts for or against negligence should be set out fairly. The knowledge that the writer of the report may have to justify his opinions to a court of law is an incentive to clear and careful thought. A well-presented, comprehensive and unbiased report, supported by reference to published expert opinion, is the best insurance against a court appearance.

Occupational Dermatitis

Nomenclature

Eczema and dermatitis are understood to be different diseases by the general public; eczema is an itchy inflammation that may be inherited and linked with hay fever and asthma, whilst dermatitis looks similar but is caused by work, and compensation for it may be paid to the worker. This oversimplified view may be partly due to the inconsistent way dermatologists use the two terms, which varies both within and between countries. If etymology and history are to be respected, eczema should be reserved for inflammations in which vesicles are demonstrable either to the naked eye or microscopically. It might avoid confusion if eczema were only used adjectivally as a description of this morphology, and dermatitis, suitably qualified, were used for the group of diseases. However the linking of "eczema" to atopic dermatitis is so ingrained that the present usage is likely to continue.

Clinical Considerations

Two main types of dermatitis are recognized, exogenous or contact dermatitis and endogenous dermatitis of various sorts, the most important of which is atopic dermatitis or eczema. These types are not mutually exclusive. Atopic dermatitis, for instance, even when quiescent, makes a worker (e.g. hair-dresser's apprentice) more susceptible to some types of occupational dermatitis [30] and atopic dermatitis may be aggravated by a variety of external influences, especially secondary infection [23], heat, extremes of humidity, and contact with wool. The primary distinction between contact dermatitis in a worker and endogenous dermatitis is, however, vital in some medico-legal cases, and the importance of constitutional factors in causation can be the cause of vigorous disputation. In cases where a worker develops dermatitis which has features that indicate that it is endogenous the question will be asked whether the worker might reasonably have been expected to contract the disease if he had not been engaged in that particular occupation and type of work [25].

Contact dermatitis may result from either allergic sensitisation of the delayed or cell-mediated type to an allergen which has penetrated the epidermis from without, or from irritation and damage to the skin and particularly to the horny surface layer, the stratum corneum, by a physical or chemical agent. The allergic response can be reproduced on normal skin by patch testing with an appropriate dilution of the agent in an appropriate vehicle. The response is eczematous and is usually delayed by about 2 days.

Various irritants may cause dermatitis by acute primary damage; chemicals may change the stratum corneum, causing a chemical burn, as with strong acids and alkalis and strong solutions of many other substances. More commonly, repeated exposure to a lesser irritant removes substances that maintain the water content of the stratum corneum [18]. The resulting dehydration, which may be aggravated by climatic factors, causes brittleness and fissuring (chapping) of the surface layer. The resistance to irritants or allergens is then much reduced and the condition becomes chronic unless the skin is allowed to return to normal.

Repeated exposure to a minor irritant can produce dermatitis that resolves without reduction of the exposure. This phenomenon is called hardening and it is the outcome for which industrial medical officers hope when machinists exposed to coolant oils, for instance, first show signs of irritant dermatitis.

There is an important distinction between irritant dermatitis and allergic contact dermatitis. An irritant can affect any skin that is exposed to it for sufficient time in sufficient strength, although there can be a great variation in susceptibility between individuals. Allergic sensitisation is, in a sense, idiosyncratic and occurs in only a proportion of those exposed to the allergen. With only a few very potent agents does the proportion approach 100%. Another distinction is in the morphology of the rash. Irritant dermatitis is typically scaly and fissured but not vesicular, whilst allergic sensitivity produces a papulo-vesicular response which may progress to scaling and fissuring but tends to retain its vesicular character.

There are other damaging external influences on the skin. Low humidity, especially when combined with draughts or winds, will cause dehydration and chapping of the surface and may be responsible for clusters of cases of occupational dermatosis within a factory [27]. Light, particularly in the ultra-violet region, may react with chemicals on the skin or circulating in the blood to produce skin changes [11, 19]. A well-known occupational example of this is the exaggerated sunburn experienced by pitch workers and called by them "the smarts".

Evidence in Favour of Occupational Dermatitis

The presence in the working environment of agents capable of causing contact dermatitis is an obvious prerequisite although the actual agent itself is not always obvious [25]. A history of the rash fluctuating synchronously with work and improving during weekends and holidays is usual but not invariable. The fact of other workers having similar skin problems may support the case but skin disorders are so common that expert corroboration of their similarity is needed.

The distribution of the eruption should correspond to the areas exposed to the postulated cause, allowing for regional variations in the permeability of the skin surface. On the hands, for instance, which are involved in a high proportion of cases, allergic contact dermatitis tends to involve the dorsal areas and sides of the fingers. Irritant dermatitis also involves these areas but may, in addition, cause fissuring of the palmar skin whilst constitutional eczema is the likely cause for a symmetrical vesicular eruption of the palmar skin. Irritants on the hands may have most effect in the finger webs and under rings. Irritating particles such as cut fragments of hair in the case of hairdressers and metal swarf in that of machinists also concentrate in the interdigital folds. Sensitivity reactions can be very localised as, for example, the fingertip dermatitis of one hand of the chef allergic to onion or garlic.

An airborne sensitiser produces a more intense rash around the eyes, on the neck, the elbow creases and scrotum, areas where the skin is thin, than elsewhere. Examples of such allergens are gases like formaldehyde, particles like aerosols, hardwood sawdust, dust from machining synthetic resins and glues, or pollen grains as from *Primula obconica*. In most cases of contact dermatitis, when all the facts are known, there is a logic to the distribution of the eruption.

The most convincing evidence comes from the details of the conditions and processes at the workplace supporting a diagnosis of irritant dermatitis or of allergic contact dermatitis, and in the latter case from confirmatory patch testing.

Patch Testing

Patch tests are a means of establishing that particular substances are the cause of an allergic contact dermatitis in the individuals being tested. To be valid, tests with the reagent must be negative in subjects who have not been sensitised. To test with an irritant only confirms that it is an irritant and does not show any causal connection between the substance and a worker who may have been exposed to it. This fact, which is self-evident to dermatologists, is not always understood by those outside the specialty.

Patch testing is a routine part of the work of all properly constituted dermatology departments [6]. Although the reagents used in testing can be prepared in a pharmacy or laboratory, it is more convenient to obtain them from one of the commercial suppliers. A standard series of reagents is used, based on the commonly found causes of sensitisation from the pooled figures of large departments in several European countries. The reagents are kept in contact with the skin of the back for 48 hours by means of special non-reactive adhesive tape. The standard series is, of course, supplemented by any special reagents suggested by the history.

Experience is needed in interpreting the results of patch tests as it is in performing them, and in the choice of reagents and the vehicles and concentration used. The literature on the subject is voluminous and has been reviewed by Fischer and Maibach [13]. The full investigation of a suspected case of occupational dermatitis may be beyond the scope of an ordinary skin department and referral to one of the centres specialising in occupational dermatitis is in the worker's best interest.

Reading Patch Tests

A positive patch test develops after a delay averaging about 2 days and the patches are removed at 48 hours. It shows as an eczematous disc, with vesicles, oedema and erythema, centred on the area exposed to the reagent but spreading beyond it in strongly positive results. If the reading is made immediately after the removal of the patches the results may be confused because of the reactive erythema from the pull of the adhesive. To avoid this, an interval of half an hour or more should be allowed before the tests are read. Some reactions develop only after an interval of three or more days and if one reading alone is relied upon the result may be falsely negative. The most common substance to react this way is neomycin. The use of an inappropriate vehicle or of too high or low a concentration of the reagent may give fallacious results also.

False positive reactions may be due to irritation rather than allergic sensitivity and have a somewhat different morphology from a true positive result. Eczematous vesicles are absent and the irritant reaction may damage the epidermis to the point of blistering. It is easier to distinguish a true from a false positive when the reaction is strong than when it is barely positive.

The possibility of false results, whether positive or negative, has considerable significance in medico-legal cases in which causation is contested. False positive results are probably commoner; fallacious results may occur particularly if the tests are carried out by an operator relatively inexperienced in industrial dermatology. Technical aspects of patch testing and the reasons for misleading results have been discussed by Hindson [20], Fischer and Maibach [13] and Rycroft [26].

Interpretation of Patch Tests

Patch tests are not just a convenient way of proving the clinician right. They may be thought provoking. Each occupation has a known range of possible sensitisers that its workers are exposed to and for each a particular battery of testing agents is appropriate. There are few agents to which both dentists and building workers are exposed, for instance. In addition to the appropriate occupational sensitisers workers are also tested to the series of general common sensitisers. An unexplained positive reaction requires further investigation as does no reaction to the appropriate series in what seems to be an occupationally caused allergic contact dermatitis. Both the workplace and home environment must be scrutinized for an unrecognised cause [29].

Some aspects of the significance and value of patch tests can be illustrated by considering two important sensitisers. The commonest sensitiser in men is potassium dichromate. Its potency is enhanced in some situations by the co-existence of an irritant effect. For instance, cement contains small amounts of chromate, varying with the origin of the rock from which it is made, and is also alkaline. When mixed with sand and ballast there is an abrasive action as well thus adding physical damage to the chemical irritation of the skin from alkali. It is not surprising that cement casting and the building industry are common sources of industrial dermatitis. In long-standing cases, cement dermatitis on the hands and forearms may take on the pattern and morphology of discoid eczema, a disorder that is in other circumstances wholly constitutional in nature.

Chromate is present in sand used for moulding in foundries and for sand blasting. It is employed as a corrosion inhibitor in heat transfer systems and to prevent rust. It is also used in tanning some leather and is present in some dyes and pigments as well as, more obviously, in chrome-plating solutions. The variety of industries which use it and the number of workers exposed to it is thus very great. Chromate dermatitis has recently been reviewed by Burrows [3].

It is probably reasonable to suspect that a chromate sensitivity in a man is occupational until proved otherwise. In women the common sensitivity to nickel is often acquired because of the skin's close contact with nickel plating on metal components of garments such as zip fasteners, hooks and eyes, studs of jeans, etc. and on costume jewellery [9]. Once acquired, nickel sensitivity can restrict the areas of employment open to the individual because so many metal objects in everyday use are nickel-plated or contain nickel in an alloy. Occupations in which women predominate, such as nursing and domestic work in hospitals, hairdressing, garment making and attending tills, all involve the use or handling of nickel-plated instruments, appliances or nickel-containing coins. In nurses, hairdressers and domestic workers there is the additional constant irritant effect of detergents, shampoos and chemical solutions, and the relative importance of the allergic and irritant actions and the question of when and where the allergy was acquired are of considerable medico-legal importance. A most meticulously taken history is the best way to get an answer.

A detailed account of the causes of dermatitis in various industries and of the agents involved can be found in texts on the subject [1, 9, 14].

Constitutional Factors in Workers with Dermatitis

As only some of the workers equally exposed to a hazard develop dermatitis there must be innate factors favouring resistance or susceptibility. One influence is the skin's thickness, which is to some extent predictable from the complexion. Fair-skinned people and freckled red-heads have a thin skin and are susceptible, as they are to low humidity dermatosis and to the damaging effects of sunlight. The belief that other predisposing causes, like the sex and race of the worker, can be identified has been part of the teaching of occupational dermatologists for the last half century, going back to Prosser White [28]. Studies to quantify the risk factors have been rather few. It may be difficult to justify the prevention of industrial dermatitis by rigorous selection at pre-employment medical examinations on the present evidence about these predisposing factors. Selection is justifiable in some other circumstances, however.

The effect of the atopic diathesis on susceptibility to irritant dermatitis is generally accepted, and a previous history of atopic eczema should make employment in, for example, the engineering industry, where there is exposure to coolant or mineral oils, in handling cement, or as a nurse or hairdresser, to name but a few occupations, very questionable [4]. Active atopic eczema should exclude almost all individuals from any occupation where there is unprotected exposure to irritants.

Discoid eczema, mentioned above as sometimes resulting from prolonged cement dermatitis, is considered usually to be due to unknown endogenous factors and is manifested as coin-size areas of vesicular or weeping eczema symmetrically placed, particularly on the extremities. It follows from the ignorance about its nature that legal debate about its relationship to an occupation hazard must be decided by the facts of the case rather than by applying a dogmatic view that it is always constitutional.

A local area of dermatitis, whether gravitational associated with incompetent venous circulation in the leg or allergic contact to a nickel-plated jeans stud for instance, may render the whole skin surface hypersensitive so that patches of eczema appear spontaneously in flexures or after minor irritation. This may be one reason for false positive patch test reactions. It may also give a vesicular morphology to an irritant dermatitis. Gravitational dermatitis is exacerbated by prolonged standing.

The possibility of developing psoriasis or the fact of having it, is likely to apply to 2% of a work force. If the reaction of other workers to red scaly patches is discounted, the main problem psoriasis presents to employers is the appearance of new lesions in areas of skin damage such as burns, lacerations or even irritant reactions. This Koebner phenomenon does not occur at all stages of the disease but if it does it may raise medico-legal questions. Psoriasis should come to mind if what has been considered a chronic irritant fissured dermatitis of the palms does not improve when the skin is no longer irritated.

A number of skin disorders are made worse by hot and humid conditions. These include seborrhoeic dermatitis, psoriasis, severe acne vulgaris and, when the humidity is caused by the footwear, tinea pedis. The lesions of eczema and psoriasis are easily colonized by staphylococci and this may make sufferers unsuitable for work in nursing, the medical profession or in contact with foodstuffs.

The possibility of acquiring a contact allergy to components of creams and ointments, whether medicinal or cosmetic, must always be remembered. Like secondary infection, this may occur as a complication of a primary industrial dermatitis. Alternatively it may have existed before the beginning of the dermatitis. In either case a reaction to a medicament complicates the clinical picture until it is recognised and eliminated. It is the first thing to consider when the course of the disease is not typical. Among the other causes of unexpected persistence in a worker on sick leave is contact with an irritant or allergen from a hobby, from moonlighting, or from contact with domestic irritants. When a worker has repeated episodes of dermatitis the later ones become more refractory.

Prognosis of Industrial Dermatitis

The behaviour of the first episode of contact dermatitis is predictable if it is recognised quickly and the cause can be avoided. With suitable treatment it will subside and the skin appear to be normal in about two weeks. The appearance is deceptive. An allergic contact dermatitis will recur in a day or two when the allergen is re-encountered. After an irritant dermatitis subsides the skin takes several weeks or months to regain its normal resistance to surface damage. Premature return to work results in relapse and each relapse is followed by a longer recovery time.

The doctor who authorises the return to work has a very difficult decision to make, the more so because the worker and the employer often apply pressure once the skin looks normal. Not only must the worker be repeatedly told that his skin is not yet back to normal but he must also be advised against contact with irritants whilst off work, whether from helping with housework or following a hobby. A dermatologist with industrial experience is in a better position than most other doctors to give the correct advice and have it followed. He is also able to suggest what is necessary to reduce the risk of recurrence.

Treatment

Irritant dermatitis requires a suitable emollient, the use of which should be continued after the skin seems normal. If a corticosteroid cream or ointment is required its strength should be dictated by the severity of the dermatitis and by its situation, bearing in mind the vulnerability of the face and flexures. Locally applied antibacterial agents should be avoided and a systemic antibiotic used to treat confirmed infection. From the worker's point of view the investigation of the cause is the essential element of the management of his case as his occupational future depends upon the advice that he and his employer are given about preventing future episodes. The advice will vary with the cause and the industrial circumstances; details are given in the textbooks of industrial dermatology.

Prevention of Industrial Dermatitis

Having tried to select workers who are not predisposed to skin disease, the employer must ensure that they know of any hazards in the workplace and have been instructed on how to avoid them. He should ensure that they use all necessary protective garments and equipment. He should update the educational and safety procedures when new chemicals or machinery are introduced [4]. It is the employer's duty to take all reasonable measures to foresee any hazards that may occur. If he has done so, he cannot be held to be responsible for an unforeseeable occurrence.

In matters of health and safety the employer's statutory obligations under the Factories Act 1961 should be the baseline on which he builds. These include ensuring the cleanliness and safety of the workplace, the circulation of fresh air and the rendering harmless of fumes, dust and other impurities such as may be injurious to health, and the provision of adequate and suitable facilities for washing. He also has a Common Law duty to care [5]. Provided he has acted as a "reasonable and prudent employer" he has a good defence against claims that he was negligent.

The worker has a duty to warn his employer of any weakness or pre-existent disease of the skin. He should also heed all the instruction given him regarding health and safety, and keep his work station as clean and tidy as possible. In the last analysis it is the worker himself who has most control over whether he contracts industrial dermatitis – by the way in which he carries out his work, uses protective measures, cleans and cares for his skin and brings to the employer's attention any hazards or shortcomings in the workplace.

The Management of Skin Diseases

The medical defence organizations (MDOs) class dermatology as a low-risk specialty. The claims relating to the skin are relatively few compared with the number of consultations for skin disorders; only 3% of the medical cases published in the last six Annual Reports of the Medical Protection Society illustrating recent problems concern skin disease. The quantum of settlements in dermatological cases is relatively modest in most instances.

The expectation, when thought to be unfulfilled, that a procedure will produce cosmetic improvement has an appreciable influence on the frequency and size of claims and this is seen most obviously in the statistically greater risk that cosmetic surgeons run. Reconstructive and cosmetic surgery will not be considered in detail in this chapter but the "cosmetic factor" will be discussed in relation to the treatment of the skin and its appendages by the various specialists to whom patients and clients go.

There are, in general, two classes of claims against doctors in relation to skin diseases. There are those in which it is alleged that an error of diagnosis led to the wrong treatment or to lack of necessary treatment. There are others in which it is alleged that the treatment given, or not given, was negligent in some respect. The circumstances that give rise to claims are varied and the possibility of defending an action may depend upon factors other than the plain medical facts of the case. Of these factors the quality of the clinical records and the question of "informed consent" are important.

Cases involving skin diseases do not often come to trial and thus get reported. In the absence of cases to be cited the author has created a series of illustrative fictional cases.

Errors of Diagnosis: the Circumstances

The most serious claims regarding errors of diagnosis concern the failure to diagnose malignant tumours, particularly malignant melanoma, in the earlier stages of their evolution when the chance of cure is greatest. The likelihood of such claims is increasing with the success of the campaigns to educate the public in the dangers of pigmented lesions [10, 12]. Because they are the first to be consulted, general practitioners are most at risk in failing to diagnose malignant melanoma. However a patient's skin can be seen by any practitioner and it is possible for an obstetrician or psychiatrist to be asked for an opinion on a pigmented mole. The temptation to give easy reassurance should be avoided by those who are not experts.

Some centres have established clinics with easy and rapid access for the diagnosis of pigmented lesions and there should be no difficulty in getting a quick dermatological opinion. The clinical diagnosis of melanoma is far from precise even when based on long and specialised experience [22] and a biopsy is required in doubtful cases. It is not negligent to fail to diagnose a melanoma but it is negligent to fail to ask for an expert opinion if that is what reasonable practitioners would do. It is also difficult to defend the destruction of a pigmented lesion, by diathermy for instance, without a biopsy if the lesion later proves to be malignant.

Basal cell and squamous cell carcinoma are relatively less likely to be subject to errors of diagnosis than melanoma and the consequences of such an error in the case of basal cell carcinoma are less dire. As the tumour does not give rise to metastases and is usually curable by one means or another, the patient is most likely to be concerned about the more extensive scars that the delay in treatment has produced. There has been the occasional claim for death due to neglect of a gross tumour that has finally eroded through the skull.

Claims based on the misdiagnosis of benign lesions are infrequent but can occur when, for instance, a benign melanocytic naevus or seborrhoeic keratosis is treated as a malignant melanoma, leaving excessive and unsightly scarring or when a lesion, curetted as a plantar wart, is later alleged to have been only a pressure callous which should not have been treated in this way.

> *Case 1.* A ten-year-old girl was referred by her GP to a surgical out-patients department because a 1 cm diameter pigmented birthmark on her left deltoid region had bled and was worrying her parents. A surgical senior registrar saw her and suggested excision under general anaesthesia without any further discussion. "We 'll cut it out for you. Don't worry," was his advice. She was put on the waiting list and operated upon 2 months later. The lesion was found to be benign by the pathologist. The scar spread and thickened and was the subject of a claim. The surgeon's defence, that excision was essential because of the risk of malignant melanoma, was considered unsatisfactory if only because he waited 8 weeks before operating. Experts thought that biopsy confirmation was needed before doing an

excision in this area. The lack of pre-operative discussion effectively denied the parents the ability to give informed consent. The claim was settled.

There are occasions when it is not the diagnosis but the prognosis that is the cause of the legal action, in that consent has been obtained on the basis of misleading information.

> *Case 2.* A beautician consulted her GP asking advice about the removal of a fleshy mole on her nose. He offered to treat it and said there would be no scar. She consented. The mole was sliced off level with the skin surface under local anaesthesia and the raw surface charred with an electrocautery. The end result was a somewhat depressed scar which she claimed could not be disguised with make up.

Negligent Treatment: Some of the Circumstances

Virus warts

A treatment that has given rise to a number of claims is that of podophyllum resin for perineal warts (condyloma acuminatum). The correct way to use this preparation and the possible adverse effects have been known for at least four decades and are set out succinctly in the *British National Formulary*. Podophyllin suspended in Friar's balsam should be painted weekly by a trained attendant on the warts only, the surrounding skin being protected from the irritating paint, and washed off 6 hours later. It is unwise to prescribe the paint and allow the patient to do the painting.

> *Case 3.* A man attended a Casualty Department with warts on the glans penis and foreskin. Podophyllin paint was prescribed and dispensed in a bottle labelled "to be used as directed". The man applied the paint liberally twice daily for 2 days and then stopped because of the pain and swelling. In his claim for damages he alleged he was not warned of the need for care in using the paint nor told how often to apply it. The doctor could not be defended as there was no evidence in the notes that he gave the instructions that he said he gave.

> *Case 4.* A man with penile warts was given a prescription for Posalfilin (Norgine), a reputable preparation for treating plantar warts only, by his general practitioner. A single treatment caused a severe reaction. His claim was not contested.

Moral: If you are not sure of the precise details of a treatment the least you can do is to check in MIMS and the BNF. For a treatment where the compliance of the patient is important a leaflet briefly giving information and instructions is a good safeguard to supplement the consultation.

The commonness of virus warts and the insistence of many patients that they want a rapid radical cure are factors behind other claims of medical negligence.

> *Case 5.* A carpenter attended a Dermatology Out-patient Department with a large wart on the radial side of his left index finger and asked for it to be frozen off. It was treated vigorously by freezing with liquid nitrogen. The following day he returned with a large blister under the wart and anaesthesia of the distal half of the side of the finger. He accepted the blister about which he had been warned but found the loss of sensation a problem as he had to hold nails with the affected finger and

complained that he had not been warned that the digital nerve might be frozen beneath the wart.

Case 6. A general practitioner saw a young girl with what he thought to be plane warts of the cheek. He prescribed salicyclic acid lotion. The pharmacist rang to say he did not have the lotion which is not marketed by drug manufacturers and asked if Cuplex (Smith & Nephew) would do. The doctor agreed that it would, apparently not realizing that Cuplex is to be used for plantar-type warts and is specifically contraindicated for use on the face or ano-genital region by the makers. The claim for damages for the severe reaction that resulted from one application could not be contested.

Corticosteroids

Psoriasis is a common disease and one where most sufferers have a strong desire to have their lesions cleared by treatments that are clean and effective, even though they may have been told that serious side effects may occur. Almost all treatments for psoriasis have a sting in their tail. The simplest and cleanest way to suppress the lesions of psoriasis is to apply a potent corticosteroid ointment or cream such as clobetasol propionate (Dermovate, Glaxo). With long-term use the psoriasis becomes less responsive, the collagen in the dermis and superficial vessels atrophies and systemic absorption may cause hypercorticism and suppression of the pituitary-adrenal axis. The BNF gives information about the untoward reactions and advice about the maximum amount of ointment that can safely be prescribed.

Case 7. A patient with chronic plaque psoriasis was referred by his GP for hospital treatment and was given ultra-violet light irradiation and tar-containing ointments. Because these measures interfered with his business activities he stopped attending and persuaded his GP to prescribe Dermovate (Glaxo) ointment. For several years he obtained amounts of the ointment in excess of the maximum recommended in the BNF with infrequent and superficial medical supervision. He continued with the treatment despite the appearance of severe dermal atrophy with striae and purpura. The grave effects of systemic absorption became evident when his osteoporotic femur fractured and he was found to have irreversible adrenal suppression. Although he contributed to his troubles by continuing to take advantage of the lax arrangements for providing repeat prescriptions after he could see that his skin was being damaged, the GP could not escape responsibility for the prescriptions he had signed.

Patients with severe atopic dermatitis may run the same risks from strong corticosteroid ointments or systemic steroid therapy, where the medical adviser may have difficulty reconciling the need to relieve distressing symptoms with the inevitable adverse effects of continuing to do so. In all such circumstances the patient must be given an adequate warning of the hazards and, where there is such a range of side effects, it is a problem to know where to draw the line. Should all possible side effects be mentioned? From a medico-legal point of view this is the ideal but the information is more than most patients can comprehend and weigh up in the time available for the usual consultation. If, however, an uncommon complication such as cataract is omitted it is probable that this will eventually be the cause for an action. There is information on the "Steroid Card" that is given to patients on systemic therapy but it is designed for another purpose and is not adequate as a way of imparting the necessary information.

Photochemotherapy

Treatment of psoriasis and other disorders such as vitiligo and chronic dermatitis by means of photochemotherapy, psoralen and ultraviolet A, (PUVA) is another source of claims. PUVA has been one of the established cornerstones of psoriasis treatment for nearly two decades but it still has a rather uncertain status in the UK as the use of psoralens taken by mouth has not yet been licensed. In the UK the treatment is supervised by a consultant dermatologist in a department where the light source is calibrated and the amount of radiation accurately recorded. Under these conditions immediate sunburn reactions are rare and the major concern must be the long-term damage to the skin and the possible carcinogenic effect. Cases of severe burns have occurred when vitiliginous skin has been painted with psoralen solution and exposed to sunlight, a state of affairs in which measurement of the amount of radiation is not possible and it is left to the good sense of the patient to judge the correct length of time.

Ugly Scars

A number of claims have resulted from procedures carried out in areas where scars are likely to become hypertrophic. The common site is near the point of the shoulder. Wrongly sited BCG vaccination may result in an hypertrophic scar, as may ill-judged surgery on benign moles, histiocytomas, etc. in this area. Further operations on hypertrophic scars are almost always unsuccessful and produce larger scars. The front of the chest is another site where scars hypertrophy and, in particular, the supramammary area in woman is one that should be avoided for all but vital surgery.

The use of a spirit-based antiseptic to prepare the skin for surgery in which diathermy or electrocautery is to be used has the foreseeable possible outcome of a fire and consequent scarring if any spirit remains on the skin. It is surprising that such cases continue to happen, but they do, and are indefensible. The scarring after diathermy of skin lesions is often deeper than seemed likely at the time of operation and reasonable skill and experience are required before using diathermy.

A possible source of litigation is the use of tattooing in medical diagnosis and treatment. In performing the Kveim test for sarcoidosis, antigen is injected intradermally and the area excised some 6 weeks later for histological examination. Unless the site of injection is marked it may be impossible to locate the area for biopsy. A properly carried out tattoo is an effective marker and is excised with the biopsy. There have been cases where the "tattoo" has not been done by pricking through a drop of dye but where dye has been injected intradermally with a syringe. The resulting tattoo may be up to a centimetre or more in diameter and is not only unsightly but does not pin-point the area for biopsy. Some radiographers use tattoos as a means of marking fields to be treated, around a breast for instance, because they cannot be washed off. When the treatment is finished the patient may ignore the successful conservation of the breast and complain of the permanence of the tattoos.

Drugs

To give a patient a drug to which they are known to react adversely is negligent and before a drug is prescribed the patient should be told its name, (preferably both official and proprietary), asked about previous reactions to it and told about any common side effects. The skin is one of the organs commonly affected by drug reactions and, although most drug eruptions are not a serious danger, a few are life-threatening. One such is toxic epidermal necrolysis (TEN) which may occur after treatment usually with butazones, sulphonamides or barbiturates [23a]. The risk, uncommon though it may be, is a factor to be considered before using these drugs.

It may be questioned whether patients need to be warned of the particular risk of TEN, but there is no doubt that a full and careful explanation must be given before prescribing a teratogenic drug such as one of the group of retinoids used to treat severe acne, psoriasis and disorders of keratinization, or thalidomide which is occasionally essential to control rare skin diseases (and which is difficult to obtain). The present custom in the UK is that such drugs should be used only under the direction of a consultant dermatologist.

Tetracyclines are frequently used on a low-dose, long-term basis to treat acne and the interaction with the contraceptive pill can lead to unwanted pregnancy if it is forgotten.

Intra-lesional triamcinolone is a useful treatment but produces atrophy of the subcutaneous fat if by accident the fat is infiltrated. Injections of steroids that were intended to be intramuscular, but were not, also produce atrophic depressed areas and have resulted in claims.

The radical changes that are being made to the National Health Service have some medico-legal implications for the treatment of skin diseases. By encouraging economic competition between GPs and by paying for minor surgical procedures only when the number per month set by the Secretary of State has been reached, the changes may tempt those minded to supplement their income in this way to operate on lesions they are not competent to diagnose or for which they lack the technique to produce acceptable scars. It is to be hoped that the GPs who offer this service to their patients will ensure that their diagnostic skill and surgical technique are of a reasonable standard and that all doubtful lesions are examined by a pathologist. Even experienced consultant dermatologists have been known to remove amelanotic malignant melanoma by curettage believing it to be a pyogenic granuloma.

Degrees of Medical Responsibility

Although a hospital consultant is, in theory, responsible for the treatment of all the patients in his department, the law recognises the fact that delegation is necessary but requires that the consultant ensures that the more junior doctor is trained and competent to do what is needed.

Consultant status has other implications besides the hierarchic and social ones. It determines whether medical insurance bodies like BUPA and PPP will reimburse their members for specialist services. It affects credibility as an expert witness and the range of a consultant's expertise is of medico-legal importance. Dermatologists may practise in areas that are within the ambit of another specialty such as pathology, radiotherapy, surgery and, occasionally, psychiatry. When they do so, it should be with the degree of skill that might reasonably be expected of a specialist in the other specialty.

Where radiotherapy is commonly given under the care of a dermatologist, in Australia for instance, an adequate knowledge of the physics and the biological actions of ionizing radiation has to be demonstrated before a candidate is granted specialist qualifications. It is generally agreed in the UK that irradiation of skin neoplasms is left to radiotherapists and that dermatologists treat only benign diseases with superficial radiotherapy. The majority of dermatologists in the UK are satisfied to leave all irradiation to radiotherapists.

In the last few decades dermatologists in many countries, including the UK, have undertaken training in the less complex reconstructive surgical procedures and carry out a lot of the treatment of skin tumours that was previously referred to plastic surgery departments and often performed there by the trainees. This change has undoubtedly led to improvement in the performance of all the surgical procedures done in dermatology departments.

Pathologists generally welcome the help of knowledgeable dermatologists in reporting sections of skin disease, as they do with other clinicians, but have reservations about reports being signed by anyone who has not had a general pathologist's training. The status of dermatologists who completely control the reporting of skin pathology does not seem to have been questioned. It is likely that, as with surgery and radiotherapy, a malpractice suit could be defended if the dermatologist could show reasonable competence.

The Cosmetic Factor

The size and wealth of the cosmetic industry is an index of the value placed on the appearance of skin and hair by people in general. For some individuals, minor blemishes may be of exaggerated importance and they consult dermatologists and plastic surgeons in search of perfection. It is the nature of such patients to be dissatisfied if the results of treatment fall short of what they desire and many of them are potential litigants. It is usually easy to recognise these perfectionists and, although pre-treatment assessment by a psychiatrist may seem an unattainable ideal, the advice given to them must be as full and accurate as possible and preferably tinged with pessimism. A photographic record is an essential medico-legal safeguard.

Beauticians and hairdressers may have claims for damages made against them if they appear to have been negligent in the way they have performed the services they offer. Medical opinion is needed to confirm anatomical damage, for instance, to hair shafts damaged by permanent waving solution applied in too strong a concentration or at too high a temperature. The details of the chemical agents used and the operator using them should be sought and, if the latter is a junior, who was supervising her.

At least one case has occurred of anaesthesia of part of the lower lip of a woman following damage to the sensory nerve by the diathermy needle of an epilationist who was removing the unwanted hairs from her chin. Cases such as this and permanent waving disasters are rarely contested by the insurers of the operators concerned.

A case from 40 years ago illustrates how lack of foresight can lead to negligence, in this instance by the maker of a new washing powder. A fashion model bought a box of Brand X washing powder and, on reading through the instructions, noticed the suggestion: "Why not add a little X to your bath?" She did so and made a "bubble bath" in which she lay up to her neck. When seen in a skin department the next day she was a bright red over her body, up to an oblique waterline on the neck, which was undoubtedly caused by the bath. She received substantial damages. The makers removed from the package the suggestion that the washing powder might also act as a toilet preparation. The irritant effect was foreseeable by anyone with knowledge about the action of the constituents of the powder on the skin. Washing powders now carry a warning about skin care.

Avoiding Medico-legal Actions

The fact that the skin can be examined closely without anything more complex than a magnifying glass is an advantage in enabling the practitioner to make an accurate morphological diagnosis. It allows the patient as well as the doctor to assess the progress of any changes. Failure to remedy a skin disease cannot be denied and does not respond to reassurance. The ease of self-examination, especially if a magnifying mirror is used, is an important factor in the anxiety and damaged self-esteem that afflict many patients with skin diseases. If the results of medical treatment are perceived to be unsatisfactory the patient can easily think the practitioner is to blame. Well-kept clinical records in which the lesions are described in as much detail as possible, (preferably with the help of diagrams), are the main defence.

Past generations of dermatologists have relied very largely on the findings at examination to make their diagnosis. For example, it is said that the great Viennese dermatologist Hebra had the patients at his hospital clinic paraded before him naked and rarely, if ever, spoke to them. Whilst it is possible to recognise many skin diseases by sight, the taking of the history serves several purposes besides giving the chronology of the signs and symptoms as noted by the patient and relatives. It also provides information about the concepts they have about disease in general and the presenting complaint in particular, and this can be relevant to subsequent discussions about the nature, cause and treatment of the illness. There seems to be an abundance of people who, undaunted by the complexity of the subject, are happy to hold an opinion on dermatological matters. A disparity between the ideas and the expectations of the patient and the doctor is a source of misunderstanding and loss of rapport and may contribute to the impulse to go to law. It is worth remembering that while the doctor is assessing his patient's personal qualities the patient is also assessing the doctor. The manner of history taking is an important factor in the rapport that should grow between doctor and patient.

Photographs are as valuable a record of skin changes as imaging techniques are of internal disorders. Any procedure or treatment which is likely to result in a change of appearance should be explained most carefully, preferably with a photographic illustration of a similar case and its outcome. Photographs should be taken before treatment to provide a basis for assessing the results of the treatment.

All explanations of what will happen should be realistic. In describing the pain or scars that are likely to result, for instance, a little exaggeration is better than the reverse. A patient's gratitude is the greater if the discomfort of the treatment is less and the cosmetic effects better than those that were originally described.

The patient wants to have three questions answered,: "What have I got? Why have I got it? What will make it better?" The consultation will be a failure if these questions are not answered in a way that the patient understands. Much of the art of the good doctor is in doing this simply and memorably.

A practitioner is risking disaster if he makes decisions and recommendations about diagnosis and treatment outside his or her training and experience. Success in the treatment of skin diseases is often dependent upon the patient following detailed instructions and the tailoring of the therapy to the individual rash. The cases of podophyllin irritation are good examples of the need to give precise instructions and to know the relevance of the different bases in which the substance can be dispensed.

In dermatology more than in most specialties the patient needs to be given precise details about the nature, cause and treatment of the disease. To rely entirely upon a verbal explanation at a consultation of limited duration is to overestimate the skill in communication of the doctor and the receptive capacity and memory of the patient. There is an indisputable case for having printed leaflets to reinforce the spoken explanation of common problems. These include the treatment of scabies and other infestations, the care of dry and cracking skin, how to avoid the common specific causes of allergic contact dermatitis (which may require a dozen or more separate leaflets), the treatment of virus warts, etc. A not unimportant advantage in using leaflets is that they can be valuable evidence of the information given to the patient if there is a later legal dispute.

There are a number of skin diseases, some common and some rare, that have prompted the formation of patient support groups. The Psoriasis Association and the Eczema Society were among the first and they set an example of co-operation with the medical profession which has been for the good of both doctor and patient. These bodies are capable of giving much closer support and detailed counselling than are provided by sporadic medical consultations and in general their advice is unexceptionable.

Those experienced in the work of the MDOs now agree that when something goes wrong it is preferable for the doctor in charge of the patient to spend time in explaining simply and truthfully what happened, without admitting liability. Most patients accept that their doctors can be fallible. What they will not accept is what seems to be a cover-up, especially if the doctors involved assume an air of all-knowing superiority.

Child Abuse and the Dermatologist

Teachers, social workers, nurses, doctors and others are alert to the possibility of physical or sexual abuse of children. Signs of injury, especially if they seem to be of bruising, scalding or burning, always raise suspicions [21]. These signs are of such everyday experience that it might be thought that no great professional skill is needed in their diagnosis. Such is not always the case.

The bluish discoloration of a bruise may be imitated if melanin pigment is situated in the dermis among the collagen fibres. This pigmentation is macular, fixed and unchanging and thus easily distinguished from a bruise if it is examined day by day. A bruise, of course, goes through a series of colour changes as the blood pigment is broken down. The most common type of dermal melanosis occurs on the back, on the lumbo-sacral region spreading to the flanks or up to the shoulders in extensive cases. The bluish-grey pigmentation increases in infancy and usually fades between the ages of seven and adolescence. It is commonly found in infants and children of a variety of races, including Asian and Afro-Caribbean. The lesion is often called a Mongolian spot. Dermal melanosis around the eye (naevus of Ota) and of the acromio-clavicular region (naevus of Ito) are conditions, largely confined to the Japanese, in which there is the same bluish staining.

The blistering due to burning with a lighted cigarette may be simulated very closely by the early stage of bullous impetigo contagiosa. The rapid outward spread, and the characteristic honey-coloured crust that appears as the disease evolves, soon indicate the correct diagnosis if the patient is followed. A less common cause of unwarranted suspicion is epidermolysis bullosa. The dominant dystrophic variety of this disease in two siblings recently aroused the suspicion of cigarette burns [8]. In this condition there is a clear family history of blistering after skin injury which is inherited in a dominant fashion and in which characteristic scars with milia are left.

The suspicion of sexual abuse of a pre-adolescent girl may be aroused by the tendency of the uncommon disorder, lichen sclerosus et atrophicus, to cause subendothelial ecchymosis and actual bleeding of the vulva. These may be the first manifestations. Vulval examination shows changes that are usually diagnostic and differ from those due to sexual assault.

In the above instances of disease mimicking physical abuse the history is likely to point strongly to the correct diagnosis. It is wise to listen to what those who care for the child have to say and consider it without prejudice before making hurtful accusations.

Ano-genital warts in infants and children are very suggestive that the human papillomavirus has been transmitted by sexual abuse and their presence is a strong indication for the child to be seen by a team experienced in child abuse. There has, however, been a clinical impression that the virus may be transmitted in a non-venereal way, for example from the fingers of those who care for the child or even of the child itself. That this can occur has recently been supported by laboratory studies [24]. In this condition the history from the carers may be questionable and the need for referral to the experts remains. Childhood sexual abuse has recently been reviewed from a dermatological viewpoint by Berthe-Jones and Graham-Brown [2].

References

1. Adams RM (1983) Occupational skin disease. Grune & Stratton, New York
2. Berthe-Jones J, Graham-Brown RAC (1990) Childhood sexual abuse – a dermatological perspective. Clin Exp Dermatol 15: 321–330

3. Burrows D (1987) Chromate dermatitis. In: Maibach HI (ed) Occupational and industrial dermatology, 2nd edn. Year Book Medical Publishers, Chicago, pp 406–420
4. Burrows D, Beck MH (1986) Prevention of industrial dermatitis. In: Champion RH (ed) Recent advances in dermatology 7. Churchill Livingstone, Edinburgh, pp 69–85
5. Bursell R (1985) Principles in dermatitis litigation. In: Griffiths WAD, Wilkinson DS (eds) Essentials of industrial dermatology. Blackwell Scientific Publications, Oxford, pp 136–144
6. Calnan CD (1978) Dermatology and industry. Clin Exp Dermatol 3: 1–16
7. Calnan CD (1987) The use and abuse of patch tests. In: Maibach H (ed) Occupational and industrial dermatology, 2nd edn. Year Book Publishers, Chicago, pp 28–31
8. Colver GB, Harris DWS, Tidman MJ (1990) Skin diseases that may mimic child abuse. Br J Dermatol 123: 129
9. Cronin E (1980) Contact dermatitis. Churchill Livingstone, Edinburgh.
10. Doherty VR, MacKie RM (1986) Reasons for poor prognosis in British patients with cutaneous malignant melanoma. Br Med J 292: 987–989
11. Emmett EA (1979) Phototoxicity from external agents. Photochem Photobiol 30: 429–436
12. Fairris GM (1988) The effect of the 1987 melanoma campaign on the workload of general practitioners and dermatologists. Br J Dermatol 119 (Suppl 33): 24
13. Fischer T, Maibach HI (1987) Patch testing in allergic contact dermatitis, an update. In: Maibach HI (ed) Occupational and industrial dermatology, 2nd edn. Year Book Medical Publishers, Chicago, pp 190–210
14. Fisher AA (1986) Contact dermatitis, 3rd edn. Lea and Febiger, Philadelphia
15. Fregert S (1975) Occupational dermatitis in a 10-year material. Contact Dermatitis 1: 96–107
16. Fregert S (1981) Manual of contact dermatitis, 2nd edn. Munksgaard, Copenhagen
17. Griffiths WAD (1985) Industrial dermatitis – a national problem. In: Griffiths WAD, Wilkinson DS (eds) Essentials of industrial dermatology, Blackwell Scientific Publications, Oxford, pp 5–6
18. Griffiths WAD, Wilkinson DS (1985) Primary irritants and solvents. In: Griffiths WAD, Wilkinson DS (eds) Essentials of industrial dermatology. Blackwell Scientific Publications, Oxford, Chap. 6
19. Harber LC, Bickers DR (1981) Photosensitivity Diseases. WB Saunders, Philadelphia
20. Hindson C (1985) Investigation of industrial dermatitis. In: Griffiths WAD, Wilkinson DS (eds) Essentials of industrial dermatology. Blackwell Scientific Publications, Oxford, pp 24–37
21. Hobbs CJ (1989) ABC of child abuse: burns and scalds. Br Med J 298: 1302–1305
22. Kopf AW, Mintzis M, Bart RS (1975) Diagnostic accuracy in malignant melanoma. AMA Arch Derm 111: 1291–1292
23. Leyden JJ, Marples RR, Kligman AM (1974) Staphylococcus aureus in the lesions of atopic dermatitis. Br J Dermatol 90: 525–530
23a. Lyell A (1967) A review of toxic epidermal necrolysis in Britain. Br J Dermatol 79: 662–671
24. Padel AF, Venning VA, Evans MF et al. (1990) Human papillomavirus in anogenital warts in children: typing by in situ hybridisation. Br Med J 300: 1491–1494
25. Rycroft RJG (1986) Occupational dermatoses. Rook A, Wilkinson DS, Ebling FJG et al. (eds) Textbook of Dermatology, vol 1, 4th edn. Blackwell Scientific Publications, Oxford, pp 580–581
26. Rycroft RJG (1990) Is patch testing necessary? In: Champion RH, Pye RJ (eds) Recent advances in dermatology 8. Churchill Livingstone, Edinburgh pp 101–111
27. White IR, Rycroft RJG (1982) Low humidity occupational dermatosis – an epidemic. Contact Dermatitis 8: 287–290
28. White RP (1928) The dermatergoses or occupational affections of the skin, 3rd edn. HK Lewis, London
29. Wilkinson DS (1980) The challenge of industrial dermatitis. Clin Exp Dermatol 5: 327–338
30. Wilkinson DS, Hambly EM (1978) Prognosis of hand eczema in hair-dressing apprentices. Contact Dermatitis 4: 63

CHAPTER 7

Ear, Nose and Throat

K.P. Gibbin

Consideration of medico-legal problems in otolaryngology should encompass discussion of cases referred for medical opinion following illness or injury as well as those instances where a patient seeks litigation against a surgeon as a result of perceived negligence or other act. It is in these latter instances that any doctor feels at his or her most vulnerable; the question of informed consent then becomes of paramount importance and a section of this chapter will be devoted to an otolaryngologist's view of this question in the light of present day practice and foreseeable developments. It is inevitable that there may be differences of opinion on certain aspects of medical management between individual doctors and this is as true in otolaryngology as in other disciplines. Nonetheless, it should be possible to agree many broad principles across a wide cross-section of doctors in any one specialty.

Otolaryngology encompasses a wide range of both surgical and non-surgical practice; patients come from all age ranges and the surgical practice itself varies from very major head and neck surgery, usually for malignant disease, to the detailed microsurgery of much of modern otological medicine. It may reasonably be questioned, therefore, whether one surgeon can be competent at all aspects of such a catholic discipline, or whether "superspecialisation" should be adopted. Traditionally in the UK, practitioners in any one discipline have been "generalists" within their own specialty unlike affairs in much of Europe and North America where there is considerable "superspecialisation". A number of otolaryngology departments in the UK are now developing a more superspecialist approach to aspects of their discipline with internal referrals between colleagues, where individuals have developed special interests.

This practice may, in the longer term, spread outside those few centres where it currently occurs and cognisance will need to be taken of this development in assessing risk factors and medico-legal aspects in the event of litigation against an ENT surgeon.

Otolaryngology covers three related specialist areas and many aspects of the medico-legal consequences of ENT practice may usefully be covered under the distinct sub-headings of Otology, Rhinology and Laryngology. However, paediatric ENT practice is becoming a subspecialty in its own right and separate discussion is needed in this field also. In the case of medico-legal reporting on behalf of a solicitor or insurance company these distinctions may be less clear cut and it is important that any ENT surgeon reporting on cases of personal injury be competent in all aspects of the discipline; where he perceives the need for more specialist opinion in a particular area he should not hesitate to recommend referral to a colleague whose interests and knowledge encompass that area.

Personal Injury and the Otolaryngologist

Most otolaryngologists receive requests for medico-legal reports following cases of personal injury, such requests emanating from a variety of sources, including solicitors, insurance companies, the Criminal Injuries Compensation Board and the Department of Social Security. Some major organisations such as British Coal may commission their own reports. The same care and attention should be given when expressing a medico-legal opinion in all instances and it goes without saying that the opinion given should not be influenced by the source of the referral – it is to be hoped that the same opinion would be given whether on behalf of the litigant or the defendant in any one case.

Otological Aspects

Much of present day otological medico-legal practice devolves around the question of noise induced hearing loss (NIHL) and a more detailed consideration may require referral to a dedicated manual. There are, however, many important points that merit discussion here; almost all cases of NIHL referred relate to occupational noise exposure, although there are also many referrals for consideration of pensions for former servicemen.

Noise Induced Hearing Loss

Noise induced hearing loss has been recognised for over 200 years [1] but its medico-legal significance has only been recognised in the last 20 to 30 years and most of the litigated cases are less than 10 years old [26]. It has been estimated that in the UK there are probably 100 000 individuals with NIHL, approximately 0.2% of the population.

In order to understand the problem of NIHL it is important to be aware of the effects of sound stimulation and associated terminology. The effects of sound on the ear are:

1. Adaption. An immediate temporary phenomenon lasting less than one second.
2. Temporary threshold shift (TTS). TTS is a more prolonged phenomenon than adaption and may be subdivided into fatigue and long-lasting TTS. The degree of fatigue increased progressively with stimulus duration and intensity. With greater noise exposure a more prolonged TTS may occur.
3. Permanent threshold shift (PTS). PTS is an irreversible elevation of the auditory threshold with permanent changes in the cochlea – the organ of hearing.

The above phenomena need consideration both in respect of the need for hearing protection and also in respect of the assessment of hearing loss in the individual. Discussion of hearing protection is outside the scope of this chapter but mostly can be considered under the headings of (1) avoidance of noise and (2) protection from noise present. Industry is now much more aware of the need to design systems and machines that are quieter and avoid an unacceptable noise environment as well as the need to provide worker awareness and hearing protection for unavoidable noise.

TTS is of great importance in medico-legal cases both with regard to the history as well as the assessment of the hearing loss. Many workers will volunteer that their hearing loss improves after a period away from the workplace, be it an overnight absence, a weekend or longer, such as a holiday period. Generally, for assessment purposes a period free of noise exposure of 12 hours is accepted as a minimum requirement. It should be noted, however, that recovery of hearing loss after noise exposure may continue for longer than this, possibly for several days.

Not all the noise involved in litigation is continuous noise and the question of explosion causing deafness must be considered, as well as the effects of two other types of noise: impact noise and report trauma. Kerr and Byrne [11] noted three broad categories accepted by the International Audiological Society:

1. Noise-induced deafness – long-term exposure
2. Report trauma – occuring in gunners where stimulus duration is less than 1.5 msec
3. Blast trauma – stimulus duration longer than 1.5 msec and middle ear damage is not uncommon.

Kerr and Byrne discuss both middle and inner ear problems of bomb blast damage having observed and managed the effects of exposure to a terrorist bomb at the Abercorn Restaurant in Belfast in 1972. The inner ear damage was variable; initially, most had some degree of sensorineural loss which was usually cleared quickly and completely.

The effects of impact noise and gunfire noise effects have been discussed by Coles [7], Ward [25] and Burns et al. [5, 6].

The diagnosis of NIHL rests upon history, examination and the results of audiometry – the demonstration of a typical hearing loss. In assessing the history of noise exposure, due account needs to be taken of both the duration of exposure and the likely noise levels experienced. During the course of employment it may take up to 15 years for permanent damage to set in [26] and individuals may experience disability only after presbycusis is added later [4]. The effects of noise are cumulative; however, once exposure to noise ceases, no further hearing loss accrues from that cause.

In assessing exposure of the cochlea to noise, account needs also to be taken of any hearing protection used; the cochlea may be protected by a voluntary act – wearing ear plugs or ear-defenders – or involuntarily as in the instance of associated middle ear pathology. A conductive hearing loss will act in the same way as an ear-defender, attenuating exposure of the cochlea to high levels of sound by the degree of middle ear deafness present.

There is a very wide range of individual susceptibility to the damaging effects of noise and there is no way of predicting this. If statistical criteria are applied relating likelihood of damage to degree of noise exposure this may still not predict for the individual as some ears are more susceptible to damage than others. Various criteria are used to establish what is a safe exposure level, a 90 dBA/4O hours exposure which is described as "safe" is safe for about 85% of the population [1]. In order to protect 95% of the population an 85 dBA level is required.

The diagnosis of noise induced deafness is often by a process of elimination, excluding other known causes of deafness. To this end a detailed and methodical history is required particularly in respect of present and past otological symptoms, past history of head injury and exposure to toxic drugs and, of course, family history. A detailed occupational history is required with special emphasis on likely noise levels in the workplace. Enquiry must be made also of social noise exposure, be this shooting or other noisy hobbies. An account of any military gunfire or blast exposure is required. Conversely, if reporting on a patient complaining of deafness due to military noise exposure, a detailed history of civilian noise exposure is required.

Examination of the ears, nose and throat is then carried out, at the same time assessing the patient's ability to understand speech both with and without lipreading and any hearing aid already in use.

Pure tone audiometry is the mainstay of the diagnosis in NIHL; the machine should have been appropriately calibrated, normally within the preceding 12 months and should provide for both air conduction and bone conduction testing and masking as required.

The presence of an assymetric sensorineural hearing loss does not preclude the diagnosis of NIHL, however, further investigations may be required to exclude other causes of unilateral sensorineural deafness including acoustic neuroma. In some industries and occupations an assymetric loss may be seen and careful history taking may then help to support the diagnosis of NIHL. Perhaps the most obvious example of unilateral loss may be seen in those exposed to rifle or shotgun fire where the left ear demonstrates a much greater loss than the right when the gun is fired from the right shoulder. The left ear in this case is nearer the explosion at the muzzle, the right being protected by the head masking it.

Whilst the majority of cases of NIHL will demonstrate a dip in the audiogram maximal at 4KHz, typical patterns of loss may vary from one industry or occupation to another and obviously will be dependent also on the period of noise exposure.

One of the major difficulties in medico-legal audiometry is the question of exaggeration of the loss. This may be suspected if there is disparity between the audiogram and the examiner's assessment of the hearing level, unaided and without lipreading. Disparity in admitted auditory thresholds on repeated testing should also raise suspicion of a non-organic element to the claimed deafness and further testing may then be instituted. Cortical evoked response audiometry is the preferred objective test as it allows threshold determination at the higher frequencies of 1,2 and 3 KHz, the frequencies most often used in assessment.

Having carried out pure tone audiometry an overall assessment of loss and/or disability must then be made and many different schemes exist. In the UK three main schemes exist, the Department of Social Security scheme being based on the hearing thresholds at 1,2 and 3 KHz being averaged for each ear separately, only those with an average of 50 dB or greater in each ear being compensated.

Coles and Worgan [8] devised a scheme for assessment of auditory handicap, grouping patients into 11 groups ranging from no significant auditory handicap to virtual total deafness. Whilst this scheme is still used the main method of determining disability is based on the "Blue Book", the result of a joint enterprise between the British Association of Otolaryngologists and the British Society of Audiology, published in 1983. This booklet ("Method for assessment of hearing disability") usefully defines the terms of hearing impairment, hearing disability and handicap.

No discussion on NIHL is complete without reference to the question of presbycusis. It is broadly agreed that for purposes of compensation no presbycusis correction factor should be applied [5] [26] even though in older patients presbycusis may account for a significant element of the deafness as can be seen from the diagram taken from Glorig's survey at the Wisconsin State Fair [9] (Fig. 7.1).

Finally, in connection with NIHL comes the question of tinnitus. Tinnitus may be defined as a sound or noise experienced by the individual but not heard by others and, therefore, may be considered to be a purely subjective phenomenon. In attributing the cause of tinnitus to NIHL the same criteria need to be applied as to the diagnosis of NIHL itself.

Head Injury and Deafness

Whilst noise exposure and deafness contribute the major element in most otological medico-legal practices, other aspects of deafness need consideration

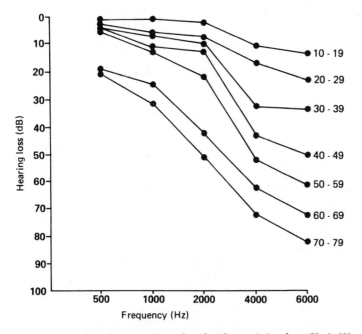

Fig. 7.1. Decade audiograms. Reproduced with permission from Glorig [9].

and the other large group encompasses the question of deafness after head injury.

Head injury may or may not cause skull fracture and, irrespective of the presence or otherwise of a fracture, may or may not cause loss of consciousness. Both skull fracture and loss of consciousness may in different ways indicate the severity of a head injury but fracture of the skull can occur without loss of consciousness and vice versa. Similarly, deafness can occur after head injury without either loss of consciousness or skull fracture.

Head injury may cause hearing loss in both the short term and the long term and the loss may be conductive (middle ear) or sensorineural. In assessing the relative factors in a case of deafness after head injury it is clear that knowledge of likely mechanisms of injury to the hearing is required.

In the early phases after a head injury a conductive loss may occur due to bleeding into the ear or to a tear in the tympanic membrane and will usually recover spontaneously. Failure to recover may suggest disruption of the ossicular chain, or the formation of adhesions and can occur from a seemingly minor head injury as in a recent case from the author's experience.

Sensorineural deafness may be partial or total and in the case of the former may be indistinguishable audiometrically from hearing loss due to noise exposure with a dip at 4KHz [10, 18] in the pure tone audiogram. More severe head injuries may cause base of skull fractures with the fracture line involving the petrous temporal bone; if there is a temporal bone fracture then its orientation will determine any likely inner ear damage, a fracture crossing the petrous temporal bone transversely being considerably more likely to produce a severe or total sensorineural deafness than a longitudinal fracture.

Whilst many patients will notice and report a hearing loss soon after the head injury, usually within a day or two of recovering consciousness and recovering from the period of post-traumatic amnesia it has been the author's experience that this is not always the case. Sometimes, several weeks or longer may have elapsed before the patient becomes sufficiently aware to report the deafness to his medical attendants.

Before giving a final opinion on any post-traumatic hearing loss it is wise to wait several months to allow any middle ear haematoma to resolve and to see if there is any recovery in the deafness. Unless a labyrinthine fistula, a leakage of the inner ear fluids into the middle ear, has developed there is unlikely to be any deterioration in hearing during this period.

Obviously, in assessing any post-traumatic hearing loss all the factors already discussed in relation to possible NIHL must be considered. The presence of other symptoms of inner ear disorder immediately after the head injury may be an important indicator of the relevance of head injury to the complaint of deafness, particularly a history of dizziness. However, such a history is likely to be absent in cases of severe head injury, being masked by the period of unconsciousness and post-traumatic amnesia.

Tinnitus may occur in association with any ear disorder and is a not uncommon concomitant of post-traumatic hearing loss. It is usually high-pitched and may be more distressing than the actual deafness. It is a purely subjective phenomenon and there are no objective tests to indicate or refute its presence.

Head injury may cause not only cochlear damage with deafness and its associated symptom of tinnitus but may also disturb the vestibular labyrinth causing dizziness. Dizziness is a common symptom after a head injury and may be caused either by damage to the inner ear or to the brain itself; it may occur without skull fracture. However, if the petrous temporal bone is fractured transversely there is likely to be severe inner ear damage and as well as the hearing loss there will be severe prostrating vertigo. This may last many days to several weeks, gradually improving with time. In the younger patient, the recovery is more rapid than in the elderly and someone over the age of 60 years may never completely recover, remaining persistently unsteady especially on sudden movement.

Less severe forms of unsteadiness often in association with headaches may constitute part of the post-concussional syndrome rather than being directly caused by inner ear damage; these symptoms usually resolve over a period of 6 to 12 months.

The symptom of positional vertigo may develop after a head injury – placing the head in certain positions usually when lying on one or other side – when certain criteria appertaining to the vertigo and its associated physical signs of positional nystagmus are present the diagnosis of benign paroxysmal positional vertigo may confidently be made and a reassuring prognosis given. The condition is usually self-limiting within a period of 1–2 years. Finally, delayed onset vertigo with a Ménière's-like disorder can occur years after certain temporal bone fractures and post-traumatic vertigo can also be caused by a perilymph leak. Thus a number of mechanisms occur causing post-head injury dizziness [16].

Trauma and Facial Palsy

Injury to any nerve may be graded according to one of several different methods of classification, Seddon [19] describing three stages of injury and more recently Sunderland [22] describing five stages. In the most severe stage described there is effective transection of the nerve. It is in these cases that the most severe prognosis is found. Head injuries both with and without fractures involving the petrous temporal bone may cause facial paralysis; when a palsy occurs without radiological evidence of a fracture the most likely cause of the paralysis is bleeding into the bony canal from the facial nerve. However, not all fractures of the temporal bone show up on routine skull radiology and further investigation such as tomograms may be requested before it can be confidently stated that there is no fracture. As already discussed, temporal bone fractures may be either transverse or longitudinal and it is the transverse ones that are more likely to involve the facial nerve.

Post-traumatic facial paralysis may be of immediate onset or delayed and may be partial or complete. Medico-legally, there is usually little doubt about the relationship between a facial palsy and an injury as long as it is recognised that a delayed paralysis may occur up to 1 or 2 days after the injury.

A complete paralysis of the facial nerve after a skull fracture will suggest possible transection of the nerve and most neuro-otologists would advocate surgical exploration, the exact technique used surgically depending on the findings at operation; if the nerve is intact but swollen or compressed a decompression should be carried out. If the nerve is severed then nerve-grafting may be required. The best results are achieved when repair is performed within 30 days of injury.

Whilst most traumatic facial palsies occur after head injury it should be noted that they can occur following surgical trauma. There are broadly two groups of operations where the facial nerve is at risk, those on the middle ear for chronic infection and those on the neck, especially on the parotid gland.

Operations for acoustic neuroma will similarly cause a total paralysis except in those few instances where the acoustic neuroma is small when it may reasonably be expected that facial function can be preserved.

Both in parotid surgery for malignant disease and operations for carcinoma and other malignancies of the ear a deliberate decision to sacrifice the nerve may have been made and discussed with the patient pre-operatively.

In general terms middle ear surgery should not cause facial nerve injury. The surgeon should be familiar with the anatomy of the ear and especially possible variations in the course of the nerve. The trainee otologist will have had the opportunity to practice his surgical craft on cadaveric human temporal bones, thus reducing the risk. However, an inadequately supervised novice surgeon presented with a chronically infected ear containing bleeding granulation tissue represents a combination likely to cause damage not only to the facial nerve but also to other middle and inner ear structures.

In most instances, therefore, a facial paralysis following middle ear surgery would be indefensible, exceptions to this statement justifying the general rule and this will be discussed further when considering consent for ear operations.

Ototoxicity

A number of drugs in use in medical practice may produce deafness as a side effect. Fortunately, this side effect of medication is well recognised and steps are normally taken to monitor and prevent such a sequel. The largest group of drugs producing deafness is the aminoglycoside antibiotics, and the importance of monitoring serum levels when administering these drugs is well recognised. It is also recognised that serum levels, and hence likely ototoxicity, will be raised in the presence of renal dysfunction. Some of the aminoglycosides are more toxic to the cochlea, producing deafness, others being more vestibulo-toxic affecting the balance mechanism within the inner ear and producing dizziness or unsteadiness. For example, streptomycin, the first of the aminoglycosides, tends to be vestibulotoxic whilst one of its early analogues, dihydrostreptomycin, was extremely cochleotoxic, such that it was rapidly withdrawn from use.

Since then, a wide range of aminoglycosides has been produced and many show selective toxicity to one or other inner ear system. Neomycin and kanamycin are very cochleotoxic, gentamicin and tobramycin vestibulotoxic. It is now recognised that neomycin can be absorbed through the bowel wall in seriously ill patients, contra-indicating its use as a pre-operative bowel sterilisa-tion preparation in such circumstances.

It should also be noted that these drugs can be absorbed through denuded skin, after burns for example, and their use as a topical agent in burns should be avoided; it would be considered bad medical practice now to treat burns topically with one of the aminoglycoside antibiotics although sadly such cases still occur and severe or profound deafness has ensued. It is important to realise that the symptoms of ototoxicity may not occur until after the drug is withdrawn and may progress after completion of therapy.

Ototoxicity may manifest itself in one of several ways, producing tinnitus, deafness or dizziness. The tinnitus is usually high frequency. Certain aminoglycosides, notably gentamicin, streptomycin, tobramycin and the non-aminoglycoside viomycin, may cause vestibular damage. One symptom of the vestibulotoxicity is bobbing oscillopsia, the sensation of objects moving on head movement. Frequently, the symptoms of vestibulotoxicity are overlooked initially as they may occur during the severe illness for which these powerful antibiotics are prescribed and may only manifest themselves during the recovery or rehabilitation period. Significantly also the toxic effects of the aminoglycosides are exacerbated in patients with renal failure and it should be noted that this group of drugs is also nephrotoxic.

A number of other antibiotics have been reported to be ototoxic but the reports of these are less frequent. The list includes chloramphenicol when used topically in the ear, vancomycin in large dosage and erythromycin.

Other drugs reported to have caused ototoxicity include the diuretics frusemide and ethacrynic acid, salicylates, quinine and its derivatives and the cytotoxic agents nitrogen, mustard and cis-platinum. Practolol, one of the early beta-adrenoreceptor-blocking drugs has been found to cause both a sensorineural and a conductive deafness; in view of this and other side effects it has now been withdrawn. Bromocriptine has been reported to cause a reversible ototoxicity whilst hexadimethrine bromide has caused severe sensorineural deafness.

It is known that many drugs can cross the placental barrier and the most notorious example of the teratogenic effects of such drugs is the experience with thalidomide. However, a number of the drugs already discussed may cause ototoxicity in the developing foetus. No drug should be administered in pregnancy unless absolutely essential and those with known ototoxicity or other side effects should be avoided altogether.

Finally, it should be noted that before administering any drug known to be ototoxic it would be wise to obtain a pure tone audiogram and vestibular assessment, however, either or both of these may be difficult in ill patients. Similarly, as in the case of the aminoglycosides, renal function should be assessed by measuring urea and creatinine levels. Dosage scales can then be used to calculate requirements based on known renal function. Monitoring of serum levels of aminoglycosides should occur both pre-administration and then one hour post-intramuscular or 20 minutes post-intravenous injections.

Trauma and the Nose and Paranasal Sinuses

The great majority of cases of nasal injury encountered both in clinical practice and in medico-legal work will involve direct trauma to the nose either by injury in a road traffic accident or by assault. Of the latter, many will present through the agency of the Criminal Injuries Compensation Board (CICB) and possibly also through the police if criminal proceedings are brought to bear on the assailant. The majority of cases of nasal injury will present with relatively uncomplicated fractures of the bony part of the nose, the bony pyramid, but the injury may also involve the soft tissue parts of the nose, the cartilaginous pyramid and the nasal septum.

The effects of injury to the nose may be considered as early and late. Early effects involve bleeding, swelling or other deformity and early functional deficit such as obstruction. One dangerous early complication of nasal trauma is bleeding into the nasal septum causing a septal haematoma; this has the potential for secondary infection with spread of infection intracranially. Because of this risk septal haematoma should always be drained surgically. The other possible complication of an infected septal haematoma is the loss of cartilaginous support for the nose with collapse producing either a saddle deformity or loss of the tip of the nose, the former being more likely.

The late effects of nasal injury may be cosmetic or functional and may include residual tenderness and discomfort in cold weather. Consideration of the cosmetic effects of an injury to the nose will be influenced by both the age and sex of the patient as a defect acceptable to a middle-aged man may not be to a young woman. As well as influencing the appearance of the nose a deformity of the nose, especially of the bony pyramid, may make it difficult to wear spectacles, another important consideration. It is essential in all cases of cosmetic deformity after injury to the nose to establish whether there is a past history of trauma to the nose and whether the patient had a perfectly straight nose prior to the injury.

The commonest functional complaint after nasal trauma is of nasal obstruction. This may be due to the nose being deviated, the nasal septum remaining relatively straight and midline; the septum itself may be injured and displaced or there may be a combined defect. In all three instances the nose may block on either side or both. It is important to recognise that although the septum may be deviated to one side the complaint may be of obstruction on either side or both sides or it may alternate. There are several reasons for this apparently anomalous situation; there may be secondary changes in the normal anatomical structure within the nose on the side opposite to the deviation, with enlargement of the inferior turbinate. Air flow through the nose is also influenced by the nasal cycle, a phenomenon of alternating vasoconstriction and vasodilatation of the blood vessels of the nasal mucosa. This produces little recognisable effect in the healthy nose but may be very apparent in the diseased or distorted nose [15].

It is not uncommon for patients to complain of nasal obstruction after a minor injury which has caused no nasal deformity and which, from the history of the nature of the blow, is unlikely to have caused any intranasal defect. The soft tissue swelling of even a minor nasal injury may be sufficient to unmask such a symptom which may then persist; even without any associated soft tissue swelling an injury to the nose may draw a patient's attention to the nose and he may become aware of a minor symptom which he had previously overlooked. It is important, therefore, always to inquire in detail about the mechanism of any injury to the nose and to relate this to the injuries sustained and the findings on examination. More severe naso-facial injuries may cause fractures which may extend to the base of the skull. Such fractures may have one of two effects: they may damage the olfactory nerves, the nerves subserving the sense of smell, and cause loss of smell (anosmia), or they may cause leakage of cerebro-spinal fluid (CSF), a potentially very serious situation in view of the risk of meningitis. When taking a history after head and facial injury one should always enquire about leakage of clear fluid from the nose. If a nasal drip follows an injury it may be helpful to collect the fluid and submit it to tests for the presence of glucose; a positive test would tend to confirm it as CSF. In such cases detailed radiology and neurosurgical opinion will be required as many cases of CSF leak from the nose fail to heal spontaneously and may require neurosurgical repair.

Anosmia may occur after any head or nasal injury and may be due to obstruction within the nose preventing smells reaching the narrow olfactory cleft in the upper part of the nose or it may be caused by damage to the olfactory nerves. These may be damaged either directly by fracture or by a shearing action as the brain moves relative to the skull in any acceleration/deceleration injury.

Associated with the complaint of anosmia may be loss of sense of taste. Careful inquiry and examination may reveal that the patient is able to recognise salt, sweet, bitter and acid items via the basic modality of taste mediated through taste buds mainly on the tongue. The aesthetic sense of taste, however, is essentially the sense of smell and it is this that allows enjoyment of the finer flavours of food and wine. It is rare for a head injury to damage the nerves of taste – the chorda tympani on either side – as well as the olfactory nerves.

There are no objective tests for the sense of smell. However, when testing the sense of smell with a variety of agents suspicions may be aroused as to the genuineness of the complaint. If there is such doubt the use of ammonia as a test agent may be of value – if the patient fails to respond to the exhibition of ammonia then doubt must be cast on the validity of his or her responses to the other test substances. The presence of ammonia is detected not by the olfactory nerves but by its irritant action on the nasal mucosa, a sensation conveyed by the trigeminal, the 5th cranial nerve.

In cases of anosmia after fractures or other head injury it is possible that there will be recovery although it is important to wait a reasonable period – say 6 to 12 months – before a final opinion may be given.

Injuries to the face and head may cause more severe damage to the facial skeleton including fractures of the maxilla and mandible, damage to dentition and, of course, soft tissue injuries, including lacerations to the face, head and neck.

Nasal deformity and nasal septal deviation may require surgical correction. Ideally, a nasal fracture with displacement should be manipulated between 5 and 10 days after the injury. It may, of course, be dealt with immediately but, often, this is rarely possible; if not dealt with straight away assessment of the need for manipulation becomes difficult due to soft tissue swelling which may take several days to settle. If left for more than 3 weeks sufficient bone healing may have taken place to prevent satisfactory repositioning of the bony fragments.

If not manipulated at a suitably early stage after an injury or if it has not been possible to achieve a satisfactory cosmetic result definitive plastic surgical correction (rhinoplasty) will be required at a later stage. Nasal obstruction may require surgical correction of nasal septal deviation either by submucous resection of the septum (SMR) or by septoplasty, both being operations to achieve the same end, a straight septum with good nasal airways. If both nasal and septal abnormalities co-exist then the more major procedure of septorhinoplasty will be required. The nature and extent of any nasal or septal operation will be determined by the pre-operative assessment and also intra-operatively and it is not possible here to discuss all possible surgical requirements in any detail. It is, however, important to recognise that nasal or septal abnormality may impair nasal function and predispose to repeated upper respiratory infections and sinusitis with the possibility of chronic sinusitis supervening. This may require further medical or surgical management although septal and nasal surgery may in some instances be all that is required; once the condition upsetting nasal function is corrected any predisposition to sinusitis will often resolve.

Fractures may occasionally involve the paranasal sinuses including ethmoidal and frontal as well as the maxillary sinuses. This will initially result in bleeding within the cavity of the sinuses but this blood clot will usually be reabsorbed. During the immediate post-trauma period there is an added risk of sinusitis developing due to this collection of blood; these fractures should be managed as compound fractures and treatment instituted with antibiotics. If a skull fracture involves the posterior wall of the frontal sinus there is a definite possibility of a tear of the underlying dura with associated CSF leak and a high risk of meningitis. As already discussed such CSF leaks may persist and require neuro-surgical intervention.

Finally, in discussing trauma to the nose it should not be forgotten that careful consideration should be given to the question of other non-related nasal pathology such as allergy and vasomotor rhinitis, the symptoms of which may be exacerbated by an injury even though the underlying disease process itself is unlikely to be directly affected.

In addition to accidental trauma to the nose, damage may be caused surgically and a number of examples will illustrate this point.

Septal surgery is usually uncomplicated but may result in septal perforation, tip depression or saddle deformity. Whilst septal perforation may occur after even the most straightforward submucous resection or other septal operation it is more likely when the surgery is carried out after fractures of the nose which have caused the septal deformity; similarly if the mucoperichondrial flaps are torn at surgery there is a greater risk of perforation. Many septal perforations are completely asymptomatic but may cause either whistling or nasal respiration or crusting and bleeding from the nose. Not all post-operative septal perforations may be blamed on the surgery; many patients poke and pick at the nose, especially after such surgery and certainly the commonest cause of nose bleeding is the patient's own index finger!

Intranasal adhesions may occur after nasal surgery causing obstruction of the nasal airway. Adhesions are most likely where surgery has been carried out both to the septum and to the turbinates; in such cases most surgeons will insert some form of nasal splint as a temporary measure in order to prevent such a development.

Antral washout rarely causes complications but occasionally the orbital floor may be partially dehiscent and the irrigating fluid may enter the orbit. This is usually easy to recognise when the procedure is carried out under local anaesthetic but may be overlooked if a general anaesthetic is used, typically in children. It is essential, therefore, that the surgeon leave the eyes uncovered by drapes in order to monitor for this possible complication. A recent case report in the Annual Report of the Medical Defence Union [13] highlights a further development of such a complication with optic nerve damage developing.

Ethmoidal surgery may place the optic nerve at risk due to its close proximity to the posterior ethmoidal air cells; the nerve is most at risk during intranasal ethmoidectomy, the relevant surgical landmarks being much easier to define using the external approach. The risks of all forms of surgery have been recently listed and discussed by Lund [12] in her article discussing developments in ethmoid surgery. Functional endoscopic sinus surgery (FESS) is a new technique for surgical management of chronic sinus disease. Proper training is the key to successful FESS but equally important is adequate pre-operative assessment including computed tomographic (CT) scans [21].

Operative complications include bleeding, cerebro-spinal leak and orbital haematoma. Blindness is a possible complication of this surgery as with other intranasal approaches to the ethmoids and this is discussed by Stankiewitz [21].

Trauma and the Throat and Neck

In order to understand the possible sequelae, both clinical and medico-legal, to injury to the nasopharynx and neck an understanding of some of the basic points of anatomy is required. Many important, if not vital, structures pass through the neck and any of these may be damaged by injury. In addition to the obvious skeleton structure, the bony spinal column, and the spinal cord contained with it, the major vessels taking blood to and from the brain and the tissues forming the upper air passages are perhaps the next most important structure.

The most prominent structures in the front or anterior part of the neck are the trachea or windpipe, and larynx, the latter forming the "Adam's apple". Lying on either side of the larynx is the carotid sheath, the major vascular bundle containing the carotid artery on either side, the internal jugular veins and running within the sheath, the vagus nerves. Lying on either side of the trachea in the neck is the thyroid gland. Closely related to this is the recurrent laryngeal nerve on each side; this is the main motor nerve to the larynx, innervating the muscles which open the vocal cords. Damage to either of these nerves may cause weakness of the voice; if both are damaged the patient is unable to open the laryngeal inlet and may experience severe breathing difficulty especially on exertion. This obstruction to the airway, typically produces an inspiratory crowing sound called stridor. It should be noted, however, that stridor may be produced by any lesion, causing obstruction to the free passage of air through the trachea or larynx. The larynx itself consists of a number of cartilages, the largest and most prominent being the thyroid cartilage; in adult life the thyroid cartilage gradually becomes bony in structure. Behind the larynx and trachea in the neck is the pharynx and upper part of the oesophagus, the food passages.

It is very uncommon for the larynx or trachea and other major neck structures to be injured in road traffic accidents in the UK; the diagonal element of the car seat belt prevents the upper part of the body from being thrown forward, the neck then flexing forward onto the chest. Where only a lap belt is worn there is a much greater risk of major laryngo-tracheal injury; the upper torso flexes forward, the neck is extended and the exposed neck comes into contact with either dashboard or steering wheel.

Injury to the larynx in these latter circumstances may vary from minor bruising to fracture of the thyroid cartilages, dislocation of intralaryngeal cartilages and even separation of the larynx from the trachea. This latter may be recognised surgically by the presence of air in the tissues of the neck producing the typical crackling sensation on palpation, surgical emphysema.

After any neck injury the larynx should be examined properly to determine the degree of damage: if there is surgical emphysema or if the patient presents with difficulty breathing then tracheostomy may be required and in such cases, the larynx and trachea should be explored surgically and appropriate repair carried out.

Road traffic accidents are not the sole cause of closed injuries to the neck; blows from a fist may cause laryngeal injury, although they rarely cause more than bruising or contusion it is not unknown for fractures to be caused. Sporting injuries to the larynx occasionally occur but it is rare for such injuries to be the cause of litigation.

Penetrating injuries are potentially life-threatening due to damage to major blood vessels or to involvement of the airway. Vascular damage may result in considerable blood loss and may result in death from this cause; penetration of any of the major veins in the neck may result in air being sucked into the vessel, carried to the heart, and causing what is effectively "vapour lock", the heart beating up a further mix of air and blood – the whole process constituting an air embolus.

If the air passages are penetrated and there is bleeding, aspiration of blood into the lungs may occur, again a life-threatening situation. Occasionally, penetrating injuries occur into the air passages with no long-term side effect.

Ingested and solid foreign bodies may result in litigation; unexpected solid foreign matter in food may implant in the larynx or oesophagus and require removal at operation. Removal of such foreign bodies is not without risk. Similarly, overlooking the presence of a foreign body may have severe consequences; apart from discomfort and difficulty in swallowing (dysphagia) the foreign body may penetrate the wall of the pharynx or oesophagus. This may result in infection in the tissues adjacent to the perforation (cellulitis) which can in turn lead on to abscess formation, in the neck if the foreign body perforates the larynx, and in the thorax if in the oesophagus. If a foreign body in the food passages is left, it is likely to be held up at one of three sites: the junction of pharynx and oesophagus, the cricopharyngeal sphincter; at the level of the aortic arch; and at the lower end of the oesophagus, the oesophagogastric sphincter. Rarely foreign bodies at the level of the aortic arch have led to perforation and erosion of the wall of the aorta with subsequent massive bleeding.

Pharyngoscopy and oesophagoscopy should only be carried out by suitably trained staff. A variety of techniques may need to be used in order to remove foreign bodies and improvisation may be required.

Finally, it should be noted that impaction of a foreign body or even a poorly chewed bolus of food may indicate the presence of other pathology such as a neoplasm of the oesophagus.

Inhaled foreign bodies are a particular problem in young children; they may cause acute, severe or total asphyxiation or their effects may be less marked. The National Safety Council of America has shown that the most common cause of accidental death in the home in children under 6 years of age is the inhalation of a foreign body. Whenever a young child presents with a history of possible inhalation of a foreign body, extremely careful assessment is required. In most cases, there is a history of choking followed by paroxysmal coughing which then subsides. If not detected and diagnosed at this stage a degree of tolerance develops and the next feature in the history may be the onset of a wheeze; the child may go on to develop persistent or recurrent pneumonia. Any of these events should trigger the suspicion of a foreign body.

Careful clinical examination may lend weight to the diagnosis of an inhaled foreign body; the presence of stridor or a wheeze, hoarseness or signs of chest infection are all possible indications.

Radiography is essential in all cases of suspected inhaled foreign body and may serve to show the object itself, or may for example, show secondary changes in the lung fields due to a blockage effect on the air passages, often producing a valvular action. This may allow retention within the lung, of a small amount of air, and cause the lung to "pump up" causing obstructive emphysema.

Vegetable foreign bodies are a particularly difficult problem and may react with the lining of the smaller air passages in which they lodge and cause intense swelling, making them even more difficult to remove. Removal of a foreign body from the air passage of a child may tax even the most experienced paediatric endoscopist.

Insertion of an endotracheal tube for an anaesthetic or to maintain an already compromised airway may cause later complications. These complications may include stricture in the area just below the larynx, the subglottis or upper trachea, where the inflatable cuff lies; this problem is much less common with modern plastic tubes with low pressure cuffs. Other complications include trauma to the vocal cords with scarring and the author has experience of two cases with a fibrous band between the two cords posteriorly [17].

A third possibility is the formation of intubation granuloma, a non-specific reaction to the presence of the tube usually occurring posteriorly in the larynx and presenting with hoarseness. The presence of such granulomata bilaterally may have caused the fibrous bands noted above.

None of these sequelae to intubation should be regarded as implying negligence or criticism of the anaesthetist but rather that endotracheal intubation has occurred.

The development of a vocal cord palsy after thyroidectomy is a recognised hazard of the procedure and in the best hands occurs in up to 1% cases [13]. The question of consent for such surgery will be discussed in the following section.

Informed Consent and Ear, Nose and Throat Surgery

The duty of care required of a surgeon involves not just the medical evaluation and surgical performance of a given procedure but also adequate explanation of the operation, its implications, risks and possible complications. It is also important to give an accurate assessment of the likely success rate of the proposed surgery. All this should be explained to the patient in suitable and comprehensive terms. It should also be made quite clear, where appropriate, that an operation is an elective one and rests in large measure on the patient's decision. Where there are strong indications for surgery such as for certain forms of active, chronic middle ear infection then the patient should be counselled more firmly and guided towards surgery. If malignancy is detected or strongly suspected then even greater pressure may need to be brought to bear.

Certain operations carry more risk than others, either due to the nature of the disease being treated or due to local anatomy or to surgical complexity.

Ear Surgery

Certain operations require special consideration when discussing consent for surgery; the three areas which most require special consideration are stapedectomy surgery, mastoidectomy operations and operations on the saccus endolymphaticus for Ménière's disorder.

Stapedectomy

The main risk in stapedectomy surgery is the development of a sensorineural hearing loss post-operatively. It is essential, therefore, that the patient receives adequate counselling before informed consent can be deemed to have been given. It must be remembered that an alternative method of treatment for any conductive deafness is provision of a hearing aid; the patient should be offered this as a possible alternative. Beales [2] has stated that there is at least an 85% chance of obtaining a good hearing improvement and 5% may expect some degree of sensorineural loss after operation. Shea [20] has suggested that 2% may develop a total sensorineural loss. The author has experience of a severe sensorineural loss developing some 8 years after a successful stapedectomy operation.

The patient should also be warned of the possibility of slight unsteadiness after stapedectomy and flying is contraindicated for at least 2 weeks.

A consent form specifically for stapedectomy surgery as used in the author's own Department is shown in Fig. 7.2; this form is not a substitute for full pre-operative discussion but it ensures that the patient is stimulated to raise questions with the surgeon.

Otomastoid Surgery

Otomastoid surgery is usually carried out for so-called "unsafe" attico-antral chronic suppurative otitis media with either a retraction pocket or a frank cholesteatoma. Typically, there may be a degree of offensive discharge present and the hearing may already have been damaged, causing a conductive hearing loss. Other possible pre-operative complications may include a labyrinthine fistula due to disease having eroded the bone containing the inner ear structures.

It has long been accepted that attico-antral disease constitutes an "unsafe" form of chronic middle ear infection with risk of developing such major complications as intracranial infections, facial palsy and dizziness due to labyrinthine fistula or labyrinthitis.

ADVICE TO PATIENTS SUFFERING FROM OTOSCLEROSIS

Deafness may be due to disease of the outer, middle or inner ear – in your case the cause is in the middle ear where the chain of three bones, conducting the sound waves from the drum to the inner ear, are attached. Your disease is called otosclerosis, which means that the 3rd bone in the chain (the stapes) is firmly fixed in its normal site and cannot move.

There are two possible lines of treatment for this particular deafness. Firstly, a hearing aid, which when worn would improve your hearing, but if discarded your deafness would relapse. The alternative treatment is for you to undergo a stapedectomy operation i.e. removing the stapes bone and replacing it with a plastic bone.

A stapedectomy operation requires you to be in hospital for about four days. You may feel a little dizzy after the operation, this does not last. The majority of patients acquire an immediate improvement in hearing, although in some the hearing does not improve and in a small percentage the hearing becomes worse. Instances have occurred when the dizziness has been prolonged and on rare occasions the patient's face has been weak on the side where the operation was performed.

Date.................................

I .... have discussed the stapedectomy operation with

.... and fully understand the nature of the operation as well as the risks involved.

Patient's name ....

and address   ....

Patient's

....   Signature...

....   Witness ....

Fig. 7.2. Consent form for stapedectomy surgery.

The decision to advise surgery must, therefore, be fully discussed with the patient and the risk of complications developing if treatment is declined should be outlined. The patient should be advised that surgical treatment is the only method open to him or her and that it has three main aims:

1. To achieve a safe ear
2. To achieve a dry ear
3. To preserve or improve the hearing.

The priorities for surgery should usually be in the above order although where the other ear has poor hearing or is similarly diseased then the priorities of surgery may alter subject to the premise that achieving a safe ear is paramount.

Care must be taken to explain to the patient that a small number of ears continue to discharge after even the most carefully and meticulously performed operations, sometimes requiring revision surgery.

Similarly, the effect of such surgery on the hearing needs to be carefully considered and discussed. Surgery is sometimes necessary on ears where the hearing is perfectly satisfactory pre-operatively, but of necessity the ossicular chain has to be disrupted with resultant conductive deafness. Pre-operative counselling of this possibility will forestall much post-operative heart searching and risk of litigation.

The question of advising the patient of possible surgical damage to the facial nerve remains a vexed one and it is not the author's practice to warn patients of this as a routine. It must be accepted, however, that some patients may ask more detailed and searching questions than others and in these instances it would be wise to raise it then as a remote possibility. Assuming the surgeon to be experienced in modern otological procedures it should not be considered negligent not to warn the patient of the very remote chance of damage occurring to the facial nerve.

Perhaps more important than failing to advise of the possibility of facial nerve damage in otomastoid surgery is failure to advise of the need for surgical treatment where there is clear evidence of attico-antral chronic middle ear disease. Such disease does not resolve spontaneously and antibiotics, either topical or systemic, will not effect a cure.

As with treatment for malignant disease the risks of failing to accept the offer of treatment, usually of necessity surgical, should be outlined to the patient.

Saccus Surgery for Ménière's Disorder

Operations to drain or decompress the saccus endolymphaticus may be considered in the management of Ménière's disorder, a syndrome comprising of episodic vertigo, tinnitus and deafness. Such surgery is established in the therapeutic repertoire for Ménière's syndrome but debate has been opened by the publication of articles on the placebo effect of operations on the mastoid without exposing the endolymphatic sac [3, 24]. Thomsen and colleagues [24] and Bretlau and co-workers [3] carried out simple mastoidectomy in one group of patients and saccus decompression on others. There was no statistically significant difference in the outcome of the two different operations. This has, therefore, raised the question of whether a surgeon should just carry out simple mastoidectomy and if he does plan such a course, whether he should advise the patient of this or whether consent should be obtained as for a saccus operation. The debate remains unsettled.

Consent for other middle ear surgery is usually less contentious although it should be stressed that the surgeon should always clearly outline the aims of proposed surgery as well as the limitations and risks.

In otological practice a considerable element of the work involves the management of conductive deafness in children, due to secretory otitis media or "glue ear". If insertion of grommets is to be carried out it should always be made clear to the parents that this does not necessarily effect a cure for the disorder but rather that the intention is to ventilate the middle ear and, thereby, allow normal hearing whilst the grommet is in situ. In many children the effusions will have resolved by the time the grommet is spontaneously extruded but a number of children will require re-insertion of the grommets. This should also be explained.

Parents will frequently raise the question of whether a child with grommets in position should be allowed to swim. There is no evidence that swimming is harmful in these cases and indeed the work carried out to investigate this question has concluded that there is no contraindication to swimming when grommets are in position.

Thyroid Surgery

Whilst not all otolaryngologists practice thyroid surgery, there is a substantial number who do; even those who do not carry out the surgery often become involved with patients for such surgery pre-operatively in order to assess laryngeal function. Some, of course, are involved post-operatively if there are any voice or airway problems after surgery or if the surgeon is unhappy about his or her exposure or identification of the recurrent laryngeal nerves.

Damage to one or both recurrent laryngeal nerves during sub-total thyroidectomy is said to occur in up to 3% of operations. It is essential that the patient is warned of this possible risk and other lines of treatment considered [14]. A thyroid surgeon needs to be aware of possible anatomical variations in the course of the recurrent laryngeal nerves and as a rule should identify the nerve (or nerves) prior to ligating blood vessels and carrying out any excisional surgery.

Tonsillectomy and Adenoidectomy

In discussing consent for either of these two procedures it should be stressed that they are two distinct operations in their own right but that indications for both operations to be carried out at the same time not uncommonly occur. Although tonsillectomy is often carried out in adults, the majority of these operations are carried out on children and, therefore, consent will be obtained from the parent or guardian.

Tonsillectomy and/or adenoidectomy carries a risk, however small, and no parent should ever be reassured that no risk exists. Tate [23] has shown the mortality of tonsillectomy to be 1 child per 10 000 operations, the primary cause of death being delay in treating any post-operative bleeding. Even when promptly treated, post-operative haemorrhage following either of these procedures can be traumatic, with possible inhalation of blood and subsequent respiratory tract problems.

Adenoidectomy presents special problems of possible post-operative palatal insufficiency with hypernasal speech (Rhinolalia aperta) especially if the adenoids are extremely large and the palate short. The presence of a bifid uvula should alert the surgeon to the possibility of a submucous cleft in which case indications for the operation should be reviewed. A submucous cleft provides a relatively strong contraindication to adenoidectomy. This should be clearly explained to the parents when discussing possible surgery for nasopharyngeal airway obstruction.

Endoscopy

The rigid oesophagoscope is probably one of the most dangerous surgical instruments used; there is a risk of perforation of the viscus because of disease, for example stenosis requiring dilatation, during the course of which the wall of the oesophagus is torn. Because a number of oesophagoscopies are carried out as a diagnostic procedure it can be extremely difficult to quantify the risk of such occurrences. Nonetheless, when obtaining consent for such procedures the surgeon should discuss possible complications. It is desirable that contrast imaging of the oesophagus be carried out before surgery and that the x-ray films be available in the operating theatre for reference during the procedure.

Nasal and Sinus Surgery

The medico-legal problems of sinus surgery have already been discussed. An honest explanation of these risks with the patient should be discussed when obtaining informed consent for surgery. In the case of surgery for acute or chronic sinusitis it is essential to highlight the risks of not carrying out the surgery, sinusitis remaining a possible cause of intracranial infection including cerebral abscess and meningitis.

References

1. Alberti PW (1979) Noise and the ear. In: Scott-Brown's diseases of the ear, nose and throat, vol 2, The ear. Butterworth, London, pp 551-662
2. Beales PH (1987) Otosclerosis. In: Kerr AG (ed) Scott-Brown's Otolaryngology, 5th edn, vol 3, Otolaryngology. Butterworth, London, pp 301-339
3. Bretlau P, Thomsen J, Tos M, Johnson NJ (1984) A placebo effect in surgery for Ménière's disease – a three-year follow-up study on endolymphatic sac surgery. Am J Otol 5: 558-561
4. Burns W (1968) Noise and man. John Murray, London, pp 84-88
5. Burns W, Hinchcliffe R, Littler TS, Robinson DW (1970) Hearing and noise in industry. HMSO, London
6. Burns W, Hinchcliffe R, Littler TS, Robinson DW, Shipton MS, Sinclair A (1977) National Physics Laboratory Report AC80. HMSO, London
7. Coles RRA (1968) Philosophical transactions of the Royal Society 263: 189-293
8. Coles RRA, Worgan D (1977) Scheme for assessment of auditory handicap. Revised 1980 (Private communication)
9. Glorig A (1957) Wisconsin State Fair Hearing Survey. Minnesota: American Academy of Ophthalmology and Otolaryngology, Rochester, Minnesota
10. Igarashi M, Schuknecht HF, Myers E (1964) Cochlear pathology in humans with stimulation deafness. J Laryngol Otol 78: 115-119
11. Kerr AG, Byrne JET (1975) Concussive effects of bomb blast on the ear. J Laryngol Otol 89: 131-143
12. Lund VJ (1990) Surgery of the ethmoids – past, present and future: a review. J R Soc Med 83: 451-455
13. Medical Defence Union (1990) Annual Report. The Medical Defence Union, London
14. Morrison AW (1989) Twenty-one years of otolaryngology litigation. J Med Defence Union 5: 27-29

15. Mygind N (1986) Essential allergy. An illustrated text for students and specialists. Blackwell Scientific Publications, Oxford
16. Rizvi SS, Gibbin KP (1979) Effects of transverse temporal bone fracture on fluid compartments of the inner ear. Ann Otol Rhino Laryngol 88: 741–748
17. Ruiz K, Gibbin KP, Moralee SJ, Abercrombie CA (1990) A rare complication of endotracheal intubation. J R Soc Med 83: 806
18. Schuknecht H, Neff W, Perlman H (1951) An experimental study of auditory damage following blows to the head. Ann Otol Rhino Laryngol 60: 273–278
19. Seddon HJ (1943) Three types of nerve injury. Brain 66: 237–288
20. Shea JJ Jr (1985) Stapedectomy technique and results. Am J Otol 6: 61–62
21. Stankiewitz JA (1989) Complications of endoscopic sinus surgery. Otolaryngol Clin North Am 22: 749–588
22. Sunderland S (1978) Nerve and nerve injuries, 2nd edn. Churchill-Livingstone, London, pp 88–97
23. Tate N (1963) Deaths from tonsillectomy. Lancet ii: 1090–1091
24. Thomsen J, Bretlau P, Tos M, Johnson NJ (1981) Placebo effect for Ménière's disease. Arch Otolaryngol 107: 271–277
25. Ward WD (1976) In: Hirsh SK, Eldridge DH (eds) Hearing and deafness. Washington University Press, St Louis
26. Wei Ping C (1986) Forensic audiology. J Laryngol Otol [Suppl 11]

CHAPTER 8

Neurology

R.B. Godwin-Austen

Neurological injury, particularly concussive head injury, is unfortunately a not uncommon event at the workplace or on the road. There is a large and increasing number of claims for compensation for injuries of this type and neurological reports are frequently required to assess quantum in such cases. This chapter will consider requirements of solicitors representing plaintiffs or defendants in actions for damages resulting in neurological injury. Claims of medical negligence, where diagnostic, neurosurgical (or radiological) mistakes are alleged, are generally either highly specialised (e.g. alleged vaccine brain damage or alleged Myodil arachnoiditis) or relatively rare isolated incidents. Neurological medical negligence will not therefore be considered in detail here.

Neurological injury separates into four main categories:

Head injury
Neck injury
Peripheral nerve injury
Psychological and psychiatric effects of organic brain injury.

The medical profession in its training as well as in everyday practice takes a fundamentally therapeutic attitude to its patients. The aim is perceived to be the diagnosis and assessment of injury or illness; and its restitution to the maximum extent possible. However, in the medico-legal context the role of the medical expert is quite different. He is seeing the "patient" in order to evaluate the effect that injury has caused and to provide a prognosis which will allow the court to come to a decision about the magnitude of compensation. By the time most claims come to settlement therapeutic aspects are generally long past. The practical therapeutic approach of medicine therefore may lead to conflicts which should be perceived by the doctor.

In clinical practice "functional overlay" tends to be discounted when an assessment of a patient's disability is made. Functional overlay is often considered irrelevant to the therapeutic process or at least a sphere of clinical activity which is the domain of the psychotherapist or social worker. In medico-legal practice anything attributable to the effects of the injury is relevant and should form a part of the claim. Similarly there will be cases where the rate (or degree of recovery from) injury is less than expected: or the contrary where the patient overemphasises to an unrealistic degree the recovery they have made.

The medical expert must be careful to adopt an impartial and objective approach in his assessment. In the former case the clinician may dismiss the disappointing recovery because it is "functional" and therefore not requiring continuing physical treatment. In the latter case most doctors will readily accept the credit for the patient's unexpectedly good recovery, whereas the court requires a realistic assessment discounting the patient's over-optimistic views. These considerations are especially important in patients with neurological injury because the recovery process is slow and brain damage may deprive the patient of the ability to objectively perceive his own disability or handicap.

In the assessment of any patient complaining of neurological symptoms some general principles must be borne in mind. Neurological symptoms may be associated with objective abnormality demonstrable on examination. But the objective signs may be disproportionate, that is, they may be less than the symptoms would lead you to expect so that wilful or subconscious exaggeration is suspected. Or the signs may seem unrelated to the symptom, for example, a complaint of paralysis when the signs indicate sensory loss. Or finally the neurological symptoms may have no corresponding sign or abnormality on examination. A lack of objective support for the organic basis of a complaint is relatively common in neurology. It occurs, for example, in many pain syndromes, especially those where the pain is associated with damage to peripheral nerve, the spinal cord or central nervous system. Migraine, epilepsy, irritability and personality change are all common post-traumatic phenomena where there is usually no associated objective abnormality. Compensation gives a motive to perpetuate symptoms previously experienced or to claim symptoms that have either recovered or never been sufficiently severe to cause disability.

The doctor must be able to recognise patterns of symptomatology associated with organic disorder of the CNS and to be able to distinguish these from symptoms that are exaggerated or feigned. Where there are abnormalities demonstrable on examination the case may appear straightforward and convincing but there should be an "appropriateness" between history, present symptoms and objective abnormality.

If there is a likelihood of organic pathology from the circumstances of the injury or the known physical damage, beware dismissing symptoms however unusual. Patients who have suffered, for example, prolonged post-traumatic amnesia after a head injury are likely to have organic brain damage as the basis for their complaints. Conversely where there are objective signs of abnormality there remains the possibility that the patient is also exaggerating or elaborating his symptoms. Assymmetry of the reflexes may be associated with little or no impairment of function in the affected limbs but claimants will not infrequently perpetuate an apparent handicap which in this case will appear to have objective evidence to support it.

Blows and injuries to the head – whether acceleration injury – as when machinery or falling object hits the head; or deceleration as in a road traffic accident, tend to cause three separate groups of neurological damage:

Injury to the brain

Injury to cranial nerves

Injury to the spinal cord and nerve roots in the neck.

Damage to the central nervous system (brain and spinal cord) is seldom fully reparable, and cranial nerve damage is usually the cause of some persisting symptomatology. Any neurological injury is therefore likely to have some permanent sequelae and the task of the medical expert is to assess the significance of the neurological damage in the context of the claim.

A poor prognosis does not necessarily apply to the psychological and affective (emotional) effects of head injury. Here the ability of the brain itself and the individual to adapt and recover can be remarkable. But the prognosis is strongly influenced by age, related injury, bereavement and a number of extraneous stress factors. Among these should be included prolonged litigation, a sense of resentment against employer or other road user, enforced invalidism and the prospect of substantial compensation.

A medical report in a neurological case must, therefore, do much more than merely record the medical facts about the case. It must give the considered opinion of the doctor about the disability experienced by the patient and the effects of that disability in terms of personal independence, suffering, need for domestic care, general mobility, ability to work, social integration and interpersonal relationships (especially with spouse) and finally life expectancy. There must always be an assessment of prospective risk of complication and in neurological practice the prospective risk of late post-traumatic epilepsy is important.

There is often genuine doubt as to what extent symptoms, especially pain, are exaggerated by the plaintiff to support their claim. In this situation the ideal is for the doctor to give a firm opinion one way or the other, that is, that the symptom is or is not genuine. And to back his view with reasoned discussion of the facts and medical knowledge that lead to this view. But opinion should go further by including comment about the effects of continuing litigation on the persistence of symptoms and in particular the doctor's view as to the likelihood or otherwise of the symptoms recovering rapidly once the claim is settled.

When expressing an opinion at the end of a report careful thought must be given as to how these opinions will be sustained in the face of the onslaught of cross-examination in court. If there is real and unavoidable uncertainty the possibilities should be spelt out in full and the reasons given for favouring one over the others.

A tactic frequently favoured by advocates in cross-examination is to imply that the doctor is being obscurantist or prevaricating in his answers when in fact the doctor is attempting to explain what may be a highly technical opinion. If that opinion has earlier been spelled out in a report the arguments supporting the doctor's view will be less easily challenged in this way.

Head Injury

The severity of the brain effects of a head injury can first be gauged by whether or not it led to concussion; and if so the duration of post-traumatic amnesia correlates well with the severity of post-traumatic brain damage [12].

Concussion

Concussion should be defined and not used loosely to describe the effects of head injury. Concussion is loss of consciousness through a blow to the head and consciousness is defined as continuous awareness of self and surroundings and the recording of continuous memory.

Concussion is associated with retrograde amnesia, that is, the absence of memory for the events preceding the blow and in this particular, concussion differs from most other forms of loss of consciousness, e.g. fainting or epilepsy.

In practical terms subjects who have been concussed have a gap in their memory starting moments (or longer) before the head injury and continuing for a variable period of time after the head injury. A post-traumatic amnesia of seconds suggests a minor injury such as might be sustained in the boxing ring and is unlikely to be associated with permanent brain damage. A post-traumatic amnesia with duration measurable in minutes (up to 1 hour) implies a moderate head injury and amnesia of hours is usually associated with severe head injury and the possibility of severe and persisting brain damage.

"Unconsciousness" in the lay mind suggests a state akin to sleep with unrousability, but it is clear from the above that a person may be apparently awake and responsive but not recording memory and thus still suffering from "concussion". If such a subject is submitted to specific tests of alertness, impairment is demonstrable. For example if they are asked to subtract 7 serially from 100 (or repeat back 7 digits or reverse the order and repeat back 5 digits) they can be shown to be unable. But questions that can be answered semi-automatically (e.g. name and address, age, etc.) may fail to indicate any abnormality of brain function.

The importance of recognising continuing concussive states is twofold. The severity of a head injury may be underestimated and a patient considered not to have suffered an injury likely to cause brain damage if they apparently woke up soon after the injury. Secondly, abnormal behaviour may be due to concussion but attributed to other causes especially intoxication. Thus the driver who behaves in an obstreperous manner (possibly refusing breath or blood analysis for alcohol) may be doing so through a state of concussion rather than as the result of alcoholic intoxication.

Retrograde amnesia is the diagnostic feature of concussion. Where unconsciousness is claimed but apparently there is memory of the impact to the head, it is unlikely that concussion has occurred. In this situation the head injury can be assumed to be non-concussive and less likely to be associated with brain damage; but also the possibility of wilful exaggeration must be considered.

Post-traumatic amnesia should be "absolute", i.e. there should be a total absence of memory. It is not infrequent for a subject to report an "island" of memory – when they were being loaded into an ambulance, for example – followed by a further gap in memory. The duration of post-traumatic amnesia is taken as the time from injury to the first "island" of memory.

Head injury, when associated with concussion, will usually have evidence of scalp or face wounds. But these wounds do not correlate well with the severity of the injury. Rather they correlate with the object which caused the blow to the head. Thus a flat yielding surface (e.g. soft earth) may cause no scalp injury but nonetheless be concussive, whereas a stab wound from a sharp instrument may cause extensive facial or scalp injuries without concussion. And a missile (e.g. a bullet) may cause a penetrating brain injury without immediate loss of consciousness.

Post-traumatic Epilepsy

The duration of post-traumatic amnesia (PTA) has relevance not only to the severity of a head injury and therefore the risks of brain damage [15]. It also correlates with the prospective risk of post-traumatic epilepsy. Any concussive head injury carries some risk of post-traumatic epilepsy. The risk is greatest in the first year following a head injury and declines exponentially thereafter; the risk approximately halving after 12 months free of fits and reducing to about 25% of the original risk 4 years after the accident (if no seizures have occurred).

While there are probably many variables that influence the likelihood of post-concussional epilepsy (for example the part of the brain injured, or the age and health of the individual), three factors are accepted as having major statistical significance in the development of post-traumatic epilepsy:

1. Intracranial haematoma identified by scan, and/or removed surgically
2. Epileptic seizures occurring during the first week after the head injury
3. Depressed fracture of the skull with tearing of the dura mater.

Where PTA is more than 24 hours the risk of late epilepsy is further increased.

In patients who have suffered concussion but in whom none of the above risk factors are present, a 1% risk of late post-traumatic epilepsy applies. Whereas where two or three of the major risk factors are present, there is a 30% immediate prospective risk and if early epileptic seizures have also occurred the risk rises to up to 60%. (For a full discussion of this subject see "Epilepsy after non-missile head injuries" by Jennett [7].)

The Driver and Vehicle Licensing Authority in the UK takes the view that where the prospective risk of late post-traumatic epilepsy exceeds 20% then that individual should be barred from driving on an Ordinary Vehicle Driving Licence [4] and any seizure (after the age of 5 years old) no matter how mild, is a bar to driving a heavy goods vehicle or public service vehicle [2].

In all neurological reports where concussion has occurred, reference should be made to the prospective risk of late post-traumatic epilepsy. Epilepsy carries the risk of accidental physical injury in an attack. And there is a risk of the order of 1 in 1000 of sudden unexpected death from a seizure. The mental effects of epilepsy are of major importance with an increased risk of psychiatric illness particularly depression and thought disorder of the schizoid type. But perhaps the most significant effects of the development of epilepsy after head injury are social. Employment is usually at risk whether or not the subject has to work at heights, with heavy machinery or open furnaces. Increasing numbers of individuals depend on their driving licence for continuing employment and the social stigma of epilepsy in personal life or at the workplace is profoundly disabling and affects marital prospects, recreation and physical rehabilitation. The prospective risk of post-traumatic epilepsy has an important influence therefore on quantum.

Likewise the actual development of post-traumatic epilepsy represents a major continuing disability. Post-traumatic epilepsy (like all the focal epilepsies) is notoriously resistant to medical treatment. Fits tend to recur with a frequency sufficient to keep awareness of the problem in the mind of the sufferer and his family and also to cause restrictions on everyday activities. There is the inconvenience and. possible side effects of anti-convulsant medication. Finally with recurrent seizures the individual cannot achieve the "two years free from an attack" necessary to requalify him to hold a driving licence.

Brain Damage

The range of symptoms and disability that results from brain damage is enormous and beyond the scope of this book. However a practical approach to brain damage as it presents in claims for compensation should address itself to answering the following questions:

1. Are the effects of brain damage improving, deteriorating or static? If static, is there marked fluctuation or variability possibly attributable to extraneous or relevant factors?

2. Is the subject suffering distress from pain or other attributable symptoms? If so, to what degree? Pain is a subjective experience and cannot be objectively measured. Its severity has to be assessed by considering the extent to which it affects the individual's behaviour, mental attitude and the extent to which it leads to physical disability. Thus however severe a patient may claim a headache or neck pain to be, if it does not prevent his leading a normal active life and cannot be shown to be affecting him psychologically or behaviourally it has to be concluded that the pain is not of a severity to be a handicap or disability.

   Similar considerations apply to patients who complain of ringing in the ears (tinnitus) or intolerable burning, tingling or pins and needles sensations.

3. Has the brain damage led to symptoms of weakness, numbness, lack of co-ordination or disturbance of balance? Also visual impairment, loss of sense of smell or taste, hearing loss or speech disturbance? And are these symptoms associated with the appropriate neurological deficit on physical examination? At the conclusion of the history taking and physical examination (with or without access to further investigation results) do the clinical features indicate focal or multifocal brain damage whose anatomical distribution is recognisable?

   A proper neurological assessment should allow clear conclusions to be drawn: (a) the brain damage has affected an identifiable region of the brain resulting in characteristic symptoms and signs; and (b) the symptoms from this type of brain damage are appropriate to the disability the patient describes and neither exaggerated nor underestimated.

4. Has the head injury been associated with subjective symptoms which are convincingly characteristic of a post-concussional syndrome?

   A large medical literature has developed arguing for and against the concept of a post-concussional syndrome. Symptoms such as headache, dizziness, fatiguability, poor concentration and irritability are often given particular emphasis by the claimant. Both doctor and the court may be led to suspect subconscious or wilful exaggeration of such symptoms for gain and the perpetuation of complaints of this type may be seen by the plaintiff not only to advance their claim but almost to be necessary because the timescale of the legal process is almost always more prolonged than the process of recovery from an injury. The prognosis for recovery from post-concussional symptoms once the claim is settled is crucial to the assessment and a clear opinion should always be given. These and related matters will be considered in greater detail later.

5. Is late deterioration of symptoms likely to occur? Or are these late complications of the injury? (e.g. late post-traumatic epilepsy or late neuralgic complications of nerve damage)

6. To what extent does this degree of incapacity deprive the patient of (a) independence for activities of daily living; (b) mobility, including ability to drive, climb steps, or transfer from a wheelchair; (c) a social life, including relationships with family and sexual relationships; (d) employment: at the pre-traumatic level, a reduced level or not at all [3]; (e) education or training (especially in children or young adults); (f) recreation; (g) a life outside institutional care?

Neck Injury

Assessment of the effects of skeletal injury to the neck is considered in Chapter 11. But in a significant proportion of patients, injury to the neck results in damage to nerve roots at one or more levels in the cervical region; or causes damage to the spinal cord itself. More rarely the vertebral or carotid arteries are injured with neurological sequelae resulting from vascular insufficiency [11]. It is not uncommon for injury to the neck to give rise to a mixture of disability resulting from bone or joint trauma (whiplash injury, disc protrusion) accompanied by damage to one or more nerve roots and bruising of the spinal cord itself. Where there is additional skeletal or soft tissue trauma to a limb (or especially if there is peripheral nerve damage in the limb) the difficulties of evaluating what symptom is due to which aspect of the injury becomes extremely complicated. However, in neurological practice it is more common for persisting symptoms to lead to litigation than the reverse and settlement of the claim seldom leads to resolution of the symptoms [5].

Root Damage

Nerve root damage in the neck is a not uncommon complication of road traffic accidents involving motorcyclists. In these cases the injuries cause varying degrees of paralysis and sensory loss in the arm. The distribution of the weakness and sensory loss will be determined by the nerve in the brachial plexus or roots affected. But whereas brachial plexus or peripheral nerve injury is potentially recoverable (when the nerve remains in continuity) there is no prospect of recovery where there is avulsion of the nerve root from the spinal cord. This fundamentally different prognosis is necessarily reflected by very different quantum of damages, because an irrecoverable neurological injury will almost always have very profound repercussions on future employment.

Furthermore root avulsion injuries are characteristically associated with a severe pain which is only treatable by potentially hazardous surgical means, whereas brachial plexus injuries seldom show these features.

In any medico-legal assessment of a case of nerve damage in the cervical region distinction should therefore be made between these two conditions and the appropriate prognosis suggested.

In some cases of post-traumatic headache the symptoms result from injury to the second cervical nerve root. This nerve gives sensory supply to the back of the scalp. When it is damaged there is usually demonstrable sensory change in the C2 dermatome. In cases of post-traumatic headache specific attention should be paid to the presence of sensory changes over the back of the head because these imply an attributable organic basis for the symptom.

Cervical Spinal Cord Injury

Flexion-extension ("whiplash") injury is commonplace in medico-legal practice but occasionally injury of this type causes damage to the spinal cord with neurological sequelae. Although most patients with neurological symptoms following neck injury show complete recovery within hours or days a proportion have persisting symptoms indicative of disturbance of spinal cord function in the neck. The distribution of damage to the spinal cord is characteristically central in the cord and gives rise to a clinical picture that is recognisable and usually described as "the central cord syndrome". Patients complain of a painful stinging, cold or burning sensation over the back of the neck occasionally extending up to the back of the scalp and usually extending down in a "cape" distribution over both shoulders (C5) and sometimes over the outer aspects of both arms (C6). Sensory testing reveals, in the same area, impaired appreciation of pain and temperature. This sensory loss is associated with variable degrees of weakness in the arms with muscle wasting and loss or reduced tendon jerks; and with spastic weakness (often mild) in the legs with brisk jerks and extensor plantar responses. There may be associated symptoms of impaired bladder control and impaired sexual function [10].

Central cord syndrome shows little improvement beyond 6 months following injury and the intractable neck pain may lead to psychological reactions that are misinterpreted as "functional overlay". In many of these cases the symptoms are far greater than the objective abnormality would suggest.

Other patterns of spinal cord damage are also seen where the main injury may affect the anterior part of the cord or one side of the cord (Brown-Séquard syndrome). The clinical features on examination are characteristic.

Peripheral Nerve Injury

Peripheral nerve injuries fall naturally into two groups. There are those which affect cranial nerves and are usually associated with head injury. And there are those which involve peripheral nerves elsewhere, the traumatic peripheral mononeuropathies. While this latter group may be the result of accidental injury or criminal injury they are a significant source of medical negligence claims when some surgical procedure has been associated with a post-operative mononeuropathy.

Cranial Nerve Damage

The cranial nerves commonly damaged through trauma are the first (olfactory), the second (optic), the fifth (trigeminal), the seventh (facial) and the eighth (auditory) cranial nerves. Damage to the olfactory or optic nerves carries a poor prognosis for recovery whereas recovery is usually good in fifth and seventh nerve lesions. Deafness from nerve damage or cochlear damage is usually persistent – although not necessarily severe; whereas the prognosis for conductive deafness depends on the nature of the injury.

Anosmia

Traumatic anosmia or loss of sense of smell is usually, but not always, noticed by the patient. It is surprising that even with total anosmia some patients are unaware of any impairment of appreciation of the flavour of food and may only realise that they have lost sense of smell when they burn food accidentally on the stove, or when tested by a neurologist. Olfaction subserves not only the perception of smell but also the appreciation of flavour (taste). Thus taste sensation is made up of (a) *primary taste:* (sweet, sour, salt, bitter), and is perceived through taste receptors in the mouth; (b) *flavour* perceived through the first or olfactory nerve; (c) *common sensations* subserving texture and temperature. Only (b) will be lost in a patient with traumatic anosmia. Patients should therefore always be tested for primary taste perception (a) (with sugar, salt or citric acid solutions) and common sensation (c) using ammonia solution which directly stimulates the mucous membrane of the nose.

It is usually accepted that sense of smell is lost through head injury causing a physical tearing of the olfactory nerves in the floor of the front of the cranial cavity [6]. Such injury is permanent with no possibility of any recovery. Some cases may lose sense of smell through damage to central structures in the brain. In these cases there may be an associated impairment of sense of primary taste and the prognosis for recovery is better. But if no recovery of sense of smell has taken place within 12 weeks of injury there is little prospect of recovery thereafter, although occasional cases have been reported to recover up to 5 years later [13].

Damage to Vision

Damage to vision results more commonly from damage to the constituent parts of the globe of the eye (and especially the retina) than from damage to the optic nerve itself. But trauma to facial bones or base of skull may cause injury to the optic nerves, chiasm or retro-chiasmal visual pathways with the appropriate neurological visual defects. The clinical distinction of hysterical blindness from bilateral optic nerve injury or cortical blindness is beyond the scope of this chapter, but any patient suspected of "functional" visual impairment has to be carefully examined for fundoscopic abnormalities, visual field defects (especially small central scotomata or "spiral" field defects) and corrected visual acuity.

Fitness to drive a car depends on a corrected visual acuity of better than 6/12 in one eye; and the absence of a lower homonomous visual field defect.

Trigeminal Nerve Damage

The fifth cranial or trigeminal nerve is commonly damaged in three situations:

1. In the region of the eyebrow (supra-orbital branch) when the forehead comes against the edge of, for example, the top of the windscreen. This injury seldom causes permanent total loss of sensation in the forehead and front of the scalp but it frequently gives rise to painful paraesthesiae and hypersensitivity of the appropriate area and may lead to persisting "neuralgic" head pains.
2. The maxillary division may be damaged where maxillary bone fracture or severe facial bruising has occurred. The former may involve branches to the upper teeth and hard palate whereas the latter will result in sensory loss confined to the cheek and upper lip.
3. Fracture of the mandible may damage the inferior dental nerve causing anaesthesia of the front lower teeth, lower lip and chin.

In all three cases the area of skin rendered anaesthetic will conform strictly to the anatomical boundaries of the affected nerve and in particular will not cross the mid-line. It is usually easy therefore to identify spurious or exaggerated nerve damage. Sensory loss in the face, as elsewhere, carries the prospective risk of accidental injury to the skin. Where the lower lip is affected there is the additional handicap of involuntary dribbling.

Injury to the seventh and eighth nerves is considered in Chapter 7.

Traumatic Peripheral Mononeuropathies

Peripheral nerve damage in the trunk and limbs will result in sensory loss or motor weakness appropriate to the distribution of that nerve.

Peripheral nerves are commonly damaged during elective surgical procedures. Indeed any skin incision is likely to damage small sensory cutaneous nerves and to result in small areas of impaired sensation close to the surgical scar. Surgical trauma of this type is less likely to cause persisting pain from sensory nerve damage than is trauma sustained as the direct result of laceration or penetrating injuries. Crush injuries or traction injuries to peripheral nerves (as opposed to nerve root avulsion injuries – see above) are also commonly associated with persisting pain and dysaesthesia as well as an area of sensory loss. There is considerable variability between individuals of the extent to which "pins and needles" sensations, tingling, hot/cold feelings or hypersensitivity are regarded. Some will find sensory disturbance of this type the source of continuing distress to the extent of disturbing concentration and leading to an obsessive attention to the experience. But many individuals ignore the feelings and will only admit to experiencing such paraesthesiae if directly questioned. The assessment of such symptoms is necessarily a subjective matter but one where some measure of severity may be gauged by the extent to which the symptoms affect the patient's personality, behaviour and emotional responses. A report based on a reasoned assessment of the effect that chronic painful hyper-sensitivity has had on an individual is more likely to command the acceptance of a judge than generalisations about the triviality of the nerve damaged. For, often, the nerve injury has affected only a small terminal cutaneous nerve perhaps in the forearm or foot, and the skin area affected may measure only a few square centimetres.

The natural history of painful dysaesthesiae after peripheral nerve trauma is variable. In most patients the initial numbness with objective sensory loss is followed within weeks or months by the development of paraesthesiae and occasionally pain [14]. These symptoms then gradually diminish so that over a timescale extending for 2 to 5 years the unpleasant sensations become less and may disappear altogether leaving only sensory loss. Occasionally this process of gradual improvement is replaced by increasing symptoms which lead to an obsessive rumination by the patient and result in a symptom complex where the pain seems to occupy the whole consciousness. Chronic pain of this type is a formidable therapeutic problem. It is also easily mistaken for the complaint of a chronic neurotic with a tendency to exaggerate or perpetuate symptoms; or the hysteric or malingerer subconsciously or consciously fabricating symptoms for gain. The proper assessment of a case of this type is among the most demanding in medico-legal practice.

Partial or complete severance of a peripheral nerve may be followed by the development of a palpable neuroma formed of sprouting axonal processes and fibrous tissue. The presence of such a neuroma provides some support for the patient's complaint of pain as these swellings are typically very sensitive to palpation and give rise to pain referred to the area supplied by the nerve that has been damaged.

The paralytic or motor effects of peripheral nerve injury generally pose fewer problems of assessment than the sensory nerve problems so far described. The functional deficit resulting from damage to, say, the ulnar or median nerve in the wrist is easily recognised and relatively stereotyped. Clearly the disability resulting from peripheral nerve damage in the hand in any individual at work is likely to be substantial.

Psychiatric and Psychological Aspects of Organic Brain Injury

Neurology, psychiatry and clinical psychology have complementary and overlapping relationships in the assessment of organic brain damage but the neurologist is probably particularly equipped by training and experience to assess the significance and prognosis of psychological sequelae from head injury. Brain damage resulting in personality change or cognitive impairment is often characterised by objective neurological abnormality which allows more firm support for neurological opinion than a psychoanalytical assessment where theory most usually takes the place of observed fact. The measurement of cognitive impairment by psychometric testing is a most valuable tool in support of a clinical assessment of impaired brain function. And similarly the psychiatric assessment of disturbed behaviour and emotion is important in reinforcing the neurological signs of focal or multifocal brain damage.

Physical injury to the brain results in a constellation of deficits which may be categorised as follows:

1. Sensory-motor physical deficit
2. Cognitive impairment; that is, focal or generalised impairment of memory and intelligence
3. Behavioural and affective (emotional) change
4. Psychiatric disease states: (a) neurotic, anxiety, depression and obsessive/compulsive disorders; (b) psychotic, acute confusional states and chronic delusional schizoid or hysterical disorders
5. Personality change, for example, apathy, disinhibition, hypersexuality

The emotional and psychological stress that inevitably accompanies the injury and the subsequent recovery process also leads to psychiatric effects which must be included in any assessment of the effects of that injury.

In this chapter three common post-traumatic states will be considered in detail (a broader consideration of the subject is presented in Chapter 14):

1. Stress reactions: anxiety, depression and psychotic (acute and chronic)
2. Post-concussional syndrome
3. The effects of focal brain damage: (a) frontal; (b) temporal; (c) parietal.

Stress Reactions

Any unpleasant experience can be said to induce a stress reaction, i.e. to be likely to cause symptoms of anxiety and depression. The extent to which this reaction is the proper subject for compensation (when it has resulted from the fault of another) is currently a matter of legal debate. But where the stress reaction is seen to form a part of the physical pain and suffering there is little room for debate, although the magnitude and importance of this part of the injury will inevitably lead to a range of opinion.

Anxiety is a phenomenon that is more common in non-concussive, than concussive head injuries. It seems that the post-traumatic and retrograde amnesias save the subject from the harmful effects of recording the experience and then reacting to the memory. In many young people a reaction characterised by feelings of tension, unreasonable fears, restlessness, insomnia and nightmares, will give way within weeks to a natural recovery and restoration of a normal mental state. However in older individuals this recovery process is prolonged, delayed or does not occur at all; and occasionally the accident or injury seems to provide the trigger for a chronic and disabling anxiety state in which there may be a specific phobia for the circumstance of the accident. Thus a plaintiff injured crossing the road may become incapable of crossing the road unless accompanied; or someone injured in a bus may develop a phobia that makes them, when they contemplate travelling by bus, exhibit all the symptoms of acute anxiety with tremor, sweating, restlessness and hyperventilation.

Depressive reactions to injury are commonplace. They do not usually bear any simple relationship to the magnitude of the injury or loss but are commoner in the elderly and in the female sex. Depression is characterised by loss of self-confidence, solitariness, uncontrollable weeping, retardation and gloomy ruminations on the future and present circumstances. Reactions of this type may develop several months after an accident when the physical effects are diminishing and the symptoms may seem to worsen by acquiring a momentum of their own, independent of any discernible connection with the accident itself, thereby giving opportunity for much legal argument. Frequently a delayed deterioration in symptoms responds to orthodox medical treatment with anti-depressant drugs but the overall prognosis for both anxiety and depressive reactions is most uncertain so that early opinions on this aspect should be given with great circumspection.

A past history of anxiety neurosis or depressive illness is an important factor in the genesis of a post-traumatic stress reaction and affects the prognosis very significantly. The likelihood or otherwise of a reaction of this type without the accident as the cause, is a matter for careful and reasoned medical expert opinion. In this situation all previous medical records are essential as it is commonplace for plaintiffs to overlook or conceal a state of chronic psychological disorder. The accident may prove, when the records are examined, to have had no discernible effect on the plaintiff's behaviour or symptomatology.

Acute psychotic confusional states are commonplace after concussive head injury and form a part of the medical management. They are seldom relevant in claims for compensation unless the individual has done himself or others an injury while so confused. Chronic psychotic reactions are rare unless by causing relapse of a previous psychotic illness. Thus severe psychotic depression or schizophrenia may follow head injury in someone who was apparently fully recovered from an earlier mental illness. The prognosis in these cases relates to the natural history of the disorder and its medical treatment rather than the severity of the injury [9].

Post-concussional Syndrome

The symptoms seen in patients after concussive head injury where no focal brain damage has occurred tend to fall into recognisable patterns [15].

Commonplace is headache which may have a migrainous pattern [1], may have features of tension headache or may have a neuralgic or spasmodic quality. In cases where a cutaneous nerve to the scalp has been damaged, lateralised episodic head pain may be characteristic [8].

Similarly, changes of mood with depressive symptoms are often associated with irritability, lethargy and disturbed sleep pattern. Limited concentration (so that the subject finds him or herself incapable of "taking in" a book or document for longer than, say, 5 minutes), absentmindedness, non-specific "dizziness" are typical and a particularly characteristic symptom is alcohol intolerance. Patients who have suffered brain injury not sufficient to cause objective physical signs may describe how very small amounts of alcohol exacerbate symptoms of headache and dizziness and create an unpleasant feeling of intoxication even when the quantity consumed is minimal.

Although symptoms of this type are not associated with any objective abnormality they probably result from a mild diffuse brain damage. In a young healthy adult such symptoms will often recover fully in a matter of months. But in the elderly or those with physical or psychiatric disorders the prognosis is very much more uncertain. In these cases severe disability may result and continue indefinitely. Such disability must be attributed to the accident unless there is good reason to suppose the individual is wilfully exaggerating or perpetuating their symptoms.

Where there is an organic basis for symptoms of post-concussional syndrome the completion of the legal proceedings and the settlement of the claim for compensation seldom leads to any discernible improvement or deterioration in the symptoms and disability.

Focal Brain Damage

Frontal

Injury to the frontal lobes commonly occurs when a deceleration injury causes the brain to shift forward within the skull. Contusions of the frontal region may be demonstrated on brain scan. But early clinical manifestations are generally obscured by associated disturbance of function in the brainstem. With recovery of consciousness the results of frontal lobe damage become manifest. The commonest associated feature is anosmia due to the tearing of the olfactory nerve beneath the frontal lobes as already described.

Frontal lobe dysfunction causes a spectrum of personality change ranging from the mildest blunting of emotional responsiveness at one extreme to a bland facile apathy at the other. The patient himself seldom has insight into the change that has occurred. He may quote others who describe him as "changed", but does so without any emotion or appreciation of the significance. Family and friends usually have great difficulty in defining or describing the personality change that occurs with frontal brain damage. Behaviour may be described as "childish" or "simple-minded", although there is no apparent impairment of intellect. The medical expert has to be alert to the possibility of frontal lobe damage and question both the plaintiff and relatives in a way that will bring out the characteristic features but without putting words into their mouths.

The spouse will often comment that the subject has lost his former sense of humour, lacks spontaneity and shows no initiative. These features are usually attributed to the physical suffering of the recovery process. Characteristically the patient is noted for a lack of any sense of consideration or thoughtfulness for the feelings of others. To social acquaintances, therefore, he seems tactless and unreliable; to his wife, lacking in affection (but not necessarily in sexual drive) and considerateness. Frontal lobe damage will lead to a formerly energetic, sociable and extroverted individual becoming apathetic, inconsiderate and lacking ability to plan for the future. Above all he lacks any apparent concern or anxiety about himself or his family. A bland acceptance of the *status quo*, if it is not discovered to be due to brain damage, may deprive the plaintiff of compensation for one of the most devastating effects of his injury.

The personality change that results from frontal lobe damage impairs the recovery process from physical injury because the patient has none of the drive and will required to obtain the greatest benefits from physiotherapy and rehabilitation. His apathy may be misinterpreted by the family (and indeed the defendant) as a hysterical reaction or "sickness behaviour" designed to maximise the quantum of damages. If he gets back to work his employer may find that all the motivation and initiative required is no longer there so that his job may be terminated. Also, sadly, many marriages fail because the spouse cannot cope with the affectionless, demanding but inconsequential individual that the husband/or wife has become [9].

In any case where frontal lobe damage has occurred the medical report should detail the behavioural changes that characterise it; and give examples that will allow an assessment of severity and therefore the likely consequences. Any physical abnormalities that are associated with the psychological changes should be carefully noted (anosmia, gait disturbance, frontal lobe incontinence, extensor plantar responses). And finally behavioural abnormalities observed by the examiner should be recorded. These may include childish or disinhibited behaviour or content of talk, or a lack of any apparent anxiety or emotional involvement with the medical examination or its purpose. (It is normal for plaintiffs to exhibit some anxiety when seeing a doctor and to show some affective response when discussing the circumstances of the accident and their own continuing symptoms.) Plaintiffs tend to emphasise (or over-emphasise) the effects of their accident but subjects with frontal lobe damage, by contrast, understate their case. It is the responsibility of the medical expert for the plaintiff to report this disability comprehensively.

Temporal Lobe Damage

The anterior and medial parts of the temporal lobes are the regions of the brain most likely to be damaged in head injury. It happens that these regions subserve memory and language function so that disturbances of memory and speech are common sequels of concussive head injury.

Where temporal lobe damage is suspected there may however be little or nothing of objective physical abnormality on neurological examination. Visual field defects due to damage to the optic radiation in the temporal lobe are rare after head injury. Damage to the internal capsule may give pyramidal weakness on one or both sides and gliotic scarring of the temporal lobe is particularly liable to result in post-concussional epilepsy often with complex focal features.

Speech defects due to dominant hemisphere brain damage (dysphasia) may be reported by the plaintiff as a defect of memory, a failure to be able to recall the names of people or places in the way he used. The family may notice he speaks more slowly and occasionally uses the wrong word. Wherever dysphasia is suspected clinical testing should be carried out and usually reinforced with formal clinical psychological assessment. The clinical tests should not only include naming tests and observations about spontaneous speech but also tests of reading ability and writing (for dyslexia and dysgraphia respectively).

Most patients after concussive head injury will claim that it has caused a poor memory and impaired concentration. But in the majority the "memory defect" is characterised by an absent-mindedness, a distractibility or a preoccupation with other mental or physical symptoms that lead to simple memory failure. For example the patient who has suffered dizziness when he gets up to answer the telephone may "forget" what the caller has told him, and the patient with a headache who goes upstairs to collect his spectacles may "forget" what he has gone upstairs for. Patients with temporal lobe brain damage causing neuro-logical dysmnesia (disturbance of memory) have a specific inability to recall from the recent or intermediate past. Remote memory and in particular events before the accident are usually relatively little affected.

At its most severe organic dysmnesia will render an individual unable to store information in their memory for more than a few seconds. This devastating disability may be concealed by a facade of affable self-confidence and often apology for being unable to give the information requested. Learnt skills such as tying shoelaces, reading or even driving a car are typically unimpaired.

More commonly the memory defect is mild and can only be confirmed as real by specific tests. Immediate recall, where the individual is asked to repeat a series of digits (or to reverse their order) is more a test of attention and co-operation than of memory. A commonly used 5-minute recall test is the "name, address and flower test" where the individual should be able to recall five out of the seven items. Tests of general information and current affairs can be used to establish that there is a real dysmnesia, and its severity. From this information the examiner should be able to give an opinion as to the likely consequences of this brain damage in terms of education and training (in the young) employment, social life, and personal independence and relationships.

The prognosis for recovery from temporal lobe damage is generally good. Thus improvement in dysphasia and in memory impairment may continue for many years. It is generally more reliable to indicate when the recovery process is likely to be complete when a period of 12 months has passed without discernible change. Whereas it used to be said that recovery was complete after 2 years it is now recognised that many cases continue to show improvement over 5 years or even longer.

Parietal Lobes

The dominant parietal lobe (usually the left) of the brain shares with the temporal lobe speech and language function. It also serves other forms of "symbolic" thought such as calculation. The non-dominant parietal lobe (usually the right) is concerned with spatial and topographical thought. Brain damage confined to one or other parietal lobes is unusual and the disorders resulting from damage to these regions generally forms a part of a complex picture of extensive brain damage with personality change, memory impairment as well as weakness and lack of co-ordination. But there must be an awareness when examining individuals with severe brain damage that loss of spatial orientation, for example, will lead to severe disability likely to prevent the individual ever being able to return to work. It may deprive him of the ability to live independently because he is unable to orientate himself with his surroundings or find his way about.

General Damages

Within the heading of "General Damages" the Law seeks to compensate the victim of injury for among other things his future needs, in terms of special appliances to overcome disability and personal care. Neurological injury is especially likely to result both in some impairment of locomotor function and commonly in some loss of personal independence. A neurological report should therefore include an assessment of the plaintiff's needs under these headings.

Table 8.1. Personal care needs in the neurologically injured

1. Mild physical or mental disability with full personal independence	Diminishing requirements for domestic care and supervision for shopping, making appointments, etc
2. Moderate physical or mental disability but where substantial personal independence has been achieved	Full domestic care with simple nurse assistance (e.g. transfer or bathing) and supervision of personal hygiene
3. Severe physical or mental disability	Full domestic care-provision of meals, laundry, cleaning etc. and intermittent nursing care on a daily (or less frequent) basis for toilet bathing and special nursing procedures
4. Moderately severe physical disability with or without mental changes	Continuous daytime nursing care or domestic supervision and night time nursing care "on-call"
5. Very severe physical disability (e.g. tetraplegia) with or without mental changes	Home care with 24-hour qualified nursing attention. Dual nursing available for some procedures, e.g. lifting and bathing
6. Gross mental and physical disability	Institutional care in a "younger chronic sick unit" or in long-stay mental hospital or nursing home accommodation

There is a hierarchy of disability due to brain damage (Table 8.1). Thus where only slight handicap has resulted from the injury the patient may only require occasional assistance in, for example, remembering appointments or making decisions. In this case employment may be perfectly possible provided there is some degree of supervision. With increasingly severe brain damage, employment at the humblest level becomes impossible and greater degrees of domestic supervision are required. The individual may be incapable of doing the shopping, attending to laundry or preparing a meal. Personal independence may be lost to the point where assistance is required with bathing, dressing or toilet and in this case increasing degrees of skilled or semi-skilled nursing care will be required – and taken into account in the assessment of quantum. Finally there is the individual who, through brain damage, is totally dependent on nursing care and where institutional care may be necessary.

The needs of the plaintiff in terms of appliances and aids should also form a part of the assessment of any neurologically damaged individual. The needs may be conveniently considered under a number of headings. Firstly mobility may be impaired but this impairment may only require the provision of a walking stick (probably of the folding variety). With increasing impairment of walking ability, two sticks, a tripod stick or elbow crutch(es) may be necessary. When a patient is so disabled by weakness or lack of co-ordination that they are partially or completely dependent on a wheelchair, a whole range of adaptations and requirements become necessary. Wheelchairs may be self-propelled or not; folding or fixed; and finally electric powered.

The disability will dictate the appropriate range of wheelchair(s) suitable for the individual and there is usually a substantial variation in the costs of these appliances especially where powered invalid vehicles are concerned. Access from the wheelchair depends on the ability to transfer, and there are a range of appliances enabling transfer to toilet, bath seat, chair, bed or motor car. In the most disabled, passive transfer may only be possible with a hoist.

Table 8.2. Appliances available to maximise independence in the neurologically disabled

For locomotion		Sticks, crutches, wheelchair. Power assisted wheelchair, stair lift, wheelchair lift, bannister handrails. Specially adapted motor car with appliances for transferring into the car.
In the home	(a) Bedroom:	Hoists, special bed, special mattress, transfer aids, e.g. "monkey pole"
	(b) Living room:	"Possum" or remote control appliances for radio, TV and answering doorbell, portable telephone, electric typewriter
	(c) Kitchen:	Appropriate height work surface, cooker and sink
	(d) Mealtime:	Non-slip mats, adapted utensils and cutlery
	(e) Bathroom:	Hoists, bathboard, bath seat, grab handles
	(f) Toilet:	Raised seat, transfer frame, sliding door and wheelchair access
	(g) General:	Accessible electric switches, electrically operated curtains. Ramps for wheelchair access, e.g. front door and garden access.
Continence		Special clothing, laundry facilities, catheters and other appliances
Recreation		Special holiday arrangements. Facilities for e.g. swimming, day centre care, apparatus (computer, snooker table, etc., etc.)

The motor car may need special and expensive adaptations for the disabled driver. And an assessment of fitness to drive should be part of any medical report where this is relevant and in doubt.

In the home a wide range of appliances are available to maximise independence in the neurologically disabled. But these appliances, and very often the structural alterations to the building that are required for their installation, are expensive and a detailed appraisal of requirements should be listed for the instructing solicitor. For a list of some of the equipment available, see Table 8.2.

The neurologically disabled may have special future needs in terms of physiotherapy to maintain optimal function. More rarely speech therapy or occupational therapy may be necessary. Special educational or training facilities are commonly required in the young. The added cost of providing for these needs must be included in the medical assessment.

Finally there is often the need to make an assessment of the likely life expectancy of the individual. Improvements in medical and nursing care and its delivery, have enormously improved the life expectancy of even the most disabled individuals. Assessment may be very difficult and indeed little more than a guess. But an opinion will be required in cases where complications of the disability may be ultimately fatal. Where appropriate, discussion of these matters may be best separated from the main body of a medical report so that its confidentiality may be better protected.

References

1. Behrman S (1977) Migraine as a sequela of blunt head injury. Injury 9: 74–76
2. Espir MLE, Godwin-Austen RB (1985) Epilepsy. In: Medical aspects of fitness to drive. Medical Commission on Accident Prevention, pp 25–34
3. Espir MLE, Godwin-Austen RB (1988) Neurological disorders. In: Edwards F, McCallum J, Taylor P (eds) Fitness for Work. Oxford Medical Publications, Oxford
4. Godwin-Austen RB, Espir MLE (1983) Driving and Epilepsy. Royal Society of Medicine, London (International congress & symposium series, 60)
5. Hohl M (1974) Soft tissue injuries of the neck in automobile accidents: factors influencing prognosis. J Bone J Surg [Am] 56: 1675–1682
6. Jafek BK, Eller PM, Esses BA, Moran DT (1989) Traumatic anosmia. Arch Neurol 46: 300–304
7. Jennett B (1975) Epilepsy after non-missile head injuries. Heinemann, London
8. Kelly R (1988) Headache after cranial trauma. In: Hopkins A (ed) Problems in diagnosis and management. WB Saunders, Philadelphia, pp 219–240
9. Lishman WA (1978) Organic psychiatry. Blackwell Scientific Publications, Oxford
10. Maxted MJ, Dowd GS (1982) Acute central cord syndrome without bony injury. Injury 14: 103–106
11. Ross Russell RW (1983) Vascular disease of the central nervous system. Churchill-Livingstone, Edinburgh, pp 375–379
12. Russell WR (1968) The traumatic amnesias. Oxford University Press, Oxford, p 84
13. Sumner D (1964) Post-traumatic anosmia. Brain 87: 107–120
14. Sunderland S (1968) The painful sequelae of injuries to peripheral nerves. Causalgia. In: Sunderland S, Nerves and nerve injuries. E & S Livingstone, Edinburgh
15. Symonds CP (1970) Concussion and its sequelae. In: Studies in Neurology. Oxford University Press, Oxford, pp 143–152

CHAPTER 9

Neurosurgery

J. Punt

The interface between medicine and the law as relating to neurosurgery encompasses two superficially different entities which in reality have an identical end point, namely, acquired damage to the nervous system. These entities are injury due to accident and injury due to alleged medical negligence. The only difference between the two lies in the medical profession's perception of the causation: on the one hand a third party is accepted as being responsible, on the other a colleague is allegedly at fault. In both cases the neurosurgeon is required to comment upon the condition of the patient, the relationship between the accident and that condition, and the prognosis. In the case of alleged medical negligence the neurosurgeon is further required to comment upon the adequacy of a colleague's performance. These aims can only be served by a thorough and totally objective review of the available facts appertaining to the case. This chapter concerns these matters as based upon the personal experience of the writer.

Head Injury

Traditionally the legal profession in England has sought medical opinions on cases of head injury from neurologists rather than neurosurgeons: this strikes the present writer as strange as neurologists have virtually no involvement in the acute practical care of head-injured patients.

The preparation of reports on cases of head injury will be considered under the following headings:

Review of essential documents
The medical examination
Preparation of the opinion
Additional recommendations.

Review of Essential Documents

It is most important to review personally the medical notes and records of the family general practitioner, wherein will be found any pre-existing illnesses or symptoms that might have a bearing on the plaintiff's present condition. Clearly any previous tendency to headaches, dizziness, epilepsy or psychological disturbance is of great importance. The notes of the general practitioner will also give some idea as to the impact of the injury on the plaintiff's state of health following the event, if only from the frequency of attendance for prescriptions for medications and for medical advice.

A review of the contemporary hospital records is equally crucial. Particular reference must be made to the plaintiff's level of consciousness at the earliest point after the accident at which it was reliably observed, on admission and subsequently during the period of hospital attendance. Of equal importance, especially in cases of severe neurological injury, is the plaintiff's general condition in terms of cardiovascular and respiratory function, and other major injuries, as these may all exacerbate the effects of the primary brain injury. In some cases it is necessary to consider the possible effects of alcohol especially if it is thought that a period of amnesia may be due to alcoholic intoxication rather than to concussion: many accident and emergency departments now estimate the blood alcohol level. Any external signs of injury should be noted. Findings on radiographs and brain scans should be sought preferably by personal review of the original films; fractures, especially if depressed, cerebral contusions and intra-cranial haemorrhage all influence the eventual outcome. Evidence for early traumatic epilepsy is critically reviewed and the extent of any surgery noted; in the case of compound skull fractures any reference to dural and/or cerebral laceration is important in relation to the risk of late traumatic epilepsy.

Motor and sensory functions and gait are examined. Reflex changes are principally of value in confirming certain patterns of organic injury and often bear little relationship to functional status. Conversely the "frontal" reflexes (theno-mental, pout and grasp) are most helpful in confirming organic frontal lobe injury.

The Opinion

The first purpose of the opinion is to confirm, or deny, that the plaintiff's neurological state is the result of the injury. In achieving this end the past history, including review of the medical records, is critical. It must be remembered that the finding of predisposition to headache or anxiety does not necessarily mean that the alleged exacerbation of such symptoms is not due to injury.

Secondly the severity of the injury must be defined. Post-traumatic amnesia is the accepted index of the degree of concussion: a few minutes being minimal and more than 1 week being very severe. The consequences of focal injury in terms of language disturbance, hemiplegia, gait disturbance and cranial nerve damage are discussed and the severity of behavioural and neuropsychological disturbance must be quantified. For all aspects of the injury the crucial point is the degree of functional disability.

Thirdly, a prognosis is required: although recovery is an individual affair, the major components of recuperation occur in the first 18 months and although the patient may learn compensatory strategies, real improvements thereafter are unusual.

Finally, an estimation of the possible future consequences of the brain injury is needed. This must include the risks of late traumatic epilepsy as indicated by the presence or absence of the established risk factors, namely, early traumatic epilepsy, intra-cranial haematoma and depressed skull fracture. The further consequences of any such epilepsy must be described. Reduction in life expectancy resulting from the injury and the potential superadded premature effects of natural ageing must be discussed.

Additional Recommendations

Many head injuries, especially those due to motor vehicle accidents, are associated with limb, pelvic, spinal, thoracic and maxillo-facial injuries. As in all fields of medico-legal practice, the neurosurgeon should not be drawn into areas outside his own specialty and should not hesitate to recommend that complementary reports be sought from appropriate colleagues. Any suggestion of altered higher mental function should be pursued by a neuropsychologist. Ophthalmological and otological opinions may be required for special tests of vision, hearing and balance. Occasionally a psychiatric opinion is necessary.

For the more severely injured a variety of aids to daily living, to mobility and to communication may be useful and even rehousing in modified or specially constructed dwellings may be appropriate. A number of organisations exist which can provide the fine details and the neurosurgeon can usefully suggest their involvement and can subsequently comment on the appropriateness of their recommendations.

Finally, the neurosurgeon can advise whether a review examination will be necessary when further recovery may be anticipated. This should not, however, be used as a method of prevarication to avoid providing a definite opinion.

Medical Negligence

The assessment of the plaintiff's medical state, its consequences and prognosis does not differ from cases of accident litigation. There is, however, the additional requirement of the neurosurgeon to comment upon causation. Alleged medical negligence may revolve around any, or all, of the following:

Failure to diagnose
Failure to explain the possible consequences of an operation
Failure to treat appropriately.

In reaching an opinion it is crucial to remember that medical management is only negligent if the standard of practice exhibited fell below a level that could reasonably be expected of the particular practitioner: a general practitioner or junior hospital doctor is not expected to display the diagnostic skills of a consultant neurosurgeon. Equally, although a particular consultant might practise in a particular way which may have led him to manage a patient in a way different to that in which the plaintiff was managed, opinion must be based upon an overview of current accepted practices, rather than his own.

The documentary evidence is of the utmost importance and all contemporary records from the general medical practitioner, from the hospital medical and nursing records, including correspondence, must be examined.

The commonest conditions to give rise to diagnostic difficulties are alleged failure to recognise raised intra-cranial pressure; presence of a brain tumour; warning subarachnoid haemorrhage; and malfunctioning hydrocephalus shunts. The neurosurgeon must reach his own opinion, based upon the documentary evidence, as well as the history obtained from the plaintiff and the family, as to when and whether the correct diagnosis might reasonably first have been reached. Not infrequently nondescript symptoms, or even symptoms of other diseases, may be taken by the plaintiff as "obvious" indications of the eventual diagnosis. Genuine failures of diagnosis usually relate to inadequate history taking. Conservative or expectant management may originally have been eminently reasonable, albeit eventually proven mistaken. Equally in the 1990s it is difficult to defend not acceding to a direct request from a patient, worried about brain tumour, to have a brain scan.

Failures of explanation of surgical procedures and potential consequences are difficult to assess unless either party has kept written contemporaneous records. It is a matter of continuing debate how much patients should be told prior to surgical procedures and there is a correct concern about causing undue distress. It could be argued that certain risks are self-evident, for example intra-cranial surgery causing death. Equally some consequences, however remote or unlikely, may be of such a grave nature that they should properly be drawn to the patient's attention; for example, paraplegia and incontinence after lumbar disc surgery. It should be reiterated that in advising upon whether the degree of consultation was adequate the neurosurgeon should take into account not only his own personal practice but that level of information that would be regarded as the norm by a body of his contemporaries. A review of the medical records should reveal whether the basic treatment offered, and its projected time course, was appropriate and comment should be made thereon. It is usually extremely difficult, if not impossible, to make useful comments upon whether a particular surgical procedure was carried out correctly. However, occasionally there may be written operative notes indicating that the surgeon had over-reached his own expertise; this particularly applies to procedures performed by unsupervised residents. The time taken may hold clues to difficulties and the anaesthetic record should be examined.

Failure to seek, or to be successful in obtaining, advice and assistance of a senior colleague is a further issue. The nursing records and observations should indicate the patient's condition immediately after operation. It is important to review the consequences of treatment: it is quite often the case that delay in diagnosis, for example in recognition of a malignant intra-cranial tumour, does not necessarily affect the eventual outcome in terms of functional capacity or even survival. For example, in the case of a large meningioma producing only headaches from the outset, delay in recognition may have caused the patient unnecessary months of headaches but the final functional result may not be altered. Conversely, the failure to identify an acoustic schwannoma while still small in size, through failure to investigate sensorineural hearing loss, may result in loss of the opportunity to conserve the facial nerve – or even the brain stem.

The failure to recognise blockage of a hydrocephalus shunt may well be negligent but the patient's abrupt deterioration with resultant permanent loss of vision may be unusually rapid.

It is again emphasised that any opinion upon the adequacies or inadequacies of a colleague's performance must be formed against a mean that is realistically rather than idealistically, achievable.

Children, Neurosurgery and the Law

With regards to accident and malpractice litigation, the general principles already outlined still apply. It should, however, be emphasised that because of the special circumstances of childhood, especially relating to the very young, it is quite incorrect for those who are not regularly involved in the neurosurgical and medical management of children to make comment.

The past history must in all cases consider the prenatal and birth history and the development of the child before the event in question. A careful family history and review of personal social circumstances is required. It is important to be fully aware of any pre-existing condition, for example febrile convulsions, that might have influence on subsequent progress. In cases of hydrocephalus it is important to consider the natural implications of the causative lesion: for example, children with congenital aqueductal stenosis may reasonably be expected to enter adult life quite normal, but a low birthweight premature baby with severe perinatal hypoxia and gross intra-ventricular haemorrhage has a high likelihood of cerebral palsy.

It is crucial to be aware that whereas major focal consequences of brain insult are relatively unusual, there is a considerable chance of loss of function in terms of learning and behaviour. Evidence must be sought not just from parents but from appropriately skilled neuropsychologists, educational psychologists, school reports and from developmental paediatricians. A simple neurological examination is rarely adequate. It must also be remembered that the time course of recovery, evolution of deficits, and of consequences is quite different as the damaged brain of the child is still developing and social circumstances evolving. The family, social and educational consequences of neurological insult must be taken into account and the prospects into adult life must be discussed. There are differences with regard to late traumatic epilepsy. Finally, it should be understood that the parents are in a unique position to influence the child's reaction to injury and may have a strong vested interest in overstating the consequences even to the point of concealing pre-existing handicaps or exaggerating acquired disabilities. It requires a skilled paediatric sense to recognise these factors.

Non-accidental Injury

The respective roles of all involved in the management of victims of alleged non-accidental injury is currently the subject of much, often very public, debate. It may well emerge that the role of the doctor is to adhere to the medical aspects and to leave the rest to the social services, the police and to the courts. The minimum requirement of the medical profession is to make the correct diagnosis and to initiate appropriate action through social services. Frequently, in cases of non-accidental brain injury, it will fall to the neurosurgeon not only to identify head injury as the diagnosis but to recognise that the injury is non-accidental. The neurosurgeon must appreciate the obligation incumbent upon him to involve social services who will institute the necessary procedures. Thereafter the neurosurgeon may prefer to confine himself to managing the surgical consequences of the injury, leaving the general care to a suitably equipped medical paediatrician. For the non-specialist neurosurgeon this is invariably the best line to follow. It is now almost inevitable that diagnoses of non-accidental injury will be disputed both in the child care proceedings and in the criminal courts. Increasingly it will fall upon the specialist opinions to explain, and possibly contest, the medical evidence. This extremely difficult, taxing and very time-consuming area may be further inflamed by spurious medical opinions provided on behalf of parental pressure groups.

It will be clear that those not regularly involved with, or strongly committed to, paediatric neurosurgical practice may sensibly avoid this contentious area.

CHAPTER 10

Obstetrics and Gynaecology

E.M. Symonds

For over 100 years, the needs of the medical profession for professional indemnity have been met by the Medical Defence Organisations. The members of the profession have, until 1990, remained independent of their employers by paying their own subscriptions, but an examination of the Annual Reports of The Medical Defence Union [5] between 1979 and 1988 shows an increase in indemnity payments from £2 million to a figure in excess of £25 million. It was apparent by 1986 that the rate of increase was unlikely to be contained on a cost basis by the profession and on this evidence subscriptions were first subsidised by the Department of Health and then followed by the introduction of Crown Indemnity in January 1990. This trend has not been confined to the UK. It had been a feature of medical practice in North America for at least a decade before it seriously affected the profession in the UK and it has now permeated into the European and Australian systems.

At the forefront of the claims, partly because of increasing frequency, but particularly for the massive increases in quantum based on life expectancy and the level of disability, birth-related injuries dominate the landscape of medical litigation. Claims settled for figures in excess of £1 million are set to become commonplace and cannot be contained within any medical insurance system where the income of the practitioners, involved in obstetric care, is fixed by the system of medical care.

Obstetric Brain Damage Claims

The majority of claims associated with birth-related injuries result from allegations that cerebral palsy and mental retardation are caused by some error in judgement or by traumatic events in labour.

Perinatal Asphyxia and Cerebral Palsy

No one knows with any certainty what percentage of cases of cerebral palsy are due to the events of labour, but large surveys, which examined perinatal events, suggest that no more than 10% of these cases has any described delivery events that could be considered to be evidence of trauma or asphyxia [3]. During the course of labour, it is common practice to provide a continuous recording of the foetal heart rate and uterine activity. This is known as a cardiotocogram. These recordings represent analogue displays of foetal heart rate and the pattern of heart rate change reflects the welfare and acid-base status of the foetus. The problem with this methodology is that it is highly sensitive but lacks specificity. The difficulty now faced by obstetricians around the world is that an abnormal outcome preceded by an abnormal tracing will almost invariably be taken to prove that the child suffered asphyxia and that this was the cause of the cerebral palsy and mental retardation. There are no national data on the number of "brain damaged" and birth-related injury claims in the UK but the likelihood is that current obstetric liability lies somewhere between £500 million and £1 billion at the present time. The author has reviewed a personal collection of 110 claims alleging brain damage for birth-related injuries over the past 10 years. Some surprising and interesting patterns have emerged. Only 8 of the 110 infants were born before 36 weeks gestation and 9 weighed less than 2.5 kg. In other words, although low birth weight infants are more likely to develop cerebral palsy, one must assume that the expectation of normality in a normal birth weight infant is higher. Forty seven per cent were delivered by Caesarean section, 24% with forceps and 6% were breech presentations. Twenty one per cent of the claims involved normal deliveries by midwives.

The general pattern of events is that the foetus develops an abnormal heart rate and a decision is made to await further developments or that forceps are applied to expedite delivery. If the child has clinical signs of foetal distress and forceps are applied, then the forceps can be alleged to have caused the damage. If Caesarean section is performed, it is usually alleged that the decision was made too late or that the time lapse before delivery was too great. Finally, if the child delivers spontaneously, vaginally, then it should have been delivered by Caesarean section.

The Statute of Limitations

Claims alleging brain damage can be commenced up to 21 years after delivery. There is, in effect, no statute of limitations in obstetric brain damage claims because, provided it can be shown that the defence is not prejudiced by the further delay after 21 years (by then defence is usually fairly hopeless) then the time limitation does not apply. Thus, very late claims may be brought where any evidence for the defence has often disappeared and where the parties to the defence have died or have long since left the country.

Defence

Example 1. A woman admitted to a general practitioner unit in the late 1970s in labour, delivered a child 8 hours after admission that was severely asphyxiated. There were no resuscitation facilities and the GP was called. The child was transferred to a special care baby unit. Subsequently there was evidence of cerebral palsy and mental retardation. In the very brief intrapartum records, the midwife had written at the time of admission, when the cervix was 3 cm dilated, that the patient should be given ergometrine maleate 0.5 mg. This was overtly crossed out and pethidine 100 mg written in its place. The plaintiff's counsel argued that she had been given ergometrine and that a tonic contraction had caused the asphyxia.

There was no evidence at all of a tonic contraction or increased uterine activity, but it was alleged that the ergometrine had caused a tonic contraction, sudden hypertension, a fit and loss of consciousness, so that none of these events could be remembered. The judge chose to believe the defence experts who argued on the grounds that there was absolutely no evidence that any such events occurred and that it would have required a deliberate and highly improbable "cover-up" by several experienced midwives for this to have been the case.

Impacted Shoulders

Physical trauma and asphyxial brain damage are common sequelae of shoulder impaction. It is a difficult complication to predict and a difficult complication to manage. Medico-legal claims arising from shoulder impaction usually allege that the condition should have been predicted by recognition that the foetus was large or the pelvis was small. In reality, birth weight is very difficult to predict with any accuracy greater than ± 300 gm and that accuracy has not been enhanced by ultrasonography. In most cases, the head is delivered spontaneously and without undue delay, but thereafter extraction of the shoulders may be difficult and traumatic, regardless of the level of expertise of the obstetrician or midwife.

Multiple Pregnancy

The birth of the second twin has always been recognised as a hazardous procedure leading to perinatal loss and morbidity. Complications of the delivery process of the second twin have led to several legal actions. The claims are usually based on the failure to diagnose the presence of a twin pregnancy or the difficulties in delivery of the second twin.

For example, if the second twin, after rupture of the membranes, presents as a transverse lie, then delivery can only be effected by internal podalic version and breech extraction of the child. In practice, as the cervix is fully dilated and as the presenting part should be easily accessible, delivery can be rapidly effected. However, if the child shows evidence of trauma or asphyxia, a claim is commonly based on delay in taking action to effect delivery, or allegations are made that the child should have been delivered by Caesarean section. As a result, it is becoming increasingly common to see the second twin delivered by Caesarean section, a procedure that has not proven to be of benefit and carries distinct risks to the mother. It would, in fact, be safer to routinely deliver all twins by elective Caesarean section.

Prenatal Diagnosis

As the demand to have a normal child and a normal pregnancy grows, the risk of litigation for an incorrect assessment grows. For example, if a major congenital anomaly is not detected by ultrasound scan, does this constitute negligent practice? It would, undoubtedly, be considered negligent if a woman having a pregnancy at the age of 40 years was not advised of the need for prenatal screening for Down's syndrome, but it would be equally important to advise her of the risks associated with screening procedures such as amniocentesis or chorion villus biopsy and to record that such advice had been given.

Advice on Avoiding Litigation in Obstetrics

The importance of good record keeping cannot be over emphasised. The effective inadequacy of any Statute of Limitations means that precise records of events, including a record of advice given to the mother, are essential. By the time the claims reach the courts it is likely that many of the persona involved in the action will have died or disappeared and the only feasible means of defending a claim will be the written record. Heart rate recordings are generally stored in the case notes and may make or break a claim. In the future, storage will be achieved by an electronic medium. The present system of paper records is unsatisfactory as the paper degrades with time. It must be said that if foetal heart rate is recorded during labour, then certain rules must be followed:

1. If the recording is unsatisfactory because of an inadequate signal or because the heart rate monitor is faulty, then the machine should not be left to record spurious information and must be changed or the electrode should be replaced. If this is not possible, then it is better to monitor with intermittent auscultation.

2. An abnormal recording requires action. There is no point in monitoring the foetal heart rate if the recording is ignored. Furthermore, all staff caring for women in labour should be adequately trained in the interpretation of cardiotocograms (CTGs).

3. It is important not to mislead mothers into believing that the cause of cerebral palsy was due to asphyxia simply because no other cause could be identified. In fact, most cases of cerebral palsy are not due to asphyxia. Arguments about the specificity and sensitivity of CTGs in predicting foetal asphyxia have not yet been effectively tested in court. There is a strong case to meet this challenge, particularly where an abnormal recording during labour is followed by the delivery of a child with a normal Apgar score and normal acid-base status, but who subsequently exhibits cerebral palsy.

Evaluation of Quantum for Brain Damage

Settlements for brain damage have risen tenfold [5] over the last 10 years. These claims are based on the cost of supporting the child over his/her projected life span. The difficulty about this type of compensation is that the settlement is not structured and the lump sum payments mean an all or nothing funding. A proper distribution of these funds without the legal expenses involved in protracted legal actions would mean reasonable support for all infants with cerebral palsy and mental retardation.

Gynaecological Problems

Failed sterilisation

One of the commonest causes of legal action is that of failed sterilisation. These actions are based on claims of negligence, trespass to the person, or breach of contract [1].

The procedure may be incorrectly performed and therefore fails to produce the desired effect. For example, if clips are used and one of the clips is visibly placed on the round ligament, then an action for negligence can be initiated and would be difficult to defend. All procedures involving tubal occlusion have a failure rate because of recanalisation and, short of hysterectomy or bilateral oophorectomy, it is impossible to be certain that sterilisation will occur. This has been generally accepted by the courts and on this basis it should be possible to defend a claim where both fallopian tubes have been demonstrably damaged. An action in trespass or breach of contract may be pursued where the operation fails to sterilise and the patient has not been warned about the possibility of failure. These arguments also apply to vasectomy as well as techniques of tubal occlusion. Until 1980, it was not uniform policy to advise a woman that there was a risk of failure, as such advice did not appear to be in the patient's interest. Indeed, it is still true to say that the only possible advantage to being told that there is a risk of failure, is that it would tend to make the patient aware of the risk of failure so that advice could be sought if the period was late and there were symptoms of pregnancy. Termination of the pregnancy could then be offered should the woman not wish to continue with it. There is commonly a claim that had the woman known that there was a risk of failure she would:

1. Have continued to use contraception
2. Not have agreed to sterilisation in the first place
3. Have insisted that the husband or male partner should also be sterilised.

In practice, no gynaecologist would recommend that both partners should be sterilised. The author has never personally known a woman withdraw her request for sterilisation on the basis that there was a risk of failure; and furthermore, it would defeat the point of sterilisation if it was still considered necessary to use other contraceptive methods to reinforce the sterilisation. In the case of *Gold* vs. *Haringey Health Authority* in 1987 [2], Mr. Justice Schumann broke new ground by saying that there was a duty to counsel the patient about alternative family planning methods, including vasectomy, despite the fact that in this case the clinical indications strongly favoured female sterilisation. It is surprising that the law should acknowledge entitlement to claim damages for the birth of a healthy child except in the context of a breach of contract in failing to achieve sterilisation. This judgement was subsequently reversed in the Court of Appeal. Argent [1] has suggested that the operation should not be described as sterilisation but should be listed according to the actual procedure such as tubal ligation or partial salpingectomy. What has actually happened is that it has now become standard practice to advise the patient of the risk of failure and the difficulties of reversing the sterilisation. As a consequence, the number of claims based on the nature of consent has diminished and most claims now relate to the technical failure of the procedure. It is common and proper practice to keep a record of the fact that such advice has been given to the patient. It could be argued that so much publicity has already been given to legal actions for failed sterilisation that such knowledge now lies firmly in the public domain, and that any reasonably informed lay person should be aware of the fact that sterilisation is not infallible. However, it is unlikely that any judge would be sympathetic to this argument.

Complications of Abortion

Termination of pregnancy is a common gynaecological procedure. It is, therefore, hardly surprising that claims arise from the complications of termination procedures. The nature of these claims has previously been reviewed by the Royal College of Obstetrics and Gynaecology (RCOG) Working Party on Litigation [4]. Allegations arise out of specific complications which follow a well-recognised pattern.

"Failed Termination"

The failure to terminate a pregnancy commonly arises in early pregnancy when the gestation sac is small and is missed by the suction curette commonly used in these procedures. It is not common practice to send material for histology and the continuation of the pregnancy is only likely to be detected if the woman is re-examined at a 6-week post-operative visit. Occasionally, the uterus may be distorted by fibroids and therefore location of the pregnancy may prove to be difficult. It is commonly argued that the uterus may be bicornuate and that the pregnancy was lodged in one horn whilst the horn curetted was empty. It is necessary under these circumstances to have evidence that the uterus is bicornuate. It is sensible to give all patients attending for termination of pregnancy a post-operative appointment, but it is common experience that these patients do not attend, even when the appropriate arrangements have been made.

Incomplete Evacuation

The common sequelae of abortion are haemorrhage and infection and these are often associated with retained products of conception. However, claims concerning retained products of conception usually arise because a portion of the foetus is passed shortly after discharge home. It is generally possible to resist such claims as they are common events and cannot be considered to indicate negligent practice.

Uterine Perforation and Damage to Viscera

The pregnant uterus is soft and relatively easy to perforate. Damage to the cervix may result from excessive or forceful dilatation but the claims commonly arise from perforation, either during the course of cervical dilatation or during the process of suction evacuation by the suction curette. Perforation may not cause any significant problems and provided the appropriate actions are taken, the claim can usually be successfully defended. However, if gross damage is inflicted, including bowel damage, ureteric avulsion and major vessel damage, it may be more difficult to argue that such actions constitute reasonable practice.

Surgical Complications of Hysterectomy

The commonest cause of legal action relates to injuries to the urinary system. It must be remembered that any gynaecologist with a substantive surgical workload is likely to damage the bladder or a ureter at some stage. Damage to the bladder sustained in a difficult hysterectomy where there is scarring from endometriosis or previous surgery may be acceptable whereas damage inflicted and unrecognised during a straightforward hysterectomy might be difficult to defend. In a similar way, it is possible to defend damage to a single ureter during the course of a difficult hysterectomy or to defend fistula formation following radical hysterectomy for carcinoma of the cervix. It may be much more difficult to defend a case where both ureters were occluded or cut during the performance of a routine hysterectomy. In other words, it is really not sufficient to say that ureteric or bladder damage is a normal complication of hysterectomy. The issues will be decided by what most gynaecologists consider to be reasonable practice.

The same arguments are relevant to bowel damage. Occasional claims arise from haemorrhagic complications, particularly where intra-peritoneal bleeding follows hysterectomy and is not recognised until the patient is "in extremis". Proper post-operative care and observation is an essential part of medical care and inadequate documentation may create great difficulties in the successful defence of such a case.

The Misdiagnosis of Cancer

Relatively few claims arise out of the actual treatment of gynaecological cancers, but a substantial number of claims are made in relation to "missed" opportunities of early diagnosis. For example, an abnormal cervical smear test that is filed in the patient's records, without being drawn to the attention of the medical attendant, may result in delay in diagnosing an invasive cancer. If a significant delay occurs in subsequent management, it will be impossible to defend the initial error. Similarly, failure to take appropriate action when a cancer is diagnosed may lead to legal action.

The wrongful interpretation of a substantial number of cervical smear tests has led to a number of claims although, in most cases, the harmful outcome generally relates to the need to implement more extensive methods of treatment than might have been anticipated had earlier treatment been instituted. Predicting the additional hazard to the patient is often impossible to assess because the original abnormal cytology may give no real indication of the extent of the neoplasm at the time of the original smear test.

Contraceptive Problems

Intra-uterine contraceptive devices have the advantage of not requiring any action on the part of the woman before coitus, but these complications include a wide variety of gynaecological symptoms, including abnormal bleeding, infection, perforation and pregnancy. Perforation of the uterus commonly occurs at the time of insertion of the device but it may initially only be partial so that the device subsequently migrates through the uterine wall. The disappearance of the coil strings demands clarification of the site of the device. Pregnancies as a result of coil failure are generally not a source of legal action, but infection and subfertility have been the source of legal action, particularly in relation to devices such as the Dalkon Shield. The problems of product liability have led to the withdrawal of devices from the market. Indeed, it has to be said that in North America, there is a real risk that product liability may substantially reduce the availability of contraceptive techniques in the future. The complications of oral contraceptive usage are well documented and legal claims tend to arise out of the failure to give appropriate advice concerning specific complications.

Conclusions

Some of the general aspects of claims relating to obstetrics and gynaecology have been outlined. There are many other variants of these themes, but the common matters giving rise to litigation have been discussed.

The need to keep clear and consistent records must be stressed. Case records are medico-legal documents and will be examined in great detail during any court action. Case note entries should be confined to statements of fact wherever this is possible and the entries should be signed. Obstetric case records must be kept for a minimum of 21 years and the present attitude in the UK now seems to suggest that records should be kept for at least 25 years.

References

1. Argent V (1988) Failed sterilisation and the law. Br J Obstet Gynaecol 95: 113–115
2. Brahams D (1987) Doctor's duty of care to give advice in therapeutic and non-therapeutic contexts. Lancet i: 1045
3. Nelson KB, Ellenberg JH (1986) Antecedents of cerebral palsy. N Engl J Med 315: 81–86
4. Symonds EM (1985) Medico-legal aspects of the therapeutic abortion. In: Chamberlain GWP et al. (eds) Litigation in obstetrics and gynaecology. Proceedings of the Fourteenth Study Group of the RCOG, London, pp 123–129
5. Symonds EM (1990) Double indemnity and obstetric practice. In: Templeton A, Cuisine DJ (eds) Reproductive medicine and the law. Churchill Livingstone, Edinburgh, pp 85–91

CHAPTER 11

Orthopaedics

J.P. Jackson

Cases involving orthopaedic problems are many and varied. Whilst many will lead to argument, in nearly all, although there may be some divergence of opinion, agreement is usually probable. In some, however there is often more difficulty, probably due to lack of knowledge of the underlying pathology, which leads to diametrically opposed views. It may well be that in time, with further research, the causation will become clearer and as a result, agreement outside the court, rather than disagreement inside, will become the rule. The first two subjects I have chosen have been extensively investigated but the site of the pain still remains an enigma. All four conditions discussed are characterised by the subjective symptom of pain which is almost impossible to evaluate. Of necessity much of the opinion expressed is the result largely of research to be found in the literature, but coloured by the views of the author. The problems reviewed are:

Repetitive stress injury
Anterior knee pain
Whiplash injuries of the neck
Osteoarthritis and trauma

Repetitive Stress Injury

The diagnosis of repetitive stress injury has been a matter of considerable contention in the past decade. These cases are largely concerned with pain in the upper limb, but the lower limb may be implicated from time to time if this is used in a repetitive manner such as in operation of a treadle. Broadly the cases should be considered in three categories:

1. Conditions which are well recognised, with demonstrable pathology, such as tenosynovitis, carpal tunnel syndrome, tennis elbow and thoracic outlet conditions
2. Repetitive stress injury (RSI, generalised limb pain of unknown etiology)
3. Malingering.

Those Cases with a Definite Pathology

These cases are mostly well recognised. They need to be excluded before a diagnosis of RSI is considered. Those most likely to cause difficulty are tenosynovitis and tendinitis in which repetition plays a significant part. Other causes of pain in the upper limb, such as tennis elbow, carpal tunnel syndrome and those conditions emanating from the shoulder and neck may also cause confusion, but often do not appear to have any relation to repetition, particularly of a rapid nature. Most complaints relate to the upper limb, since the lower limb is much less frequently used in a repetitive fashion. Tenosynovitis and tendinitis do occur in the lower limb, but are more likely to be associated with sporting activity rather than industrial problems and are, therefore, less often the source of litigation.

Tenosynovitis and tendinitis are both easily recognisable conditions, which can be excluded by eliciting the physical signs, particularly those of an objective nature. Inflammation of the tendon sheaths and tendons is apparent because of the swelling, which is visible and palpable in relation to the structures affected. Since the changes occur as the result of a specific movement, only one tendon sheath or a group of tendons (such as the flexors or extensors of the fingers) is likely to be affected. A knowledge of the anatomy of these structures will indicate which tendon or tendon sheath is affected. The swollen area is usually well circumscribed and is related to the inflamed structure. An increase in temperature and crepitus may also be apparent. The latter sign is most often felt in the condition which affects the tendons of the radial wrist extensor and the abductor pollicis longus, just above the wrist. Because of the frequency with which crepitus is present at this site, it is known as peritendinitis crepitans.

The causation of these conditions is still a matter of some conjecture. No studies on the etiology have been made with an adequate control group or indeed with any controls at all [12]. The most common causes are thought to be over-exertion, sprain or local blunt trauma. Reports have accumulated during the past hundred years, mostly indicating that the disease is caused by exertion with or without trauma [14]. The type of work which mostly precipitates the condition is described as repetitive or strenuous without any more precise ergonomic analysis. In the hand and forearm there is no doubt that in many cases the causative factor is found in industry, but even so, the employer may be unjustly blamed. There is evidence to implicate the inexpediency of movement and muscle. New workers and workers resuming after an absence, such as a holiday or sick leave, have been reported as more at risk. However, in 78 cases (13%) of a large series, Thompson et al. were unable to ascribe a cause [19]. In half of the cases reported out of 544 the condition occurred after unaccustomed work or a return to work after a long absence. Blunt trauma was the precipitating cause in half of 78 patients described by Howard [12].

In all these cases of tenosynovitis a definite pathology can be found. Exudation into the sheath with a deposition of fibrin occurs. The tendon becomes thickened and loses its lustre. In tendinitis there are changes in the paratenon, especially at the muscle tendon junction. Oedema and accumulation of fibrin may be seen.

Whatever the etiological factors causing the onset of tenosynovitis or tendinitis it would seem that stopping work results in the cessation of symptoms, particularly when accompanied by partial immobilisation. Using this regime Thompson et al. [19] recorded a recovery period of 10.5 days in their large series. A relapse rate of 6.2% was recorded. Delay in starting treatment did not affect the outcome.

Pain in the Neck, Shoulder and Arm

Pain in the upper part of the limb tends to enter the realm of hypothesis rather than fact. Most workers are agreed that degenerative changes in the neck may be associated with symptoms. These changes start after adolescence and progress continually with increasing age. They are accepted as physiological and become increasingly apparent in the radiographs of patients over forty years old. Their association with symptoms is, however, much more problematical. Ergonomic analysis has not been very thorough nor indeed very helpful, but static and kinetic stress and minor injuries have been incriminated [1]. Symptoms may be confined to the neck, but pain in the arm occurs from time to time. Pain is rarely continuous but most often comes in attacks which last days or weeks but rarely months. Neurological signs in the limb aid in making the diagnosis.

Thoracic Outlet Syndrome

Nerve pain in the arm may be caused by compression at the thoracic outlet. Various causes have been cited, such as scalene compression and cervical ribs. Arterial compression can occur, giving rise to Raynaud's phenomenon and even on occasions thrombo-embolic episodes. Various tests such as Adson's manoeuvre, the costo-clavicular test and Allen's hyperabduction test can be employed, but a number of observers have commented unfavourably on these manoeuvres. Wright, indeed, found that Allen's test gave 80% false positives [23]. Telford and Mottershead found that they were able to demonstrate positive tests in 38%–68% of normal persons [18]. Cervical ribs have been implicated (present in 6/1000 persons) but their role is problematical, being symptomless in as many as 90% of cases [2]. Symptoms from these conditions are usually mild. Postural and occupational factors are not thought to be important in their etiology [22].

Work-related Upper Limb Disorders

When all clinical syndromes with objective physical signs have been excluded, a group of patients with limb pain of unexplainable origin remains. Attempts have been made to categorise them [21]. Once all conditions with objective findings are excluded, all that remains may be classified as "Tension neck syndrome". Waris et al. [21] state that the diagnostic features are confusing because there are no generally accepted criteria to follow. Indeed they go on to say that the diagnosis is made by exclusion of other conditions. They test what they describe as "objective" findings: muscle tenderness and spasm, often associated with nodules and swelling. They further add "weakness, limitation of movement, decreased lordosis and drooping of the shoulder" as described by other authors. Most of these findings are in fact subjective. Nodules are often palpable in normal persons and are of doubtful significance. Loss of lordosis in the cervical

spine may be found in routine films and can in many cases be a normal finding
[5]. What remains after exclusion of recognisable conditions is therefore a
collection of patients who have unexplained symptoms in the limb with no
objective signs which might suggest some pathological process. Attempts have
been made to group these under the diagnostic umbrella of repetitive stress (or
strain) injury. Much has been written about this syndrome, both for and against
its existence as a pathological entity. In some cases it would appear to follow a
recognisable condition such as tenosynovitis. Long after the objective signs have
disappeared complaints persist. There seems every probability that union
literature [8] and suggestion from those treating the patient may well play a part
in the continuance of symptoms. The notion that failure to obtain treatment may
end in complete crippling, as indicated in much of the advice, is certainly
enough to persuade any patient to cease work.

This condition has been cited as occurring in commerce and is said to follow
a predictable course, whether treated or untreated. The patients are divided
arbitrarily into various grades on the basis of the severity of the symptoms [6]:

1. Pain in one site on causal activity
2. Pain in multiple sites on causal activity
3. Pain with some other uses of the hand, tender structures demonstrable, may
    show pain at rest or loss of muscle function
4. Some pain with all uses of the hand, post-activity pain with minor uses, pain
    at rest and at night, marked physical signs of tenderness, loss of motor
    function (loss of response control), weakness
5. Loss of capacity for use because of severe, continuous pain and loss of
    muscle function, particularly weakness, gross physical signs.

Fry in his article [6] describes the physical signs that are present. These are
however all of a subjective nature. He does allude to tenderness as "semi-
subjective", but this is of course purely subjective since it cannot be assessed in
an objective way. Indeed it can in the author's experience more often than not
be shown that these patients who complain of pain even on the lightest touch
have no complaints when pressure is applied to the same muscle by producing
intra-muscular tension. This can be done by various active and resisted
movements that do not immediately alert the patient's awareness. Another
factor is that pain and discomfort in a limb associated with work is a common
occurrence. Hadler [9] states that at any given time approximately 10% of adults
experience some discomfort in the neck with or without arm pain and 35% of
adults can recall such an episode. He goes on to say "arm pain is a ubiquitous
recurring experience responsible for mild to modest transitory nuisance;
medical advice is seldom sought. Reproducible objective signs of inflammatory
or dystrophic abnormality are not associated with this discomfort". Enquiries at
Australian Telecom showed that 40% of telephonists in Sydney complained of
unreported work-related back pain and 20% of neck pain [4]. Furthermore,
Lawrence found neck and arm pain present in 9% of males and 12% of females
as part of the activities of daily living [15].

The term repetitive stress injury which has been applied to the condition in
itself raises difficulties. Injury implies damage to tissue, though this has never
been demonstrated, despite wide-ranging tests. These tests include such investigations as biochemistry, radiography, electromyography, nerve conduction

studies, radio-isotope scanning, thermography and haematology [13]. The adjective repetitive implies repeated damage to tissue. No evidence is, however, forthcoming about such damage.

As a consequence of adverse literature and the example of other "sufferers", patients expect to feel pain under circumstances which offer no threat to tissue damage. This is in contradistinction to the usual function of pain, which is to protect tissue from damage. Pain can of course be extended by anxiety and financial compensation worries. These may well be a factor in some cases of this syndrome.

The pain which occurs in this condition may be consistent in one patient but there is no consistency when compared with other patients; nor indeed can the area of pain be explained on the basis of any known anatomical pathway.

Of further interest is the investigation carried out by Horal [11] in which two large groups were matched for age, sex and occupation presenting to their family doctors. One group complained of low back pain, and the other of symptoms unrelated to this. Enquiry revealed that 60% of the second group also had low back pain with similar symptoms, signs and radiographic changes. Magora [17] found that back pain and work incapacity were linked by the patient in a belief that their work had injured their back. They also had job dissatisfaction.

The role of repetition, in RSI has to some extent been supported by the observation that the introduction of more sophisticated electronic machines has increased the rate of working and fuelled the numbers of sufferers. Enquiry amongst typists revealed that almost without exception, they find their work easier, since they have graduated from the mechanical to the electronic via the electrical model. Investigation of the Australian Telecom epidemic does not support repetition as a cause. Telegraphists whose work involves 12 000 keystrokes per hour had only 17 cases in 5 years from 500 employees and no reports of telegraphist's cramp. Telephonists on the other hand with a key-stroke rate of a few hundred per hour sustained 343 cases in 5 years in 1000 employees [10].

Poor ergonomics has been cited as a further cause of this condition coupled with a demand that employers consider this aspect and make every effort at improvement. Whilst ergonomics has made the workplace more comfortable and the work less arduous, there is no evidence that the incidence of RSI has been lowered by any improvements [17]. Furthermore, comparison of two Adelaide telephone areas, one handling international calls and the other local, showed that there were 10% of cases in the former but 45% in the latter. This was despite the fact that the ergonomics of the international group were significantly poorer. They did however have greater job satisfaction [7]. The probability is therefore that uninteresting work may be a significant psychological factor in the aetiology of RSI [3]. Ferguson indeed found that neurosis was high in both the groups complaining of cramp and myalgia in the telegraphists that he studied [3]. He was of the opinion that psychological factors both in work and social environment were important. Wallace in an uncontrolled study of 197 complainants found non-work stress such as family strife to be important [20].

In summary therefore, it should be stated that there is no objective evidence for this condition being due to injury and much of the investigation tends to exclude repetition as a cause. Most observers would concur that repetition, particularly if rapid does play a part in the aetiology of tenosynovitis; a condition which is well documented with a known pathology and which responds to suitable treatment within a short period of time.

The balance of evidence at present available would not implicate employers of negligence in causing RSI, nor is there any real proof that ergonomics play a significant part. Job satisfaction should be improved if possible, but in the majority of cases this may not be feasible, since some activities are intrinsically boring. It would seem likely that RSI is largely a psycho-social problem often related to family and domestic difficulties, beyond the control of the employer.

Malingering

Since repetitive stress injury does not produce any objective signs, malingering must inevitably be considered. In some patients there may well be a desire to exaggerate a discomfort or minor pain for the sake of financial gain. There may have been, initially, a perfectly genuine attack of tenosynovitis or possibly the normal aches and pains of physical activity. In addition the impact of literature representing this as a serious disease and possibly the success of a workmate in the courts may also play a part. Unfortunately without evidence that the patient is able to carry out activities incompatible with the complaints, malingering is difficult to prove.

Anterior Knee Pain (Chondromalacia Patellae)

Pain in the front of the knee is a common complaint. When the onset is associated with trauma, medico-legal problems may arise. Frequently it is introduced under the diagnosis of chondromalacia patellae. This is a condition about which there is considerable doubt, both as to its origin and its ability to cause pain. That articular cartilage may become malacic is unquestionable: that the patello-femoral area of the knee may be the site of pain is also true. Whether or not these two facts are connected is less certain. Anterior knee pain is common in young people, especially those actively engaged in sport. Abernethy et al. [24] questioned 123 first year medical students and found that 29% had had transient discomfort and 3% chronic patello-femoral pain. If indeed there is a painful condition of chondromalacia of the patella, in all probability it is only one of the many conditions that give rise to pain in the front of the knee. Certainly it can only be considered after such complaints as meniscal tears, osteochondritis dissecans, synovial entrapment, patellar subluxation and a host of other lesions have been eliminated. Good routine history taking and clinical examination will often need to be followed by radiography, NMR scans, etc. Arthroscopy may be needed to exclude many of the more easily recognisable conditions. That some articular cartilage degeneration will be seen on arthroscopy is highly probable, since this is the rule rather than the exception in most knees. Of itself, it cannot give rise to pain since articular cartilage is insensitive.

If indeed chondromalacia exists as a separate entity, then it could be described as a syndrome characterised by retropatellar discomfort, exacerbated by certain activities such as stair climbing, squatting and getting up from a seat. The condition may be associated with patello-femoral crepitus (asymptomatic crepitus was found in 63% of Abernethy's series). As the name implies, there are changes in the patellar articular cartilage.

The assessment of anterior knee pain is made more difficult by the appearance of the ageing articular cartilage on the patella. Degeneration is universal, but in most cases is completely asymptomatic. This has been established by many authors, notably Emery and Meachim [37]. They examined 98 white subjects ranging in age from 4 weeks to 94 years. All those with evidence of previous disease were excluded. They reported that overt destructive change involved practically the whole of the patellar surface in the course of time. The rate of development was relatively slow, but on average in 50% of males and 55% of females the patellar surface was clearly damaged by the age of fifty. Changes are often already apparent in teenagers. They also made the suggestion that in the elderly, ageing in itself sometimes causes sufficient patello-femoral damage to constitute osteoarthrosis. The area most frequently affected was the medial part of the medial facet and the periphery of the patella. When full thickness loss was developed, this was usually sited on the lateral and central aspects of the patella. Unfortunately many of the reviews of chondromalacia fail to take full account of this ageing phenomenon. Ficat et al. [29] states that chondromalacic changes were visible in 63.26% of single contrast arthrograms. Most of these must have been "normal" changes.

The high incidence of cartilage degeneration of the central medial facet and the low incidence of symptoms suggests that the degeneration should be regarded as an incidental finding in most of those patients who suffer from anterior knee pain.

There appear to be two separate pathologies acting on the patella associated with malacic changes, both of which may cause pain. Firstly, degeneration on the central ridge and lateral facet is probably associated with some abnormality of patella tracking. The changes may well be due to increased lateral pressure of the patella on the femur. This has been proposed as a frequent cause of anterior knee pain with the diagnostic label of excessive lateral pressure syndrome (ELPS) by Ficat et al. [29]. Insall and colleagues [35] are of much the same opinion, suggesting that patella malalignment is a frequent cause of pain. He states that the pain is reproduced by applying firm pressure against the lateral border of the patella. When pain is present, he explains this as being due to the abnormal shear loading on the subchondral bone, even when the cartilaginous surface is intact. Hallisey et al. [32] have suggested that the source of the increased pressure is the excessive lateral pull of the vastus lateralis obliquus muscle. Fulkerson et al. [30] have produced some evidence that the pain is due to sensory damage in the lateral retinaculum. There does seem to be the possibility that all these hypotheses may be linked. Nonetheless there is considerable confusion as to the causation and even the existence of chondromalacia as a cause of anterior knee pain. Many surgeons have sought to relieve the pain by release of the soft tissues on the outer side of the patella. The results of this procedure have tended to be good in the short term, but with relapse not infrequently in the longer term [43]. Insall, although initially an enthusiast of the operation, writes in his "Current concepts review of patella pain" that "his experience has led him to become less sanguine and only about half the cases are improved" [33]. A placebo effect or even the period of rest associated with any surgical procedure cannot easily be eliminated as a cause of the improvement.

A rather different approach to the problem has been put forward by Goodfellow et al. [31]. They have pointed out that there is, in a number of these cases, a lesion astride the odd and medial facets. They described these changes in 23 young patients (aged 14–27 years) all of whom had suffered pain for 2 to 3 years. The interesting difference in the lesion described, compared with those on the lateral facet, was the manner of its formation. Goodfellow and his co-workers found that their lesion commenced with basal degeneration and first appeared as an apparent blister with a smooth surface. Ogilvie-Harris and Jackson [41] showed similar changes. Later the blister ruptured and the appearances became indistinguishable from those that commenced with surface degeneration. They further pointed out that the area in which the blister appears is under pressure when the knee is flexed to 90 degrees and beyond, in which posture the typical pain of "chondromalacia" is felt. The patella was tender over the medial area in many cases. Eighteen of the 23 patients were treated by full-thickness excision of the lesion with complete relief of their symptoms. The other five who had the same treatment had no relief and the cause of their pain remained a mystery. Goodfellow and his co-workers also found changes on the odd facet in half the youthful population, but did not think that these were the associated with pain. Other hypotheses to explain these changes on the medial part of the patella have been made, but have not stood the test of time. Wiberg [45] thought that the shape of the patella was important and Outerbridge [42] incriminated the ridge of cartilage on the femoral condyle.

Relationship to Osteoarthritis

Claims are frequently made in court that plaintiffs who suffer anterior knee pain as the result of an accident would be liable to develop osteoarthritis. Most of the evidence is against this outcome. Firstly, progression from anterior knee pain to osteoarthritis has not been recorded in any clinical study of adolescents. Secondly, those patients who present in later life with symptoms of osteoarthritis seldom recall any symptoms of chondromalacia when young [25, 35]. Karlson [36] followed a series of patients for 23 years and found no incidence of osteoarthritis.

Meachim and Bentley [39] found that the changes of osteoarthritis were on the lateral facet and contrasted this with chondromalacia which they believed mainly appears on the medial facet. If there has been some disturbance of the joint surface such as a fracture producing irregularity, then osteoarthritis would be a reasonable outcome. Articular cartilage surface damage alone, would in all probability not be enough to cause osteoarthritis, since Meachim [38] has shown that surface scarification of mammalian cartilage does not result in this condition. Moreover, cartilage damage can heal by fibro-cartilage. Anything more traumatic would in all probability produce an osteochondral fracture, visible radiographically.

Relationship to Trauma

Clearly any blow on a knee may produce pain due to soft tissue damage. The proximity of bone to skin renders the area very liable to bruising, as any child will confirm. Happily, resolution of the complaint is the almost invariable sequela. Only in those cases in which there has been a fracture, patellar dislocation or ligamentous tear producing instability is there likely to be long-continuing disability.

Insall et al. [34] in a review of chondromalacia stated that 40 out of 105 knees had suffered a direct blow before complaining of persistent anterior knee pain. However many of these cases suffered from malalignment or even recurrent dislocation and might well have had symptoms in any event. Furthermore it is interesting to note that in his review of patellar pain written some six years later [33], Insall states that "the assessment of these injuries is often complicated by litigation and compensation considerations". Bentley [26] stated that of 140 patients reviewed for treatment of chondromalacia, 17 gave a history of direct trauma and 14 of a twisting injury. No loose bodies were seen and he concludes that the "role of trauma in producing chondromalacia remains unclear".

Of interest in relation to knee pain following trauma is the total lack of mention of its occurrence as a complication of dislocation of the hip [27, 40, 44]. This injury is most frequently the result of direct trauma to the knee. The force is transmitted up the femur causing the joint to be dislocated often with fracturing of the acetabular rim. Although there are a number of reviews of long-term follow-ups of this condition, none mentions either pain or osteoarthritis of the knee as a complication, although as many as 500 or more cases may have been considered. It might be argued that the problem of the hip overshadows the knee, but many of the patients are reported as being asymptomatic. As the blow on the knee must be very considerable in order to dislocate the hip, it seems likely that if direct trauma to the knee causes pain in that joint, it cannot be very severe.

Summary

Degenerative changes on the patella are common. They are mostly age-related and asymptomatic. There are two conditions which may give rise to pain and are associated with articular cartilage changes. Firstly, a basal degeneration occurring mainly on the medial surface of the patella is a lesion found in young people and symptoms from this cause are probably uncommon. The condition is benign and most often self-limiting within a few years. Young athletes are more liable to this complaint and it probably results from a shearing stress. Secondly, a surface change occurs more often on the lateral facet. This is not uncommon and may be seen at all ages. The cause is probably an increase of the lateral pressure, notably from subluxation or an increase in the Q-angle. Surface change may progress to osteoarthritis but it is improbable that basal changes on the medial facet do so. Whilst articular cartilage changes could give rise to pain indirectly by some disturbance of the subchondral bone, by pressure changes or some alteration of the vascularity, the pathology remains a matter of some conjecture.

Direct injury, unless it produces irregularity of the joint surface, is no more likely to lead to progressive pain than a blow elsewhere in the body.

Whiplash Injuries of the Neck

Cervical Spondylosis

Before the long-term effects of whiplash injuries can be assessed it is necessary to consider the symptoms and radiographic changes caused by pre-existing degeneration and the likely course that these would have followed in the absence of any injury.

Most "normal" persons will at some time or another suffer from the symptoms of this condition, i.e. local cervical pain, neck stiffness, brachial neuralgia and headache [48]. In addition other symptoms may occur, such as paraesthesiae in the fingers, pseudo-angina and shoulder pain. Hult [53] reviewed 1137 men engaged in industry, 471 on light work and 666 on heavy work. He found little difference between the two groups. He reported that 10% of complaints in the group aged 25-54 occurred as a result of injury. These tended to be more troublesome than the more common spontaneous attacks. In the younger patients (25-29) 25%-30% had had one or more attacks of neck stiffness. Brachialgia had afflicted 5%-10%. Over the age of 45, 50% had had neck stiffness and brachialgia. Indeed the numbers suffering from neck stiffness and brachialgia showed a linear progression, reaching 95% between the ages of 55 and 59. Clearly the symptoms are extremely common in the "normal" population; a fact that should be borne in mind when assessing the effects of injury. Although the symptoms are often mild, there are patients who are severely disabled.

Radiographic Changes

These do not give a great deal of help in deciding the cause of neck pain. Friedenberg and Miller [49] reviewed patients with and without neck pain and brachialgia and found little difference between the degree of degeneration in the two groups. Changes were apparent in as many as 25% in the fifth decade rising to 75% in the seventh decade, whether or not symptoms were present. Changes were predominantly present in the C5/6/7 disc spaces.

Loss of the normal cervical curve is not infrequently interpreted as evidence of muscle spasm following injury. Whilst this may be the case, changes in the curve are not infrequent in asymptomatic patients. Fineman et al. [47] reported that out of 330 routinely obtained lateral radiographs, made with the neck in neutral position, 61 (19%) showed a straight or slightly kyphotic spine. Of these patients, 49 gave no history of previous trauma, 29 had evidence of degenerative change, but 27 had neither signs of spondylosis nor a history of trauma; 7 of these latter being kyphotic. They further investigated the effect of lowering the chin slightly in 129 unselected patients. This simple variation produced 53 (41%) with loss of lordosis (75% had no history of trauma). This variation in posture they described as slight and comparable with many films taken in the "normal" way. It is clear therefore that radiographs give little help in determining the severity of symptoms after an injury and may actually be misleading.

Mechanism of Injury

Whilst a variety of accidents may result in neck symptoms, the most common injury leading to litigation is damage arising from motor vehicle crashes, particularly the rear-end shunt. These types of injury were first recognised following the introduction of catapult assisted take-offs from aircraft carriers. The increase in motor cars during the past few decades has made this a common injury and the rear-end collision has become the villain of the piece. In North America this kind of accident constituted 20% of all vehicle collisions in the 1950s [55].

Basically there are two main types of injury, both related to the direction of the applied force. That in which the patient is travelling in a vehicle which is bought to a sudden halt has the effect of throwing the patient forwards. If the body is anchored by a seat belt then the head continues to go forwards. This movement can only continue until the chin comes in contact with the sternum. This range is within the normal physiological limits and in the majority of cases results in little lasting damage. Car drivers may to some extent control forward movement of the body by gripping the steering wheel. McNab [54] in his review of 575 patients with a flexion acceleration injury found that none had significant disability. Of 69 patients who sustained lateral flexion injuries, in which movement is arrested by the shoulder, 7 reported neck pain and only 2 minor disability continuing for more than two weeks.

More troublesome, however, were the complaints of those patients suffering from a rear-end shunt. In this collision the head is thrown backwards, whilst the trunk is anchored by the back of the seat. Crowe [46] attached the name "whiplash" to the acceleration extension injury and this may have exaggerated its effects in the minds of the public. Only the extension-acceleration type of trauma justifies the term whiplash, indeed after the initial backward movement, the head may be rapidly flexed. Severy et al. [57] estimated that the head was, accelerated backwards with a force of 10 g in a 15 miles per hour collision. In McNab's study [54] 266 patients suffered in this manner. Of these, 145 were seen personally at review. He assumed, perhaps not entirely correctly, that those that did not attend were unaffected by continuing symptoms. Of those seen, 121 (45%) were still having symptoms 2 or more years after settlement of any court action. In the majority, the residual complaints were a continuing nuisance rather than a significant problem. Further account should be taken of the fact that these cases were referred for specialist opinion. Those who were seriously affected, therefore, would be an even smaller number, since many were treated by their family doctors only.

The reason for the more serious symptoms following a rear-end shunt is the excessive range through which the head travels. Movement may continue until the head is stopped by the back of the trunk. This involves an unphysiological range. As a result, there is considerable tearing of soft tissue. MacNab [55] makes further interesting observations in relation to the extension injury.

Extension of the neck can only occur up to a point at which the occipito-mental line is 45° to the horizontal. This figure is approximately halved when the neck is in 45° of rotation. The older patients will also have a more restricted range.

Paradoxically the extension movement of the neck may be limited by higher speeds (over 20 mph). This causes the trunk to slide forward on the seat (even with a seat belt) and converts the hyperextension movement to traction, due to the body being more horizontal. Breaking of the seat back may have a similar effect. McNab conducted experiments in which the necks of monkeys were forcibly extended by sudden arrest, after dropping from a height, simulating a rear-end shunt. He found that the sterno-mastoid muscles were torn, and with greater force, the longus colli were also damaged. Retro-pharyngeal haematomata were found and on occasions the sympathetic plexus was affected. The anterior longitudinal ligament and even the discs could be disrupted. Despite these injuries, after 6 months no radiographic evidence was visible in the disc spaces.

The acceleration–extension type of injury may cause, in the acute phase, swelling of the sterno-mastoid muscle due to haemorrhage and oedema. This may result in difficulty in raising the head. Both the upper and lower cervical plexus roots may be damaged giving rise to sensory disturbance in their distribution. A positive Tinel's sign may be found over the posterior auricular and supraclavicular nerves as they issue from the sterno-mastoid and this may persist for several years. In most cases, continuing neck pain and occasionally brachialgia are the main symptoms. Occipital headaches are not uncommon and these may radiate forwards to the temporal region. More unusual complaints are dysphagia, tinnitus and dizziness. Blurring of vision can occur and if associated with Horner's syndrome may indicate serious soft tissue damage.

In summary it can be concluded that flexion and lateral flexion injuries should only infrequently cause persisting physical problems. Those injuries resulting from extension, however, are rather more serious and may give rise to chronic complaints in a number of cases. McNab found that 45% continued to have symptoms after litigation. The majority suffered no more than a continuing nuisance. This figure should perhaps be revised down, since these were a special and more troublesome group, having been referred for consultant advice. Gotten [50] in his survey after litigation, came to the conclusion that 88% had largely recovered and this approximates to McNab's figures when all the factors are considered. Gotten found that 3% were still off work or conversely that 97% had returned to full-time activity. The percentage seriously affected may well be fairly small.

Hohl [52] reported the results of a review of 743 patients. Unfortunately, only 146 (27%) attended for a follow-up review. Of the remaining 73% not seen, the probability is that the majority were symptom free. Follow-up was not less than 5 years. Symptomatic recovery occurred in 57% of 146 patients. Poor prognostic factors were thought to be advanced age, severe initial complaints and brachialgia. Unfortunately, there was no assessment of the severity of symptoms nor of the type of accident. Radiographically it was noted that sharp reversal of the cervical curve was a harbinger of degenerative change, but whether or not this pre-empted the injury is not known. Hirsch et al. [51] found that neurologic deficits were particularly unfavourable.

There is little factual medical evidence in any review of the effects of either seat belts or head restraints. The provision of head restraints should theoretically prevent excessive extension of the neck and reduce the numbers of seriously affected patients. A seat belt may anchor the body but can exaggerate the forces on the head and neck, particularly in a flexion acceleration injury. Neither presumably was fitted in any numbers in the cases cited by McNab or Gotten since these occurred before such safety measures were used routinely. Norris and Watt [56] found more recently that belts and neck restraints had little effect in rear-end collisions. The numbers quoted, however, were not large and the evidence is not very conclusive.

Osteoarthritis and Trauma

The aetiology of osteoarthritis is still a matter of some conjecture. There is no doubt that any joint in which the loadbearing characteristics are significantly altered by congenital or acquired disease may develop osteoarthritis. Trauma can certainly be a cause in these circumstances. Whether it initiates degenerative changes in the absence of recognisable damage is a matter of considerable doubt. Doctors are commonly asked as to whether or not a plaintiff has developed osteoarthritis as a result of injury or, alternatively, whether the underlying condition, which was dormant, has been aggravated by trauma so that symptoms have arisen. Most will give a positive response to both questions if there seems to be a relationship in time between the onset of symptoms and the presence of radiographic osteoarthritis. Whilst there may be good reason for relating the two in some cases, there is a doubtful connection in most. Indeed, the etiology of osteoarthritis described in most textbooks does not mention trauma as a precipitating cause, except in special circumstances.

In order to answer the questions concerning trauma, it is necessary to have some understanding of the basic condition, its epidemiology and symptomatology.

Osteoarthritis is a non-inflammatory disorder of a synovial joint, characterised by deterioration and abrasion of articular cartilage. New bone formation also takes place at the periphery of the joint. This latter feature is not of itself evidence of osteoarthritis, though is apparent in most osteoarthritic joints. Osteophytes have been recorded as being present for as long as 10 to 15 years, without full development of the disease [60].

Epidemiology

There is some degree of degeneration of articular cartilage in the major joints of any individual over the age of 30 and these changes are progressive [59]. Peyron [68] in 1986 confirmed the ubiquitous nature of the disease and gave the following figures of its presence:

Age	Male	Female
45	2%	3%
46–64	30%	24.5%
Over 65	68%	58%

Even by middle age, therefore, the condition is well established and over 65 almost three-quarters of the population is affected. Kellgren et al. [65] in their review of the population of Leigh, Lancashire, found that over 80% had one joint affected and that 23% of males and 20% of females complained of pain. They also noted that a history of injury to the knee joint was not uncommon, especially in males. After analysing a number of the patients affected in this way, they concluded that injuries of the type likely to be remembered were not responsible for the symptoms of osteoarthritis. Although changes are not visible radiographically until fairly advanced, Kellgren [64] found that 11.1% of male knees in a population survey of the age group 55-64 showed radiographic changes of osteoarthritis. Only a quarter of them complained of pain. Lowman [67] reported that after the age of 40, 90% of patients have degenerative changes in weightbearing joints, though not necessarily symptomatic. Although there may be some argument as to the exact numbers of the population suffering from osteoarthritis, there seems no doubt that the condition is extremely common, both with and without symptoms.

Clinically osteoarthritis is characterised by pain which is aching in character and probably results from synovitis, caused by fragments of articular cartilage, abraded from the joint surface. These accumulate in the synovial recesses and secondarily cause capsulitis [66]. Some episodes of pain may result from microfractures which are produced by overloading as a result of loss of normal incongruity. Hypervascularity and venous congestion have also been blamed for the pain by some authors [58]. As the condition progresses the joint capsule becomes contracted and joint movement is lost. Lloyd-Roberts [66] thought that the contracted capsule was the most likely cause of pain although he considered a number of other possibilities.

Joint Incongruity

In the normal joint there is now wide recognition of the fact that incongruity of joint surfaces is necessary to spread the load. As the articular surface takes weight, its elasticity produces deformation so that congruity occurs, allowing the load to be spread over a much larger surface, thus evening out the stress. Once the load is removed, the cartilage rapidly returns to its normal shape. The menisci in the knee perform a similar function. Their removal results in degenerative change consequent on the increased loading over a small area of articular cartilage [63]. Inevitably the question arises as to why some joints become osteoarthritic and others, which slowly degenerate with age, do not seem to be afflicted in a similar manner. Many authors divide osteoarthritic joints into two groups, in one of which there are obvious deformities resulting from deformity and disease. This distortion results in mechanical imperfection of the joint and more rapid wear. Joints in this group are considered to be secondarily arthritic. Most observers believe that they are roughly half of the total of hips affected. Lloyd-Roberts [66] estimated that only 20% fell into this group. Harris [62], on the other hand, was of the opinion that almost all cases fell into this category. If care was taken to measure the joint accurately, he stated that evidence could be found of previous disease. Solomon [69] was of much the same opinion. He reported on a series of 327 cases and in all but 27 found an identifiable cause. In 33 of these he identified trauma, but in all these cases there was an initially identifiable change such as avascular necrosis or at least some visible subchondral damage.

A study of the literature does not incriminate trauma as a cause of osteoarthritis. Durman [61] stated that no authority has come forward with the claim that a single trauma to a joint, even severe, has anything to do with the production of degenerative arthritis or exacerbation of a pre-existing arthritis. He gave the following exceptions to this rule:

1. Permanent impairment of the circulation of the subchondral bone
2. Malalignment of the joint
3. Irregularity of the articular surface or a combination of these three.

Impairment of the circulation does raise problems of immediate diagnosis, since there may be no obvious radiographic signs. An example is avascular necrosis of the femoral head which may follow a subcapital fracture. In most cases there is a long latent period following the initial pain of the injury, before further osteoarthritic pain develops, secondary to bony collapse of avascular bone. This phenomenon of avascular necrosis is uncommon and limited principally to those sites in which there is an arrangement of end vessels supplying the affected bone.

Articular cartilage damage without fracture of the bone can occur. Should this be the case, then the resulting deformity is usually small and cartilage has adequate healing properties. Loose bodies consisting only of cartilage may grow and cause interference with the joint mechanics, but this is an uncommon outcome. Where the fragment is of any size, there is almost invariably some bone in its composition, which can be identified radiographically.

Aggravation of Osteoarthritis

Finally the possibility of aggravation of pre-existing osteoarthritis needs to be considered. Clinical experience supports a view that a joint which is affected by marked degenerative change but asymptomatic may become painful and those joints which are already painful may become worse as a result of injury. The cause of this exacerbation probably stems from the capsule, which as Lloyd-Roberts [66] has pointed out is the likely cause of most, if not all, of the pain in this condition. Since the capsule is contracted, it is more likely to be injured because the joint movements are limited. The pain that results from the injury is similar to that following a sprain. Recovery is likely to be similar to that following the sprain of a normal joint, i.e. it will clear up within a matter of weeks. Occasionally, discomfort may persist for some months or even much longer periods although any significant pain should pass within a matter of weeks.

If serious pain persists, then in all probability the natural progression of the osteoarthritic process is responsible rather than the injury. Pain in osteoarthritic joints may perhaps be caused by pressure on the subchondral bone which has been exposed by the osteoarthritic process. This feature is possibly responsible for the boring type of pain which may result in disturbance of sleep. If this is exacerbated, then it is probable that the cause is a fracture producing bone distortion. The likelihood of this is not great without the presence of a haemarthrosis or radiographic change being visible. Furthermore, it should be remembered that the subchondral bone is stronger in osteoarthritic joints in response to the abnormal loading which has occurred. Indeed, fracture of an osteoarthritic hip is infrequent, presumably due to the unusual strength of the bone.

In order to study this problem further, the author questioned 73 patients who had been admitted for joint replacement. Between them 100 joints were affected with 56 patients undergoing hip replacement and 44 knees. Surprisingly, since these were elderly patients, only 22 admitted to any injury. As might be anticipated, the majority, 16 of these, were knees. Of those suffering trauma, in 9 joints no history was obtained of exacerbation and in 11 the interval between injury and the onset of symptoms was more than 2 years. This interval was considered too long to be associated with the osteoarthritis. One patient had symptoms in both knees for about 3 years and during this time there were two separate falls. In one knee there was no significant difference but in the other joint the patient considered there was an exacerbation after 6 months. Another patient suffered osteoarthritis in both hips and fell off his bike. One hip was exacerbated but the symptoms were much the same after 2 months. A third patient who had had pain in both knees for 40 years stated that he had suffered some eight falls but without any deterioration in his condition. This investigation did not produce any very convincing evidence of either commencement or exacerbation as a result of trauma.

In summary, therefore, it can be said that osteoarthritis is only precipitated by recognisable circumstances. Although injury may cause pain or temporarily increase it in osteoarthritic joints, there is no evidence that the pathological process is accelerated thereby, unless recognisable changes occur as enumerated above.

References

Repetitive Stress Injury

1. Caillet RD (1971) Shoulder Pain. FA Davis, Philadelphia
2. Dale WA, Lewis MR (1975) Management of thoracic outlet syndrome. Ann Surg 181: 575-585
3. Ferguson D (1971) An Australian study of telegraphists cramp. Br J Ind Med 28: 280-285
4. Ferguson D (1987) R.S.I. Putting the epidemic to rest. Med J Aust 147: 213-216
5. Fineman S et al. (1963) Transformation of normal lordic pattern to linear pattern in normal posture. J Bone Jt Surg [Am] 45A: 1179
6. Fry AJH (1986) Overuse syndrome alias tenosynovitis/tendinitis: The terminological hoax. Plast Reconstr Surg 78: 414-416
7. Graham G (1985) Job satisfaction and repetition strain injury (Dissertation), Adelaide; Elton-Mayo School of Management. South Australia Institute of Technology, 32 pp
8. General Municipal, Boilermakers and Allied Trade Unions (1986) Tackling Teno. GMU, London
9. Hadler NM (1985) Illness in the workplace: The challenge of musculo-skeletal symptoms. J Hand Surg 10A: 451-456
10. Hocking B (1987) Epidemiological aspects of repetition strain injury in Telecom. Med J Aust 147: 218-222
11. Horal J (1969) The clinical appearance of low back disorders in the City of Gothenberg, Sweden. Comparison of incapacitated probands with matched controls. Acta Orthop Scand 188: 1-109
12. Howard NJ (1937) Peritendinitis crepitans. J Bone Jt Surg 19: 447

13. Ireland DCR (1988) Psychological and physical aspects of occupational arm pain. J Hand Surg 13B: 5–10
14. Kurpa K, Waris P, Rokkanen P et al. (1979) Peritendinitis and tenosynovitis: A review. Scand J Work Environ Health 5 [Suppl 3]: 19–24
15. Lawrence JS (1961) Rheumatism in cotton operatives. Br J Ind Med 18: 270
16. Lucire Y (1986) Neurosis in the workplace. Med J Aust 145: 323–326
17. Magora A (1973) Investigation of the relation between low back pain and occupation v. psychological aspects. Scand J Rehab 5: 191–196
18. Telford ED, Mottershead S (1960) Pressure of the cervico-brachial junction; An operative and anatomical study. J Bone Jt Surg [Am] 42A: 392–407
19. Thompson AR, Plewes LW, Shaw EG et al. (1951) Peritendinitis crepitans and simple tenosynovitis: A clinical study of 544 cases in industry. Br J Ind Med 8: 150–158
20. Wallace M (1986) Factors associated with occupational pain in keyboard users In: Wallace M (ed) Occupational pain (R.S.I.). Melbourne Brain Behaviour Institute, La Trobe University, Melbourne, pp 15–18
21. Waris P, Kvorinka I, Kurppa K et al. (1979) Epidemiological screening of occupational neck and upper limb disorders. Scand J Work Environ Health 5 [Suppl 3]: 25–38
22. Waris P (1980) Occupational cervico-brachial symptoms. Scand J Work Environ Health 6 [Suppl 3]: 3–14, 21
23. Wright IS (1945) The neurovascular syndrome produced by hyperabduction of the arm. Am Heart J 29: 1–19

Anterior Knee Pain

24. Abernethy PJ, Townsend PR, Rose RM, Radin EL (1978) Is chondromalacia patellae a separate clinical entity? J Bone Jt Surg [Br] 60B: 205–210
25. Bentley G (1978) The surgical treatment of chondromalacia patellae. J Bone Jt Surg [Br] 60B: 74–81
26. Bentley G, Dowd G (1984) Current concepts of etiology and treatment of chondromalacia patella. Clin Orthop 189: 209–228
27. Brav EA (1962) Traumatic dislocation of the hip. J Bone Jt Surg [Am] 44A: 1115
28. Epstein HC (1974) Posterior fracture dislocation of the hip. J Bone Jt Surg [Am] 56A: 1103–1127
29. Ficat RP, Philippe J, Hungerford DS (1979) Chondromalacia patellae. Clin Orthop 144: 55–62
30. Fulkerson JP, Tennant R, Jaivan JS, Grunnet M (1985) Histologic evidence of retinacular nerve injury associated with patello-femoral malalignment. Clin Orthop 197: 196–204
31. Goodfellow J, Hungerford DS, Woods SC (1976) Patello-femoral joint mechanics and pathology: Chondromalacia patellae. J Bone Jt Surg [Br] 58B: 291–299
32. Hallisey MJ, Doherty N, Bennett WF, Fulkerson JP (1987) Anatomy of the junction of vastus lateralis tendon and the patella. J Bone Jt Surg [Am] 69A: 545–549
33. Insall J (1982) Current concepts review of patella pain. J Bone Jt Surg [Am] 64A: 147–151
34. Insall J, Falvo KA, Wise DW (1976) Chondromalacia patella. J Bone Jt Surg [Am] 58A: 1–8
35. Insall J, Bullough PG, Burstein GH (1979) Proximal tube realignment of the patella for chondromalacia patellae. Clin Orthop 144: 63–69
36. Karlson S (1940) Chondromalacia patellae. Acta Chir Scand 83: 347–381
37. Emery IH, Meachim G (1973) Surface morphology and topography of patello-femoral cartilage. Fibrillation in Liverpool necropsies. J Anat 116: 103–120
38. Meachim G (1963) Effect of scarification on articular cartilage in the rabbit. J Bone Jt Surg [Br] 45B: 150–161
39. Meachim G, Bentley G (1977) The effect of age on the thickness of patella articular cartilage. Ann Rheum Dis 36: 563
40. Nicoll EA (1952) Traumatic dislocation of the hip joint. J Bone Jt Surg [Br] 34B: 503–504
41. Ogilvie-Harris DJ, Jackson RW (1984) The arthroscopic treatment of chondromalacia patellae. J Bone Jt Surg [Br] 66B: 660–665
42. Outerbridge RE (1961) The etiology of chondromalacia patellae. J Bone Jt Surg [Br] 43B: 752–757
43. Radin E (1979) A rational approach to the treatment of patello-femoral pain. Clin Orthop 144: 107–109
44. Upadhay SS, Moulton A (1981) Long-term results of traumatic dislocation of the hip. J Bone Jt Surg [Br] 63B: 548–551
45. Wiberg GG (1960) Roentgenographic and anatomical studies on the femoro-patella joint. With special reference to chondromalacia patellae. Acta Orthop Scand 12: 319–410

Whiplash Injuries of the Neck

46. Crowe HE (1928) Injuries to the cervical spine. Paper presented to the meeting of the Western Orthopaedic Association, San Francisco
47. Fineman S, Borrelli FJ, Rubenstein B, Epstein H, Jacobson HG (1963) The cervical spine: Transformation of the normal lordotic pattern into a linear pattern in the neutral posture. J Bone Jt Surg [Am] 45A: 1179-1183
48. Frankel VH (1971) Whiplash injuries to the neck. In: Cervical pain symposium, 1971, Wenner-Gren Centre, Stockholm. Pergamon Press, Oxford, pp 97-112 (International symposium series 19)
49. Friedenberg ZB, Miller WT (1963) Degenerative disc disease of the cervical spine. J Bone Jt Surg [Am] 45A: 1171-1178
50. Gotten N (1956) Survey of 100 cases of whiplash injury after settlement of litigation. JAMA 162: 865-867
51. Hirsch SA, Hirsch PJ, Hiramoto H, Weiss A (1988) Whiplash syndrome: Fact or fiction. Orthop Clin North Am 19: 791-795
52. Hohl M (1974) Soft tissue injuries in the neck in automobile accidents. J Bone Jt Surg [Am] 56A: 1675-1682
53. Hult L (1971) Frequency of symptoms for different age groups and professions. In: Cervical pain symposium, 1971, Wenner-Gren Centre, Stockholm. Pergamon Press, Oxford, pp 17-20 (International symposium series 19)
54. MacNab I (1964) Acceleration injuries of the cervical spine. J Bone Jt Surg [Am] 46A: 1797-1799
55. MacNab I (1971) The whiplash syndrome. Orthop Clin North Am 2: 389-403
56. Norris SH, Watt I (1983) The prognosis of neck injuries resulting from rear-end vehicle collisions. J Bone Jt Surg [Br] 65B: 608-611
57. Severy DM, Mathewson DH, Bechtol CO (1955) Controlled automobile rear-end collisions: An investigation of related engineering and medical phenomena. Can Serv Med J 11: 727-759

Osteoarthritis and Trauma

58. Arnoldi CC, Lempry RK, Linderholm H (1975) Intraosseous hypertension and pain in the knee. J Bone Jt Surg [Br] 57B: 360-363
59. Bennet GA, Waine H, Bauer W (1942) Changes in the knee joint with particular reference to the nature and development of degeneration joint disease. Commonwealth Fund, New York
60. Daniellson LG, Hernborg J (1970) Clinical and roentgenologic study of knee joints and osteophytes. Clin Orthop 69: 302
61. Durman DC (1955) Arthritis and injury. J Mich Med Soc 54: 301-303
62. Harris WH (1986) Etiology of osteoarthritis of the hip. Clin Orthop 213: 20-33
63. Jackson JP (1968) Degenerative changes in the knee after meniscectomy. Br Med J ii: 525-527
64. Kellgren JH (1961) Osteoarthritis in patients and population. Br Med J ii: 1
65. Kellgren JH, Lawrence JS, Bier F (1963) Genetic factors in generalised osteoarthritis. Ann Rheum Dis 22: 237
66. Lloyd-Roberts GC (1955) Osteoarthritis of the hip. J Bone Jt Surg [Br] 37B: 8-47
67. Lowman EW (1955) Osteoarthritis. JAMA 157: 487
68. Peyron JG (1986) Osteoarthritis: The epidemiological viewpoint. Clin Orthop Rel Res 213: 13-19
69. Solomon L (1976) Patterns of osteoarthritis of the hip. J Bone Jt Surg [Br] 58B: 176-183

CHAPTER 12

Litigant's Backache

J.H.S. Scott

In ordinary medical and surgical practice malingering is relatively uncommon, indeed its very existence as an entity is not accepted by many clinicians. The more involved in medico-legal practice one becomes, however, the more frequently is this problem encountered.

Trimble [6] has traced historical references to it down the ages and gives examples of both the negative and positive forms in the Bible. For example, King David feigned madness to avoid danger, and Amnon, son of David, "lay down and made himself sick" to lure his sister-in-law to his bed. Later accounts of malingering were mostly found in literature relating to the prisons and armed forces.

With the advent of the Industrial Revolution a new dimension was added to malingering and fresh impetus was provided by the Employers' Liability Act of 1880 and later by the Workman's Compensation Act of 1906. The advent of the railway produced "railway back" and the motor car the "whiplash" injury. Now in the computer age we have repetitive stress disorder.

Back injuries spearheaded this upsurge of industrial malingering which is still with us today. Each patient presenting with such a back problem does so in an astonishingly similar manner, so much so, that one is justified in postulating a special syndrome, "Litigant's Backache".

Recognition of this syndrome is helped by this uniform presentation. The patient is most frequently found in social groups four and five and malingering is most likely to occur after industrial accidents rather than traffic accidents or sporting injuries. Miller [4] highlights this by suggesting that the response of a workman recovering consciousness after being struck on the head by a brick is not "where am I?" but "Whose brick was it?".

We will now trace the progress of a typical patient from the moment he enters the consulting room. Hopefully on this occasion female readers will forgive me if the patient from now on is referred to as he or him; indeed, it is my impression that this sort of behaviour is commoner in the male.

Presentation

The patient enters the consulting room slowly and apparently in great pain. He is usually accompanied by his wife or a friend who carries a container or plastic bag weighed down with bottles of painkillers, anti-inflammatory drugs, hypnotics and tranquillisers. Later the supporter will testify to the patient's great courage, will describe the moments of agony which she recognises by dramatic changes in the patient's complexion, and the number of pills he then surreptitiously swallows, trying not to cause her any anxiety. Incidentally, this drug regime apparently fails to control the patient's pain.

Accoutrements

The patient wears at least two or more of the following items: dark glasses, a collar and a wrist support. On disrobing a surgical corset is revealed and possibly also tubigrip supports on the knees. One or more sticks are used. If a single stick, it is used on the inappropriate side, the side on which the pain exists. Occasionally the ultimate malingerer presents in a wheelchair.

Gait

The patient usually has a limp which does not have the characteristic rhythm of a painful gait. In the presence of genuine pain, weightbearing on the painful member is reduced as far as possible and the rhythm of the gait is painful normal, painful normal (quick slow, quick slow), and so on.

The malingerer has the opposite rhythm, weight is sustained on the apparently painful member allowing time to dramatise the agony. The rhythm is therefore "painful" normal, "painful" normal (slow slow, slow slow). As previously mentioned if a single stick is used it is deployed on the same side as the pain. Incidentally it is wise, when observing the patient's gait not to walk too close to the patient who has a tendency to collapse on the examiner, perhaps to make the maximum impression on him.

History

The most striking features of the malingerer's history are his astonishing recall of every last detail of the accident which may have happened a long time ago; coupled with this is an amazing vagueness when questioned in detail about the influence his present daily routine has on his symptoms. This detailed questioning makes the patient initially uneasy, then irritable and finally aggressive. As mentioned later, care must be taken not to incite this reaction.

The pattern of pain which finally emerges is of constant pain throughout the day, even at rest, with dramatic exacerbations resulting in stabbing, shooting and burning pain. If time allows, pain drawings will give a permanent record of the patient's conception of his pain. On reviewing the details of the accident it may be noted that the mechanism of alleged injury was inappropriate and may have involved a direct blow to the back.

The alleged accident is always the fault of some other agency, often a large and impersonal one. Since the accident the patient's resentment has gradually increased and the clinician must be aware of this and do nothing to antagonise the patient during examination.

Despite a long period of inactivity, rest and many forms of treatment, the patient's alleged symptoms have not improved and if anything are still allegedly deteriorating. Inappropriate symptoms are offered, including pain radiating upwards to the neck and arms from the lumbar region, pain or numbness involving the whole of the limb, weakness involving the whole of a limb and sudden giving way of a leg or legs without warning and without any discernible pattern.

This history contrasts with that of the hysteric, who may present the same illness behaviour. The long-term history is, however, vague but detailed questioning about the present situation is apparently welcomed and less than expected concern about an apparently disastrous state is evident [2].

Finally the patient or his spouse will recount the number and variety of drugs consumed daily in a futile effort to control the alleged symptoms. As previously mentioned the actual drugs may be on display.

To summarise this section the striking feature in the history is the contrast between the detailed recall of the accident and the vagueness of the patient's account of his present situation. Next we note the tendency to deteriorate despite inactivity and continued treatment, the constancy of the pain throughout the day and the inappropriate symptoms offered. Finally we note the tendency of the patient to become flustered and irritable under close scrutiny.

Examination

One must be resigned to the fact that examination is likely to take some time. Attempts to hurry such patients are counter-productive as this fuels their carefully fostered resentment. One can be consoled by the knowledge that the longer the examination takes the more likely it is that the patient's attention will begin to wander and his guard relax [3]. Ideally the patient is observed undressing and subsequently dressing. If the consultation has been conducted in a calm and friendly atmosphere, for the reasons given above, there may be a marked contrast in the two performances at the beginning and the end of the consultation.

The following examination routine is recommended, individual tests are described in more detail in the Appendix.

The patient's gait is checked particularly for its rhythm and the patient is then examined standing. Note is made of his posture and of his spinal movements. All will be restricted in the malingerer. The range of flexion is noted, the level to which the patient can reach with his fingertips and more importantly the direct measurement of flexion with a tape measure of the lumbar movements. Simulated rotation and axial loading are then checked. The patient is then examined supine on the examination couch, his performance getting on to the couch is also recorded. Straight leg raising is noted and also the response to the ankle dorsiflexion tests and the bowstring sign. There are often discrepancies in the patient's response to these two latter tests, both of which put tension on the sciatic roots.

Sensation is recorded but only in general terms as to whether the distribution of sensory deficit is anatomical or non-anatomical and of a stocking distribution.

Motor power is checked, and most important, accurate measurements of girth of both the calf and the thigh on both sides should be recorded. This is particularly important where there is asymmetrical weakness, which is not accompanied by corresponding wasting of the affected muscles in the malingerer.

A quick check on the hip joints is carried out simply by rotating the legs on the bed. In the malingerer this may allegedly aggravate his pain. If rotation is normal no other hip movement need be checked. It is sometimes difficult to check the other joints because of the patient's resistance and it is normally a waste of time to attempt to do so. The patient is then examined prone. Normally one would expect the patient to have great difficulty turning over but if a request to turn over is made in the middle of a relaxed conversation the patient may do so before he has realised what he is doing. If he does it, it is interesting to note that sometimes the pain remains on the same side of the table in relation to the examiner despite the patient having turned over. If the patient has apparent great difficulty in turning over it is adequate simply to request him to lie on whichever side he is more comfortable and this will give access to the back for assessment of local tenderness, performance of the femoral stretch test and of a further test on the ankle jerks.

As the patient is getting off the plinth he is invited to rest while sitting with his hips and knees at right angles. The opportunity is then taken, ostensibly, to re-check the knee and ankle jerks. The latter are checked with the knees in full extension. While doing this one is surreptitiously carrying out the flip test which checks the authenticity of the patient's spinal flexion and straight leg raising.

When the patient is once more on his feet he is asked whether walking on tiptoe or walking on his heels aggravates his back pain. He is not asked whether he can stand on tiptoe or walk on his heels.

Finally as the patient dresses his performance is compared to his undressing. One then ascertains that he is wearing his own shoes and, as long as they are not new the wear pattern on the sole of the shoes is noted.

Having completed the examination, including radiographs, the clinician is sometimes faced with a dilemma. This is particularly the case when he suspects that the appellant has been coerced into litigation by friends, relations or trade union officials.

The impulse may be to give the patient some hint that his deception has been unsuccessful. On the other hand in medico-legal practice the doctor has no therapeutic responsibilities towards the patient. However, if kindness prevails, the message can be gently passed by expressing puzzlement about the diagnosis and a pious hope that one will never have to stand up in court to explain the patient's complaints on anatomical grounds.

Comment on Examination

By carrying out the above routine one should be able to assess all five of the non-organic physical signs in low back pain described by Waddell [7]. It must be emphasised that abnormal responses do not necessarily prove that the patient is malingering, they only do so if it can also be proved that the patient is consciously fabricating these signs for personal gain. Objective rather than subjective observations have more impact on the legal mind and remembering this perhaps it would be helpful to run through these five groups of non-organic clinical signs:

1. *Tenderness.* Assessment of this is subjective and may vary from observer to observer. These findings, although they should be accurately recorded, may not carry great weight as evidence.

2. *Simulated rotation and axial loading.* Both these observations are objective and repeatable findings.

3. *Distraction.* This entails assessment of spinal movements in different postures and again is an objective finding and therefore useful.

4. *Regional weakness and sensory change.* Assessment of sensation is obviously subjective and therefore not too much time should be spent on delineating the pattern except to note whether it is anatomical or non-anatomical. The assessment and gradation of motor weakness is subjective but the mere fact it is present coupled with the presence or absence of measurable wasting makes the two combined findings an objective and useful contribution.

5. *Over-reaction.* Again this is a subjective finding and depends largely on the observer's reaction to the patient. These findings should be recorded, but again they may not carry great weight.

At the end of the clinical examination, which will of course include assessment of radiographs, one should have a battery of inappropriate and inconsistent responses on the part of the patient. While this does not prove that he is malingering it establishes the fact that he is not a reliable witness.

Radiographic Examination

X-ray film of the lumbar spine requires special assessment. The presence of degenerative changes in the discs, osteophyte formation and even spondylolisthesis can be quite irrelevant as their presence does not necessarily indicate painful lesions. What is important is the assessment of the general posture of the spine.

Painful lesions in the lumbar spine produce spasm of the related muscles and this in turn flattens or reverses the normal lordosis, and produces a lateral tilt seen in the antero-posterior view. Having said this, the presence of these abnormal postures does not necessarily indicate that the patient has a painful back lesion. However, if the normal lordosis is preserved, even when associated with disc changes or spondylolisthesis and there is no lateral tilt on the antero-posterior view, one can presume the alleged back pain has no physical source in the lumbar spine.

Isthmic spondylolisthesis presents special problems. It is sometimes claimed that a specific injury caused the lesion. In the rare event that the patient presents within a year of the alleged accident a bone scan should resolve this problem. If the scan is hot at the appropriate level one could argue that the accident had caused an acute fracture of the pars interarticularis.

Most authorities accept that this lesion occurs before the spine is fully mature and is therefore present by late adolescence. It is, however, often claimed that an alleged accident has destabilised or aggravated a pre-existing spondylolisthesis. If radiographs are available from the time of the accident and a significant period has passed before current radiographs have been taken, careful measurement of the degree of displacement is useful. The amount of displacement should be expressed as a percentage of the anterior-posterior diameter of the vertebra above. This will allow a comparison of the two findings and allow an opinion to be expressed as to whether or not the lesion had been destabilised.

Finally if the patient gives a long history of unilateral and disabling leg pain, an antero-posterior radiograph of the pelvis or antero-posterior views of both knees on the same plate are indicated.

If the complaint is genuine and weightbearing has been restricted on the painful side for a significant period disuse demineralisation of the skeleton on that side will be noted. If this change is not present one can presume that the apparently painful leg has been subjected to the normal stresses of weight-bearing and indicates that the patient has been walking normally over that period of time.

Special radiography, such as radiculograms, computed tomography (CT) scans and magnetic resonance imaging (MRI) studies require careful assessment. If they are negative they are of positive value. If they are positive these changes must be carefully correlated with the patient's symptoms. Unless they fit into the clinical picture these findings may be irrelevant.

Summary

When considering all the information we have accumulated following examination of the patient we should keep in mind the definition of malingering of Miller and Cartiledge [5]. They state that the term "malingering" is used to encompass all forms of fraud related to matters of health. This includes the simulation of disease or disability which is not present; the much commoner gross exaggeration of minor disabilities and the conscious and deliberate attribution of a disability to an injury or accident that did not in fact cause it, for personal advantage. The key phrase is that the behaviour must be a conscious and deliberate effort to deceive on the part of the patient.

It could be argued that the clinician can only provide a selection of subjective and objective findings which indicate that the patient's behaviour was inconsistent and inappropriate. This would indicate that the patient is an unreliable witness. The most a clinician can state is that, in his opinion the patient's behaviour fulfils the criteria for malingering as laid down by Miller and Cartiledge.

The only uncontroversial evidence of malingering is the observation of the patient carrying out activities which he alleges he is unable to do, or a confession that he is malingering [3]. The patient may be induced to provide this evidence when under examination or cross-examination and Trimble [6] gives two classic examples of this. The first concerned a man with an apparently paralysed arm. When being cross-examined by the defendant's counsel he was asked how high he could raise his arm before the accident and he, without a moment's hesitation thrust his arm high above his head. The second even sadder tale involves an apparently helpless patient who on hearing of a generous award for her alleged injuries made a violent and apparently muscular demonstration of joy when the jury announced her good fortune. I am sure most clinicians could match or cap such episodes; however, they do not happen often.

The provision of such evidence is not a medical commitment and I note it is becoming increasingly common for the patient to be put under surveillance either by special Investigators of the DHSS or agents employed by the defending lawyers. The development of more sophisticated videocameras has accelerated this development.

Occasionally, if the medical evidence has raised doubts about the veracity of the patient's account of his accident, a detailed review carried out on the actual site of the accident occasionally provides evidence that the mechanism of the alleged accident would have been physically impossible at that site.

One therefore has to accept that the final and most conclusive evidence may be non-medical and we should perhaps keep in mind Richard Asher's comment [1] that the pride of a doctor who has caught a malingerer is akin to that of a fisherman who has landed an enormous fish and his stories (like those of a fisherman) may become somewhat exaggerated in the telling!

Thus reminded we must strive to be as objective as possible and ensure that the information we provide is similarly objective.

Appendix. Examination Techniques and Tests

Assessment of Spinal Flexion

The patient is observed standing and then two marks are placed over the lumbar spine, the upper 10 cm above the lumbo-sacral level and the lower 5 cm below that level.

The patient is then asked to try and touch his toes keeping his knees straight.

The level he reaches with his fingertips is recorded and also the increase in the distance between the two marks. The normal range is 5 cm more or less, depending on the build of the patient.

Forward flexion, of course, is a combination of hip flexion and spinal flexion. The malingerer characteristically can only reach his mid-thigh or knee level with his fingertips but the actual range of flexion measured by a tape measure on his spine is within normal limits. This indicates that the patient is voluntarily avoiding hip flexion, as he has previously been noted with his hips flexed to a right angle when sitting.

Simulated Rotation

Again with the patient standing the pelvis is held firmly on each side and the trunk as a whole is rotated on the hip joints, no significant motion taking place in the spine itself.

If this reproduces the patient's symptoms the test is positive.

Axial Loading

Again with the patient standing, gentle pressure is placed on the top of the patient's head. If this produces pain in the lumbar region this test is positive.

Sciatic Stretch Tests with the Patient Supine

With the patient in this position passive straight leg raising is carried out. At the tolerated extreme the ankle is passively dorsiflexed. If this causes pain to radiate up the leg to the back the stretch test is said to be positive.

The bowstring test is carried out by flexing the knee when the patient reaches the limit of passive straight leg raising. This relaxes the sciatic roots and the hamstrings and the patient should then tolerate further hip flexion with the knee flexed. The malingerer, however, almost invariably continues to resist hip flexion.

Having achieved flexion of the hip and knee the knee is then extended until the patient resists. At that stage pressure is placed on the nearer hamstring tendon the middle of the popliteal fossa and over the opposite hamstring tendon; the patient is asked which is painful, the first, second or third pressure. If the patient selects the second he is asked where the pain is. If the pain and discomfort is localised in the popliteal fossa the test is negative. It is only positive if the pain radiates up or down the leg on pressure over the posterior tibial nerve in the middle of the popliteal fossa.

The malingerer presents with limited straight leg raising a positive ankle dorsiflexion test but a negative bowstring sign.

The Flip Test

This is a simple way of performing a distraction test and is best delayed until towards the end of the examination when the patient's attention span is almost spent.

As the patient is getting off the table and is sitting with the hips and knees at a right angle he is invited to have a rest and at the same time a further check is ostentatiously carried out of the knee jerks. This rivets the patient's attention and he does not register the fact that one then has extended his knee to test the ankle jerk.

The malingerer will tolerate full extension of the knee in this posture, the equivalent of forward flexion to touch the toes when standing or straight leg raising of 90° when supine.

The patient with a genuine sciatic root tension will "flip" over backwards and at the same time flex his hip and knee. If the tension is less extreme he will simply flex the hip and knee without changing the sitting posture in general.

Measurement of Muscle Weakness

In addition to assessing the weakness it is very important that the girth of the calf and thigh should be measured. This is particularly important if the weakness if asymmetrical. The characteristic finding in a malingerer is weakness unaccompanied by muscle wasting.

If there is bilateral weakness the measurements may be less helpful. In this instance it is important, as the major weakness generally presents around the ankle in the malingerer, that when he is once again on his feet he is asked if walking on tiptoe and on the heels makes his pain worse. He should not of course be asked if he can walk on tiptoe and heels.

The malingerer generally proceeds to walk on his tiptoes and on his heels but in apparent agony. This would be an activity impossible to achieve if the marked weakness noted on formal testing with the patient supine was in fact genuine.

Check on Shoe Wear

As mentioned in the text this is only likely to be helpful if there is a unilateral complaint of leg pain.

The point in asking the patient if the shoes are his own was prompted by an experience of the author. The patient had allegedly been partial weightbearing with elbow crutches for a number of years, her shoes however showed absolutely symmetrical wear. When confronted with this the patient claimed that she was wearing her sister-in-law's shoes which she had borrowed for that special occasion.

References

1. Asher R (1972), Talking sense – a selection of his papers. Ed. Sir Francis Avery Jones. Pitman Medical, London
2. Engel GL (1970) Conversion symptoms. In: MacBryde CM et al. (eds) Signs and symptoms, 5th edn. Saunders, Philadelphia, p 650
3. Hurst AF (1940) Medical diseases of war. Edward Arnold, London
4. Miller H (1961) Accident neurosis. Br Med J i: 919
5. Miller H, Cartiledge N (1972) A simulation and malingering after brain and spinal cord injury. Lancet ii: 580–585
6. Trimble MR (1981) Post-traumatic neurosis from railway spine to the whiplash. John Wiley, Chichester
7. Waddell G (1980) Non-organic physical signs in low back pain. Spine 5: 117

CHAPTER 13

Paediatrics

D. Hull

We are all sad when a child is hurt and damaged for whatever reason but it is particularly painful if we, who were trying to care for the child, are thought to be at fault. Legal conflicts about a damaged child are distressing whatever the rights and wrong of the issues. When we are involved in such conflicts it is important that we remember that it is the child who is at the disadvantage and it is his or her caring family who have the burden of care. Whilst we may sympathise with the family, it is difficult for a stranger to appreciate the full weight of the burden that they carry.

When children are left damaged, their families, and later the children themselves if they are able, will ask questions of their medical advisors. They will want to know amongst other things why it happened, whether it could have been avoided and was anyone at fault. Parents often blame themselves. Recently I stood by as a father said farewell to his five-year-old son. His child was unconscious, the ventilator had been switched off and the tracheal tube removed after tests had shown that the brain had been extensively and irreversibly damaged by a fulminating attack of bacterial meningitis. He said sorry to his son for letting him down. Telling him that neither he nor anyone else was at fault would not have eased his feelings then. The issue was not one to be answered by medical science or legal proceedings. Later perhaps he and his family will reflect upon what happened. In Nottingham we offer all parents who experience such events the opportunity to discuss the experience with us some 6 to 8 weeks later. It is then that the questioning begins. If a child survives and is left damaged, then questions of cause, fault and the future are bound to arise, sometimes again and again.

What we say on these occasions is very important, we naturally wish to help in whatever way we are able, but perhaps we should reflect more on all the consequences of what we say, and that includes the legal implications, for in the long run it will not help the parents if we mislead them on that issue as in any other.

Advising Parents After a Tragedy

What Was the Cause?

Sometimes the cause of the damage is clear and sound advice can be given, but often the cause is not obvious and all we can do is offer an opinion based on possibilities. Perhaps we do not always emphasise that it is *only* our opinion. We have to be aware that parents may interpret our views in a way we do not intend. It can be difficult at times to avoid observations which are open to more than one interpretation. All too easily misunderstandings develop.

The questioning process can itself become harmful to the child and the caring family, and they may lose confidence in their medical advisors. In the face of the "need to know" it is tempting for us to give firmer answers than the evidence justifies. Any short-term comfort that follows may be far outweighed by the lasting damage. For example, in the absence of any other explanation, birth asphyxia and vaccine damage have been extensively used in the past to "explain" brain damage. Parents on the advice they have been given, have sued obstetricians and vaccine manufacturers. As a result Caesarean section rates have increased and vaccination rates have fallen to the detriment of many. There have been major and very expensive trials in both areas. Yet the evidence is that birth asphyxia is not a common cause of cerebral palsy and it has not been established that the pertussis vaccine ever caused permanent damage [8, 10].

Could It Have Been Avoided?

It is to be expected that parents will wish to know whether the damage could have been avoided. We will also want to know that, but for different reasons. Only by making such enquiries can we hope to avoid similar tragedies in the future. It is one way to improve our practice. In the language of the time, it is an important form of audit. It is probable that in future such enquires into why an infant dies or is left unexpectedly damaged will be subject to more structured analysis in the same way as confidential inquiries are made into maternal deaths.

There is a risk of confusing what we are seeking with what parents want to know. It is not difficult to think of scenarios whereby the damage resulting from some illnesses could have been avoided. If the parents had not done this, if the child had not gone there, if the GP had arrived sooner, if that medicine had been given earlier etc. etc., then, yes, the tragedy would have been avoided. That is the answer to our question. We use the answers to inform ourselves, to modify our therapies and to direct our service developments.

The parents' question is far more specific. They want to know if the damage could have been avoided, given the specific sequence of events which resulted in *their child's problems*. This is a far more testing question and should not be attempted until all the facts are known. The initial discussion may be all important because it is the parents who will give doctors who subsequently have care of their child the "history". All too often when negligence is being investigated statements appear in the notes about the "cause" which are reaffirmed by consultants and specialists who have not themselves examined the original facts. They have accepted what the parents have said which is what the parents have concluded from what they have been told. In this way the parents' misunderstandings can be reinforced and they are not unreasonably upset when they seek legal advice, and that advice is that experts looking at all the information on their behalf are of the view that they have misunderstood or been misled. Sometimes, of course, it is the judge who has to reach that conclusion having heard all the arguments in court.

Even with all the information before us it is still difficult for us to be objective about what actions might have avoided the damage because *we know what happened*. It is impossible for us to put ourselves into the position of those who had to make the decisions at times when the outcome was not clear. It is natural for us to give ourselves the benefit of any doubt and to assume a diligence that we would wish to achieve but which in reality we often do not.

Even those with the greatest integrity, insight and humility can still have difficulty assessing whether any action would have avoided the outcome. Our medical knowledge whilst useful in answering the "audit" questions on causation, is far more limited when we are addressing the parents' questions. It is tempting to assume that the *particular* child followed the usual or average clinical course. How can one make allowance for the virulence of an infection or the peculiar vulnerability of an individual or an exceptional sequence of circumstances. The phrase "in my experience" is said to impress the judges but in truth many of the tragedies that come before the courts are not within the experts or anyone's experience, they are frequently examples of the unexpected.

Before we conclude that some remedy should have been administered sooner, we should reflect on how confident we are that it would have been effective. Again in these matters we tend to give our therapies the benefit of the doubt. If a child gets better we take the credit. It can be unfair to conclude that a medicine if it had been given would have almost certainly have worked, or because the child did not recover fully it had not been properly administered, without very good evidence that that is the case. Modern medicine does not always work, antibiotics do not always avoid brain damage in meningitis, a delay of 20 minutes in performing a Caesarean Section (CS) may have made little or no difference to the outcome.

None of these are reasons for not answering the parents' questions as openly and as honestly as we are able, but it is as well for us to reflect that if they conclude that a doctor is a fault, what we say will be examined and cross-examined in court. If it does not stand up to scrutiny we will have let the parents down.

Was Anyone at Fault?

The parents may say that we have told them the cause, we have said it could have been avoided if this or that therapy was applied, it is then very reasonable for them to ask why it was not. Could they or their medical attendants have done better? It is always difficult to judge the actions of others. Many claims are placed because of loose comments made to parents by doctors, not infrequently by doctors in specialist centres who receive the children once the illness is established and the damage has been done. For example, a teenager with a rare condition developed an even rarer complication resulting in arterial occlusion of the blood supply to the leg, the vascular surgeon to whom the child was referred said words to the effect that "If only the child had arrived sooner we could have saved the leg". That may be a perfectly valid observation. In the face of a tragedy it is perfectly understandable why an able doctor should say it, but the parents have every right to conclude that the doctors who had previous care of their child should have acted sooner, that they were at fault. One may ask the question, would the outcome have been different if for some unlikely reason that child had been from the beginning under the vascular surgeon's care? The real question in the legal setting is, however, was it reasonable to expect the clinicians who had the care of the child to recognise the early signs?

At this stage in the interview it is correct to be extremely cautious for it is wrong to accuse anyone falsely and yet it is usually important for us to face the question so that the family do not get the impression that our reluctance arises out of a wish to protect ourselves, our colleagues, our profession or our hospital. Our contributions to the defence organisations and the hospital insurance arrangements are intended to recompense, as far as money can, those damaged by medical negligence, as well as defend doctors when they are falsely accused.

Was It Negligence?

The family after reflecting on what they have been told, and burdened, as they are, with the continuing care of a disabled child, may seek a remedy in law. They decide to sue the doctor for medical negligence. Doctors cannot be expected to get everything right, or to avoid every potentially avoidable tragedy. Negligence means that the doctors failed to fulfil their duty of care to the child. To succeed in their claim the parents have to show that their child is damaged, they have to demonstrate the cause of that damage and then to prove on the balance of probabilities that damage was due to negligence of a doctor. When the negligent action is clear, for example, if the doctor simply did not turn up when on duty, the matter is settled out of court and little is heard of it. When the doctor believes that he or she behaved properly then the demands on both parents and defending doctor are considerable. Adversarial combat in court may well be necessary to assist the judge to resolve the matter in his own mind, but it is painful and damaging to the child and family and to the accused doctor whatever the rights and wrongs of the matter. It seems to me that parents should have access to an independent panel of experts who could advise them, not on causation but on whether they had reasonable grounds for proceeding. Lawyers from either side should not be allowed to go on seeking expert opinion until they find one which suits their case.

The assessment of the duties and proper actions of others has to be within the context of the time, place, attitudes and expectations of the carers, resources available, knowledge and understanding of the condition, and in paediatrics, an appreciation of the inherent problems which relate to the age of the child.

I have begun by discussing the initial interview because that is often where the seeds of medical litigation are sown. It has also allowed me to highlight some of the problems in pursuing a course which is fair to all sides.

When the injured person is *a child* there can be special problems. In the remainder of the chapter I shall try and illustrate some of them. The illustrations themselves are contrived, but the issues are real enough.

Problems of Causation When a Child Is Injured

Cause: Unknown

There are still a number of disorders in childhood, for example encephalopathies which cause devastating brain damage, whose aetiology and pathology are not well understood. This was clear from the National Childhood Encephalopathy study. There is a temptation to ascribe resulting damage to those aspects of the clinical course that we do understand.

> *Example.* The parents of a 12-month-old child called their doctor because he had not "been himself" for 24 hours and had begun to vomit and pass frequent loose stools. The GP visited and recommended oral fluids. Over the next 12 hours the child became dehydrated and shocked and was admitted to hospital on a 999 call. On admission i.v. fluids were commenced. On the second and third days the serum sodium level was above 160 mmol/l, and the child began to fit. Recovery was slow and incomplete.

Was the GP negligent? Earlier admission to hospital might perhaps have avoided the development of dehydration and subsequent brain damage due to shock. Did the GP underestimate the severity of the illness or miss early signs of dehydration? Alternately were the hospital doctors at fault for allowing the serum sodium to rise and to stay high for over 24 hours? Might not that alone have been responsible for the encephalopathy?

Both these claims rest on interpreting the clinical course only in terms which we understand. They make no acknowledgement of the many illnesses about whose pathology we know very little. Some of the haemorrhagic encephalopathies present with diarrhoea and vomiting. The children develop dehydration and become shocked very quickly. Correcting these would not necessarily avoid the damage. Presuming that failure to correct them was the reason for the resulting disability has been the basis for a number of claims of negligence.

Sometimes in the course of such illnesses moderate hypernatraemia develops. The reasons are not always evident. Again to ascribe any resulting disability to failure to detect, or when detected to correct hypernatraemia, is tempting because of the earlier work which showed an association between hypernatraemia and brain damage in children with severe dehydration. It is a presumption to conclude that the high serum sodium level was the cause, or the major cause and that correction of the high level would have avoided brain damage. Of course, a high serum sodium level is not desirable and when it is identified attempts should be made to correct it. It is a mistake not to be aware how much sodium is being administered not only in the rehydration and maintenance fluids but also alkalis given to correct acidosis (8.4% Na Bicarb contains 1000 mmol/l of sodium). Nevertheless without more information it would be wrong, in my view, to conclude that any different action by the doctors would have avoided the tragic outcome. We must acknowledge that often we do not know why a particular child either dies or is left with residual brain damage after a serious illness and others are not. The issue of whether the doctors were negligent also rests on whether they acted properly at the time in the light of what they knew or should have known.

Incorrect Presumption of Cause

No one doubts that severe birth asphyxia can cause death or permanent brain damage. It is all too easy to conclude that if a child suffered birth asphyxia and has cerebral palsy that the one caused the other. The majority of infants at the time of birth experience asphyxia to some degree. The causation argument rests on the severity of the asphyxia [7]. If severe asphyxia is defined by a low Apgar score at one minute after birth, then it has to be said that by far the majority of those with Apgar scores of 2 or below at one minute do not develop cerebral palsy and that by far the majority of those children with cerebral palsy did not have Apgar scores of 2 or below at one minute. It then gets very difficult at any level of proof to assert that birth asphyxia caused the cerebral palsy [9].

Nevertheless the "association" of birth asphyxia and cerebral palsy has led paediatricians and others to advise parents that their child's handicap was probably due to birth asphyxia on the lightest of evidence; it follows that the parents then ask why if midwifes and obstetricians were overseeing the pregnancy they did not take steps to avoid such damage. Obstetricians have responded by devising increasingly sophisticated systems to detect fetal asphyxia and when they detect it, to control delivery. The hidden message is that the fetal asphyxia was responsible. Small maternity units without a 24-hour expert team on call have closed, they are no longer safe. More cynically, they are too great a legal risk. The consequences of these events are still unfolding.

> *Example.* A 25-year-old mother at 39 weeks gestation became aware of decreased fetal movements. The obstetrician admitted her to the antenatal ward at her GP's request. 24 hours after admission fetal heart rate irregularities were detected and a Caesarean section (CS) was performed 2 hours later when the operating theatre became free. The infant at birth was pale, the heart rate below 100 beats/minute. With tracheal intubation and lung infection the heart rate accelerated so that the Apgar score at 1 minute was 2. By 5 minutes the infant was pink and making respiratory efforts, by 10 minutes the tube had been removed and the baby was crying. The subsequent newborn period was uneventful. When he was 18 months old the child was found to have cerebral palsy.

Was the cerebral palsy due to intra-uterine asphyxia? Would a CS on the day of admission have avoided brain damage? Was the obstetrician at fault for not performing a CS on admission, or at least immediately the fetal heart irregularities were recorded?

We collect evidence of associations by defining an initial episode and a clinical outcome. From it we may conclude that a child experiencing the initial episode is at increased risk of suffering the undesired outcome. It does not follow from this that by avoiding the initial episode the outcome would be avoided. The two may be both expressions of an underlying pathology. If the infant's brain was damaged, say by rubella infection in early pregnancy, then such an infant is more likely to show signs of fetal distress in late pregnancy or when the uterus begins to contract strongly and is likely to have residual neurological damage from the intra-uterine infection. Performing a CS to avoid fetal distress would not avoid the outcome. How can we decide whether asphyxia was or was not responsible?

The Clinical Features of the Outcome

Little it appears can be gained by studying the brain of the damaged child, though EEG and CT recordings may in rare instances suggest other diagnoses, for example congenital toxoplasmosis. The clustering of the disorders and their development over time may help. For example, it is most unlikely that isolated mental retardation is the outcome of birth asphyxia for such damage appears to invariably involve the motor centres. Again on current evidence it would seem that isolated deafness or epilepsy are most unlikely to be the sole outcome of birth asphyxia. Obviously *developing* hearing loss or visual difficulties or *progressive* mental deterioration cannot be ascribed to asphyxia. However children with spastic quadriplegia can become increasingly disabled without evidence of further brain damage. Problems of interpretation arise when the child shows unusual dysmorphic features or a number of minor congenital anomalies. A child with Down's syndrome is as vulnerable to birth asphyxia as any other, perhaps even more so.

The Clinical Features of the Initial Event

These can be more helpful. It would be wrong on these matters to rely on the parents' recall of the events. There is no alternative but to look at the original records. Sadly these are often not as helpful as they might be. They are, of course, written by doctors to assist in the management of the child at the time and not primarily for experts trying to tease out the causes of handicaps which at that time were unforeseen. Often those reading the notes seeking enlightenment have not only more experience and a wider knowledge but also have the benefit of medical information published after the event. They also have far more time to study the notes than the doctors had to write them. I have been troubled on many occasions when experts and lawyers alike have concluded that because the notes are inadequate for their requirements that that reflects in some way the care the child received. Excellent note keeping has a disproportionate value when matters are in dispute. If hospital authorities are to stay in business they would be wise to require more precise collection of data to meet their legal obligations.

Given good record keeping of the event at the time it is often possible to reinterpret what happened in the light of the outcome. Thus the obstetric events may record fetal distress in early labour with recovery, the resuscitation record may indicate the need to assist the infant to establish independent existence, the neonatal records may describe an encephalopathic illness and the infant clinic records document poor post-natal brain growth as indicated by skull circumference. Given that sequence then we can be fairly confident that the infant suffered an insult in the early stages of labour.

However, any one of those episodes in isolation is a far weaker ground for establishing the cause. The signs of intra-uterine asphyxia are poor predictors, babies after birth can have many apnoeic episodes without residual damage, children can be unconscious with encephalopathies or after head injuries and make a full recovery.

Asphyxia immediately after birth and the need for active resuscitation are equally unhelpful. The Apgar score is not a measure of birth asphyxia but a guide to resuscitation, if the infant is flat at birth then immediate resuscitation is indicated, thus an Apgar at 1 minute tells you how successful you have been, which might be a commentary on the state of the infant or the skill of the operator. Likewise if the infant has not been resuscitated then an Apgar score at 1 minute tells whether the infant has begun to breathe; he or she may have failed to do so for many reasons including maternal sedation as well as birth asphyxia. If this is true for the Apgar score at 1 minute it is even more the case at 5 and 10 minutes. Nelson and Ellenberg [9] have reported the association between the Apgar score and brain damage. Not surprisingly the correlation is weak. In their analyses we have no information on the skill of the attending staff.

Neonatal encephalopathy, sometimes called asphyxial encephalopathy is a stronger predictor of outcome, but even so it is not very helpful. The name "asphyxial" encephalopathy is an assumption for in some there is no previous history of fetal asphyxia or resuscitation problems immediately after birth. In the studies reported, infants with grade III invariably die, infants with grade II usually die but may survive with severe damage, infants with grade I make a full recovery. Grade I encephalopathy is not a guarantee of intact survival but it does mean that Grade I encephalopathy in itself is not a sufficient cause.

A head circumference, after the swelling caused by the birth process has subsided, which falls across the centile charts over the first months of life, is strong evidence of a damaging event around the time of birth; on the other hand normal growth in head circumference does not exclude the possibility.

Inadequate Evidence

There was no doubt at that time, and there is no doubt now, that a small percentage of those vaccinated with the smallpox vaccine suffered a reactive encephalopathy [1]. Some died, the others after an unpleasant illness usually recovered fully. Smallpox is such a devastating illness that no one doubted the benefits of protection when balanced against a rare adverse reaction. Happily the immunisation programme against smallpox has been so effective that we no longer have the dilemma of the benefit–risk ratio for smallpox vaccination.

It was very reasonable and proper for Dr Wilson and colleagues [6] to be concerned that the pertussis vaccine might cause a severe encephalopathic reaction in certain vulnerable children. They published their clinical experience in which the two events, DTP vaccination and an encephalopathic illness, were chronologically associated. Both before their observations and since, every effort has been made to define a clinical course, to identify a characteristic pathology, to establish diagnostic tests, to produce animal models and to seek effective precautions and remedies, all with no success. The reaction if there was one was not like the encephalopathy that followed smallpox vaccination.

Once the question was raised that pertussis vaccination might cause an encephalopathic reaction with or without resultant brain damage it was inevitable that the Authorities would advise caution [6]. Alas the consequence was a loss of public confidence not only in immunisation against pertussis but the other vaccines as well, including the very successful poliomyelitis vaccine. The government advisory committee, the Joint Committee on Vaccination and Immunisation [JCVI] concerned by this development, initiated a nationwide study of brain damaging events in infancy. Of over 1000 such episodes only 32 were chronologically associated with pertussis vaccination. One important conclusion from this study was that many infants suffer from encephalopathic responses whose pathogenicity is not understood. Establishing that a small number occurred after vaccination did not establish that the vaccine was responsible. It might have been chance. In fact it was calculated that it was three to four times the number expected. That is worrying, but in itself it still does not establish cause and effect. What was also clear, however, was that the whooping cough itself was associated with a far larger number of brain damaging events and that it still occasionally caused death. The report strengthened the view of the Joint Committee on Vaccination and Immunisation that whether or not the vaccine, on extremely rare occasions, caused encephalpathic reactions, the benefit–risk ratio in favour of the vaccine was clear [3].

What were parents to think when their child was left severely damaged and their medical advisors, for want of an alternative, told them that the illness was probably due to the vaccine?

> *Example.* An 18-year-old young man is severely disabled with spastic quadriplegia, mental retardation and fits. His parents recall that he had a severe illness with fitting which developed 2 days after his second DTP [diphtheria, tetanus, pertussis] jab, and that he was never the same again. On questioning they reported that he had a difficult birth and required special nursing for a few days and that they nearly did not give him the vaccine because he had the snuffles at the time. They sought compensation under the Compensation Act and were awarded £12 000.

Was the vaccine at fault, and if so, does a liability rest with the company that made it, the government who recommended it, the Health Authority who supplied it, the GP who signed the prescription or the nurse who injected it? Were there contraindications to the vaccination which should have been heeded?

As a result of the public concern about the possible damaging effects of vaccination the government passed a bill to recompense those who could establish a chronological relationship between the brain-damaging illness and the administration of the vaccine. It is a form of no-fault compensation. All the parents had to demonstrate was the chronological association. The amounts over the years have been relatively modest, £10 000 rising to £20 000. One effect of this legislation was to reinforce the public view that the vaccine was culpable. It was inevitable that parents would seek fuller compensation through the courts. Thus it was that Mr Justice Stuart Smith heard evidence from world experts on causation, and produced a judgement which should be mandatory reading for all those wishing to establish causation [5]. He found the case unproven. It might be asked why the scientific facts of the matter had not been subject to similar scrutiny by the Authorities and the medical profession many years earlier. Much of the evidence related to the interpretation of the national childhood encephalopathy study, some of which had not then been published. The previous assumption of causation was based on inadequate data.

Questions about contraindications complicated the issues further. Recommendations listing contraindications suggest that under certain circumstances the vaccine can cause damage. They were initially based on what was considered to be clinical common sense. They were not based on any scientific inquiry. Happily the UK list of contraindications has been adjusted. There was a time in the UK when it was recommended that infants known to have suffered brain damage should be given the pertussis vaccine because they were thought to be at greater risk of adverse reactions, whilst in France a special effort was made to vaccinate infants with brain damage because they were particularly vulnerable to the infection. The teams of experts came to contrary recommendations on the benefit–risk ratio. The UK position is now closer to that in France. In another country, doctors and authorities are being sued because they withheld the pertussis vaccine on the basis of contraindications. The child in question was damaged by the whooping cough illness.

Circumstances Long Passed

The law allows claims with regard to children to be made long after the event, for at the time of the incident it may not be apparent that damage has been done, or it may not be possible to assess its full consequences. This also means that parents can repeatedly review their grievance in the light of a better understanding of the condition and increasing expectations of the success of medical care. Establishing causation for brain damage which occurred many years ago is complicated not only by the difficulties of knowing what the practice was at that time, but also because the medical and nursing records are often lost or have been destroyed.

> *Example.* A 27-week infant was delivered 20 years ago in a gynaecological ward. The nurse attended to the mother; the aborted foetus was placed in a kidney dish; some minutes later a noise was heard; the infant was still alive. He was taken round to the nursery and placed in an incubator and given oxygen. Amazingly he survived, but was left damaged.

Delivering infants at 27 weeks gestation in a gynaecological ward is not acceptable practice now, but was there anything that they might have done which damaged the child or which they should have done to protect the infant according to the standards of the time? When it was explained to the lawyers that 20 to 25 years ago it was often the practice to place the foetus under 28 weeks gestation with the other extruded products, it was their firm opinion that there was no defence for medical or nursing staff who did that. Would it be possible to find an expert to go into court to assert that that was a practice that he or she recommended 25 years ago? Only in the last 20 years have infants under 28 weeks gestation survived [4].

Delayed Outcome

Whilst the idea that we should be judged by the standard of 20 years hence seems inherently unfair, it is not difficult to sympathise with parents who believed that their child had fully recovered from a serious illness only to discover later that that was not so. During the formative years much of the developing brain is silent. It is only as the child grows and the brain begins to do its work that underlying defects may become evident. Evidence of permanent damage may only become clear many years after the damaging illness. That is the reason why a child can seek remedy in law up to 21 years after the event (see Chap. 17). It does however present particular problems in establishing causation.

> *Example.* An infant 4 months of age went off his feed and his parents called their GP. The GP examined the child and finding nothing specific prescribed a teething powder. The infant was reluctant to take the powder but the parents persisted. He began to vomit and became increasingly drowsy. They called the GP again, who advised them to take him straight to hospital. The Casualty doctor saw him and wrote "?meningitis" in the notes and arranged admission to the ward where lumbar puncture (LP) was performed and antibiotics were given. The records indicate that the time of arrival in casualty was 12.00 h and the cerebro-spinal fluid (CSF) report was timed at 16.00 h and the prescription chart indicated that the first antibiotics were given at 17.00 h. The medical records did not give the times. The Senior House Officer (SHO) was fairly confident that a bolus dose of antibiotics would have been given much earlier but would not necessarily have been written on the prescription chart. The parents were told at the time that the illness was so severe their child might not survive. But the child survived and made good progress, so much so that the paediatrician reassured the parents that all was well and discharged him from follow-up clinic 3 months later. When he was 2 years old the finding of mild spasticity, poor speech development, and a short attention span suggested that their child was disabled. They gave the child all the love and care that they were able. Problems for them arose when their child became an adult, they were getting older and they saw the time coming when they would no longer be able to protect and care for him. They wished to ensure that their child received care in the future. The welfare state meets only some of the needs of disabled adults. The parents took the one route open to them to get extra resources, they sued the doctors on the grounds that the damage should not have occurred in the first place.

Meningitis is a potentially damaging disorder, happily most children survive and are undamaged but it was not always so. However there is now the expectation that all children should survive unharmed. Claims of negligence are not uncommon when they do not. Resolving the question is not easy. Sometimes the claim is against the GP who had seen the child the day before admission, sometimes it is against the hospital doctors for prescribing antibiotics which by present standards are considered inadequate, or because they were slow to perform the necessary test, or delayed antibiotic administration. On reflection, in the example, did the GP miss early signs of meningitis? Would he be able to defend teething powders? As for the hospital team, is a 5-hour delay between hospital admission and the administration of antibiotics acceptable in the absence of any explanation in the hospital records for the delay?

To read the records written 20 years ago and to try and interpret what was in the mind of those who wrote them can be very difficult. Often the senior doctors concerned are dead and therefore cannot help, but even if they are alive they are unable to recall an event 20 years ago. Any recollections they may have will be distorted by the passage of time. When a doctor is challenged with respect to events long ago, they end up saying what they would have done. That, of course, would be what we would have liked to have thought we would have done and the judge knows that. In such circumstances it does not help to claim a standard of practice which whilst appropriate in later years would not have been possible at the time of the event in question. To be wrong and unreliable on one matter undermines any confidence the judge might have in our general competence. There is no substitute for good contemporaneous records.

The general question of meningitis and resulting brain damage is also more complicated than it first appears. Without treatment meningitis in childhood is usually fatal. It is tempting to conclude that with delayed or inadequate treatment, life may be preserved but damage remains. However there is plenty of evidence that, in some instances at least, once the disease presents the damage has already occurred. Deafness has been found on presentation. The main argument for the introduction of a vaccine against *Haemophilus influenzae* infections in the UK is that neither a better health care delivery service, nor more effective antibiotics will significantly, if at all, reduce the mortality and morbidity that follows *H. influenzae* meningitis. The cost–benefit analyses are based on this assumption.

The question of causation when the child is assessed many years after the damaging event becomes particularly testing when the brain has not been extensively damaged. Concepts of minimal brain damage, a cognitive performance below what was expected, hyperactivity, uncontrollable behaviour, whilst they are open to clinical definition are not obvious clinical entities. The causes are many and multifactorial, they may include a genetic contribution, an unfavourable intra-uterine environment, limited early nutrition, hypersensitivity to food additives, limited parenting skills and instability of the social environment. Whilst "minimal" brain damage, limited cognitive performance, and hyperactivity suggest trivial problems this is far from the case. Both with regard to education and success in life they can have major consequences for the individual and the family.

Who is to say whether or not in the future, in the light of discoveries in the next 20 years that such affected persons might not consider that doctors should have taken more care in the light of what is already known.

Multiple Causes

It is always easier when everything is simple. There are powerful forces which operate in legal settings to keep it simple. I was a little nonplussed when a judge said that what I was trying to say, which depended on an understanding of the oxygen dissociation curve, was too difficult to follow. To me, it was central to the point I wished to make. He did not understand it and did not accept my conclusion. The truth of the matter is that the causes of disease are rarely simple, the clinical expressions and complications reflect a complicated interaction involving many factors and we are aware of only some of them.

> *Example.* A mother delivered her baby at 28-weeks gestation. Both she and her husband believed that being given the blood of another is wrong. The doctors who had care of the child in the neonatal unit in deference to their wishes limited the number of blood samples they took to monitor the child's condition over the first few critical days to avoid the need to give top-up transfusions. The baby had cyanotic episodes and was given oxygen-enriched air to breath. The infant survived and is progressing well except she is blind due to scarring as a consequence of retinopathy of prematurity (ROP).

Were the doctors in error giving extra oxygen when they were unable to monitor the infant's blood gases according to their usual practice? This raises many questions. The first is, does extra oxygen cause ROP? It *was* the clinical accepted view that oxygen *was* the major contributor to ROP, but a scrutiny of the original studies indicates that this was far from established. Many premature infants who were given oxygen in excess of their requirements did not become blind, and some children who became blind did not receive added oxygen. If infants are examined routinely then a large percentage of those under 28 weeks' gestation develop ROP even when blood oxygen pressures are monitored continuously. ROP is still a common development despite our efforts to avoid oxygen excess. Only a very small percentage of those who have ROP go on to have scarring with loss of vision. Why some infants advance to this unhappy outcome is not known [12]. Analysis of the clinical records of those infants who develop ROP or have residual visual loss has indicated that many adverse factors are associated with the development of the condition. The one required factor is immaturity, the associated conditions include birth asphyxia, post-natal hypoxia and hypercapnoea, patent ductus arteriosus, intracranial bleeds, cyanotic and apnoeic episodes, etc. To say that there is any one cause would be wrong. In my view to assert that excessive oxygen is a sole cause is also incorrect. Can it be claimed to be a significant cause?

In the example there was another issue; in their duty to the infant patient should the doctors have compromised their clinical practice to accommodate the parents wishes? It has left them unable to establish that they did not give excess oxygen. It has been argued that the fall in incidence of blindness due to ROP, after oxygen administration was curtailed, established that excess oxygen damaged the retina. Alas, subsequent studies showed that as a consequence of limiting the supply of oxygen to very sick immature infants more of them died. It is the sickest infants who are most likely to develop the severest forms of ROP, it was therefore to be expected that the number of children left blind by ROP would fall.

If it is accepted, as some assert, that oxygen excess is a significant cause, where then lies the limit of the duties of those who have care of these very sick infants to monitor the infants blood oxygen pressures? Frequent checks in the first days are possible. Often, however, infants have cyanotic attacks and occasionally respiratory failure persists into the fifth and sixth week of life when serial blood oxygen tensions often cannot be measured for technical reasons. Are transcutaneous oxygen tension values or oxygen saturation levels sufficient? It is as well to remember that another common reason for litigation by parents of prematurely born infants is because of residual injury which follows damage to arteries and veins.

Fault

Duty of Care

This is a legal notion. If a doctor is to be found at fault it has to be established that he or she had a duty to care, but there are some grey areas. House officers on appointment are not skilled in neonatal care, but they are often left to manage without cover because experienced staff are simply not available. Consultants covering neonatal units are not as skilled as the younger registrars in performing the technical procedures; it may be the unsteady hand and the failing vision or it may simply be a lack of practice. So those who stand in a duty of care may not always be as competent as they should be.

Who has the responsibility to ensure that an SHO, especially a locum, knows the policies and where everything is? Is it the consultant in charge or is it the administration of the hospital who appointed the doctor? Doctors should perhaps speak louder when they believe the cover to be inadequate. It is recommended that we put our concerns in writing to the administration with a copy to their and our defence organisation.

Omission: A Service That Is Not Good Enough

Negligence implies neglect, that the doctor simply failed to act. Deciding when a doctor should attend or not, and if he is to attend how quickly, are often central to the question of negligence. They cannot be decided on the basis of the clinical facts alone. Any expert opinion is concerned with what that expert considers to be an acceptable service. However, most experts called to give evidence work in fairly privileged settings and are hardly in a position to give a reasonable assessment of what is the norm elsewhere.

For example, how long should it take to perform an emergency CS , how quickly should a neonatal SHO attend an apnoeic infant, how long should it take to perform an intubation? The next question is would the delay have materially contributed to the infant's injuries?

> *Example.* A 2-year-old child was admitted to the paediatric ward with croup. On the first day he remained reasonably well, he drank sufficient to meet his needs and played happily in the ward. On the second day of his admission he was eating well and was observed carefully by the nurses but suddenly collapsed. He stopped breathing and his heart slowed then stopped. Cardiac massage was commenced. During resuscitation the contents of his stomach filled his pharynx frustrating the nurses' efforts to artificially ventilate him with bag and mask. The emergency bell was pressed and the emergency team called. They arrived in 4 minutes. The trachea was intubated without difficulty but he did not begin to respond for a further 10 minutes. He has now got evidence of residual brain damage.

Should all nurses be able to effectively resuscitate any infant who collapses? Should the emergency team have arrived sooner? If it had arrived on the ward within one minute would it have made any difference to the outcome? These are all reasonable questions but they are very difficult to answer.

We hear much these days about standards of practice, quality of care and of audit. It is a delusion to imagine that these, when they are in place, will enable us to do things which we cannot do at present. Just because we have a policy, it does not mean that at all times it will be possible to maintain it. If a woman with triplets delivers them unexpectedly at 28 weeks' gestation in the Accident and Emergency department, then the resources of the largest neonatal services would be severely taxed, if two mothers so behave then we would all fall below our accepted standard. Negligence is below the lower limit of what is permitted in our standards, so the question of how long it should take the emergency team to arrive depends on knowing more than whether their bleep systems were working or not.

Audit will not remove the need for clinical judgement. Sometimes the judgement is when to call and see a patient, or when to invite them to contact you again, or when to go back and check. It is always easy to say after the event, "if only I had gone back and checked". The legal yardstick is whether the majority of doctors in that position, given what was known at the time, would have done so.

Making a Mistake

By contrast when doctors have done things which cause harm the position can be much clearer.

> *Example.* An SHO in a neonatal unit inserted an intravenous line into a sick newborn infant. He wished to wash the line through with saline (NaCl) and asked the nurse for saline. The nurse handed him a phial and he took the top off, drew up the clear fluid and injected it. The baby died. The fluid was potassium chloride (KCl).

No one would suggest that the doctor did it deliberately, nor that the nurse was to blame because she handed it to the doctor. In this instance the doctor is at fault. He made a mistake and is negligent. There can be few of us who cannot remember an experience involving ourselves in which we did not check the phial handed to us, or wrote the wrong dose on a prescription chart, but in which happily there was no adverse outcome. We need to be continuously reminded that in certain activities of clinical medicine we must always follow the rules. Check what is written on the phial before injecting its contents. Check that the dose written on a prescription chart is appropriate. Do not take other people's word for it.

Experience and Training

It is true that a doctor qualified in medicine and surgery and registered can legally practise a whole range of modern therapies. In paediatrics the question of qualification to do the job is brought into sharp focus in the neonatal service. Considerable skill and sensitivity of care are required for success, failure can mean prolonged tragedies. It is an intense 24-hour service where the workload cannot be controlled other than to elect to withhold care. Even in this area the law has intruded; in the USA it is required that everything is done to preserve life by which is meant the legal definition of life, a pulsating heart. Consciously or unconsciously this cannot be considered the sole standard if the good of the individual and the good of the family are put into the equation. Blind obedience to a pulsating heart may represent an abdication of our wider responsibilities. When legal and moral judgements conflict it is as well for us to remember our duty is to the child and family. In these matters we all stand equal, family, house officers, nurses and consultant alike.

Example. A baby was born at 28 weeks' gestation and developed respiratory distress. At 8 hours of age the SHO inserted an umbilical artery catheter and performed a chest X-ray to determine the position of the tip. It was in the left upper thorax. The oxygen sensor at the tip gave irregular results and the Registrar removed the catheter and inserted another. He performed a chest X-ray, the tip was still in the left upper thorax. It transpired that both were in the umbilical vein, not the artery. In both instances the tip had come to rest in the pulmonary vein, and sampled blood returning from the lungs.

Were the doctors negligent for not identifying the catheter was in the wrong vessel? A judge in a similar situation reached the conclusion that the SHO was not, but the Registrar was because he had more experience. For my part I would not distinguish between the two, for in my view anyone who inserts a catheter must know of the necessary checks irrespective of their appointment. It is not expected that a doctor on qualification and registration should know all the answers, but he should know his or her own limitations and seek help when it is needed. It is a wise practice in this as in other matters to record in the official medical records the decisions made and when advice was sought. As with all such notes there should be a date and a time and they should be signed. Then the duty of care on the matter passes to the responsible doctor. If the consultant was not told then he cannot be involved. If he was told and knowing all the facts made a decision which in the event proved to be the wrong one, he is far less likely to be found at fault than an SHO who made the same decision on the basis of less knowledge and less experience.

It takes on political overtones when the issue is one of the size of the establishment needed to provide a safe service, or the need for new and better equipment. All the law requires is that we respond appropriately with what is provided. It would be wrong to attempt an elaborate procedure which puts the patient at risk when it is known that the equipment is inadequate. On the edge of this territory doctors may again be left to make some hard decisions.

In the example given the catheter came to lie where blood samples would have given reliable values of oxygen tensions. No injury flowed from the negligent act.

Negligence and Consequence

In the legal debate it is not only necessary to establish that the doctor was negligent but also the injury resulted from that negligence.

Example. A doctor was called to see a sick child. He did not interpret the call to be urgent but when he arrived some hours later he found the child to be irritable with a petechial rash. On admission to hospital the diagnosis of meningococcal septicemia was confirmed but the child suffered irreversible brain damage.

Would the outcome have been better if he had called earlier, say 3 hours before? The hospital paediatrician is bound to say that the damage might have been avoided if the child had been diagnosed and treated earlier. Well that might be true although there is little evidence to show that earlier diagnosis has significantly reduced the complication rate now that effective antibiotics are available. Nevertheless it has to be said that without any treatment most children would die so there must be some truth in the assertion.

But the scenario is open to another interpretation. If the doctor had arrived sooner the rash might not have been so florid and recognisably petechial, or it may not have been present at all and the doctor could have prescribed for an upper respiratory tract infection and awaited developments. So the tardy attendance though unsatisfactory may not of itself have made any difference.

There may be the claim that in such a situation the doctor should have given an intra-muscular injection of penicillin because that is what government circulars have recommended. The doctor may not have been aware of such advice and for that he could be found to be at fault, but there would be many who would give evidence to the effect that they have read the directive and having given it full consideration have elected not to inject penicillin in such circumstances.

It often seems wrong to me when the whole burden of the outcome is laid upon a single phase in the therapy which can be shown to be due to an action or inaction which fell below an acceptable standard. I have the same feeling when I read the name of a junior doctor who has been selected from a team of doctors who were involved with the care of a child critically ill for many days, simply because it is thought that a case can be made against him on the evidence available. In such matters some noble registrars and consultants state unequivocally that they share the responsibility but to the lawyers this is an irrelevance because they have not been named in the claim and they cannot be shown to be at fault, if fault there is. It is the professional responsibility of lawyers to present their client's case to the client's best advantage whatever the rights and wrongs of the wider issues might be.

Shared Responsibilities: Parents as Partners

In paediatric practice we are increasingly involving the parents as partners. We rely on their observations, we depend on them to seek help when they need it, and we bow to their assessment of their child's wellbeing. It is a matter of judgement how much we should depend on the parents. One family doctor knowing the mother was a sensible and professional person depended on her good sense to call him again if the infant deteriorated. In the event she did not, was the doctor then at fault, as she thought he was? Who made an error of judgement? In this instance the judge sided with the doctor. One family demanded of the family doctor that their child be referred to hospital and the SHO after a careful examination elected not to admit the child. He informed the general practitioner. Ten days later the child died and was found to have evidence of pneumonia. Was the SHO at fault, as the GP and family thought he was? In the intervening 10 days the GP had not visited and the family had not called him. Some parents may call the doctor too often. Others believe the doctor knows more than he actually does about what is happening and do not call him often enough. It is very difficult when a doctor is charged with not acting promptly, to argue that the parents fell short of what might reasonably be expected or that it was inaction on their part that was largely to blame.

Quantum, Assessing the Future

Quantum refers to how much compensation the families receive and relates to the consequences of the illness itself and the degree of residual disability. To assist them in making their assessment on how much money must be paid, lawyers ask medical experts for advice on the child's future. As with cause and fault, there are special problems when the injured person is a child. How will the injury limit the child's education, achievements, family life, longevity and happiness? What was the child's potential and what is the child's potential now? These are all difficult matters so it is not surprising the size of the awards appear somewhat arbitrary. Usually the award takes the form of a lump sum, as it is meant to provide for the child without regard to any support the child might receive from the State. Anyone who reflects upon the overall fairness of the current legal arrangements whereby people injured as a result of medical negligence seek compensation are bound to wonder whether no-fault compensation schemes might not be more acceptable. This issue is the subject of a recent report of the Royal College of Physicians [11].

References

1. Conybeare ET (1964) Illness attributed to smallpox vaccination during 1951-1960. Monthly bulletin. Ministry of Health and Public Health Laboratory Service, HMSO, London, 23: 126-133, 150-159, 182-186
2. Department of Health and Social Security (1981). Whooping cough. HMSO, London
3. Department of Health, Welsh Office and Scottish Home and Health Department (1990) Immunisation against infectious disease. HMSO, London
4. Hull D (1988) The viable child. The Croonian Lecture. J R Coll Phys Lond 22: 169-176
5. Judgement in Loveday v. Renton by Right Honourable Lord Justice Stuart-Smith, 1988
6. Kulenkampff M, Schwartzman JS, Wilson J (1974) Neurological complications of pertussis inoculation. Arch Dis Child 49: 46-49
7. Levene MJ, Sands C, Grindalis H et al. (1986) Comparison of two methods of predicting outcome in perinatal asphyxia. Lancet ii: 67-68
8. Nelson KB (1988) What proportion of cerebral palsy is related to birth asphyxia? J Pediatr 112: 572-574
9. Nelson KB, Ellenberg JH (1981) Apgar scores as predictors of chronic neurologic disability. Paediatrics 68: 36-43
10. Paneth N, Stark K (1983) Cerebral palsy and mental retardation in relation to indications and perinatal asphyxia. Am J Obstet Gynecol 147: 960-962
11. Report of the Royal College of Physicians (1990) Compensation for adverse consequences of medical intervention. Royal College of Physicians, London
12. Silverman WA (1980) Retrolental fibroplasia. Grune and Stratton, New York

CHAPTER 14

Psychiatry

G.L. Harrison

A practical approach to medico-legal problems in psychiatry depends upon a sound grasp of the theoretical principles involved. We shall therefore deal briefly with the principles of torts, liability and compensation, before examining in detail the special problems involved in evaluating the claims of victims who have suffered psychiatric injury. The growing field of medical negligence claims in relation to psychiatric treatment will not be dealt with here, although many of the principles and practical points outlined in this chapter will also apply to these cases.

Some Legal Principles

Law of Torts

The word "tort" derives from the latin "tortus", meaning "twisted" or "crooked". It provides a vivid description of the wrong-doing which in civil law may result in a claim for damages. The law of torts essentially provides a legal framework for compensation where the interests of one party have been harmed by acts, whether of omission or commission, of another.

The purpose of the criminal law is to protect the interests of the general public by punishing those who break the laws which regulate our social behaviour. Criminal proceedings are initiated by the Crown, or by the State. In contrast, the law of torts protects the interests of *individuals* on the basis that society does not accept that the consequences of unreasonable behaviour should be borne by innocent victims. The victim, as the plaintiff, therefore seeks to attribute *liability* for his losses to the party he holds to be responsible for his misfortune (the defendants).

Liability

In many cases the problem of establishing the fault, or liability, can be easily solved. For example, there is likely to be little debate about liability where one party to an accident has failed to stop at red traffic lights. In many instances, however, the issues may be less clear cut and liability may be the first matter needing to be settled by the court. The court may decide in certain cases that the plaintiff has a degree of *contributory negligence*, and his or her claim for damages will be reduced accordingly.

Although this aspect of the civil action is a legal matter not involving the psychiatrist, he should be aware of the possible effects of mental disorder on the plaintiff at this stage in the proceedings. A depressed plaintiff, for example, haunted by a sense of guilt and self-blame may be reluctant to pursue a claim for an incident in which he can only perceive his own culpable actions.

Compensation for Pain, Suffering and "Psychiatric Injury"

Once liability has been established, claims may be contested on the basis of *quantum*, i.e. the amount of damages thought to be appropriate to the injury involved. This may be relatively straightforward when dealing, for example, with a simple and straightforward injury such as a broken limb.

Recent major disasters in the UK such as Zeebrugge and Hillsborough have focused public attention upon the psychological repercussions of trauma. In the past, lawyers have been reluctant to pursue psychological aspects of their clients' injuries, because of the complex problems involved. "Nervous" problems and emotional difficulties are still stigmatised in the public mind, and often equated with weakness, dependence or "low moral fibre". The courts are understandably suspicious of claims for disorders which seem to depend so much upon the history given by the plaintiff. Nevertheless, the courts are now beginning to accept that emotional pain, and the suffering associated with psychiatric disorders, may in some cases involve far greater distress for victims than a straightforward physical injury, and indeed continue to afflict them for many years after the event. Compensation for psychiatric injury is therefore a growing area in the field of civil litigation, but demands careful consideration of the special problems involved. In particular, there are problems of reliable definition of "illness" or "disorder", and difficulties in establishing causality and in differentiating the genuine from the fraudulent. These particular issues will be dealt with separately, before going on to consider some of the common disorders encountered in medico-legal practice.

Psychiatric Injury: Some Special Problems

Causation and Vulnerability

Legal problems of causality are among the most complicated and controversial issues of the law of torts. This is especially so for psychiatric problems. For example, consider the case of a patient who sustained a physical injury as a result of a road traffic accident and loses his job. Supposing that he becomes depressed and takes an overdose of medication, sustaining a degree of permanent brain damage. To what extent can this train of events be considered the "fault" of the defendant? Could the defendant have reasonably foreseen such an outcome to his actions and taken steps to avoid it?

In these circumstances, the wrong-doers liability must somehow be limited. Under common law, this is achieved by the doctrine of *"proximate liability"*, which attempts to exclude those consequences of the defendant's liability which are considered to be too remote from the incident of wrong-doing. However, because of the complicated nature of some incidents, it may be necessary to ask a court to make a judgement on the basis of each individual case.

Although sometimes an extremely complicated matter, the issue of causation is crucial to the success of a claim for compensation. The plaintiff may recover damages only for those problems which can be shown to have been caused by the defendant's wrongful actions. In considering causality, the psychiatrist or psychologist must take several factors into account, including vulnerability of the plaintiff, any pre-existing condition and the role of other life events around the time of the accident.

The question of vulnerability is particularly relevant where the severity of the emotional or psychiatric symptoms after an injury appears disproportionate to the stress associated with the incident itself. Psychiatrists are of course aware that vulnerability to breaking down under stress results from a complicated interaction of genetic and constitutional factors. Where such factors exist, the defendant may argue that they can hardly be held responsible for the patient's idiosyncratic and unusual response to a trauma which would have been negotiated with relative ease by the vast majority of "normal" individuals.

Fortunately, this issue has been simplified by an important legal precedent: the "thin skull principle". This ruling says that a plaintiff who suffers greater injury in an accident because of his thin skull cannot be held responsible because a person with a normal thickness skull would have suffered lesser damages. In other words, "you must take a victim as you find him".

The thin skull principle was further extended in 1970 when Judge Lane ruled:

> The defendant must take [the plaintiff] as he finds her and there is no difference between an eggshell skull and an eggshell personality. [*Malcolm* v. *Broadhurst* 1970.]

On the basis of this judgement, if the psychiatrist can demonstrate that, but for the injury, the psychiatric difficulties were unlikely to have occurred, then the plaintiff is entitled to be compensated, regardless of his vulnerability at the time. This introduces the "but for" principle which may also assist in disentangling factors of causality:

> If the damage would not have happened but for a particular fault, then that fault is the cause of the damage; if it would have happened just the same, fault or no fault, the fault is not the cause of the damage [15].

There is a compelling logic here which appears to clarify the central issues for the legal mind. The law wishes to identify the factor that "tips the balance" or the "straw that breaks the camel's back". Unfortunately, the psychiatrist and physician is more used to dealing with complex relationships between the human body and mind, and may often take a multifactorial and interactive view of causality, in which no one event can be singled out as the overriding factor. Consequently, in many contested cases the defendants may obtain an expert witness prepared to identify a different "final straw" to that of the plaintiff, or to argue that, given the background of the patient, the condition would have occurred regardless of the accident. It is important in these circumstances that the psychiatrist, whether appearing on behalf of the plaintiff or defendant, makes himself fully aware of the previous history and background of the patient and is prepared to offer an informed and reasonable judgement and to remain impartial. It is often necessary to offer the court a judgement based upon the "balance of probabilities".

Pre-existing Conditions

Psychiatric *vulnerability* must be distinguished from a *pre-existing* condition. Inevitably, a degree of judgement is required: a few minor symptoms of anxiety could hardly be considered to constitute a pre-existing condition compared with symptoms of a severe post-traumatic stress disorder or major depressive illness following a major trauma. On the other hand, consider the case of a victim of a road traffic accident complaining of panic attacks and agoraphobic symptoms who had similar symptoms, but present to a lesser degree, prior to the accident. The victim here is considered to have suffered an *aggravation of a pre-existing condition*, and compensation will be adjusted accordingly. In these circumstances, defendants may attempt to "play up" the change in their symptoms following a trauma and the court requires an accurate assessment from an expert witness of both the pre- and post-accident condition of the patient, corroborated by a history from informants and all available case notes. For certain patients, the nature of a pre-existing condition may be such that it is more than likely that the victim of an accident would have developed his symptoms anyway. For example, a patient with a unipolar affective disorder shows no discernible change in either the frequency or severity of depressive episodes after an accident. The psychiatrist must make clear the nature of this pre-existing condition, whether instructed by the plaintiff or the defendant. In certain cases, the pattern of the illness may suggest that its progress has been *accelerated* by a trauma, and damages may be awarded accordingly.

Problems of Defining Illness Boundaries

> The court has to draw a line between sorrow and grief for which damages are not recoverable, and nervous shock and psychiatric illness for which damages are recoverable. [Lord Denning: Hinz v. Berry 1970, Court of Appeal].

The courts recognise that psychiatric disorder must be distinguished from general pain and suffering. Significant psychiatric symptoms were first referred to as "nervous shock" and entitlement to compensation for such was accepted in 1910 in *Yates* v. *South Kirkby and Company Collieries Ltd*. It was said that "nervous shock" causing incapacity for work was as much "personal injury by accident" as a broken limb or other physical injury. The term "nervous shock" subsequently became something of a hallowed expression, but the difficulties of defining its boundaries have always been acknowledged:

The basic difficulty of the subject arises from the fact that the crucial answers to the questions which it raises lie in the difficult field of psychiatric medicine. The common law gives no damages for the emotional distress which any normal person experiences when someone he loves is killed or injured. Anxiety and depression are normal human emotions. Yet an anxiety neurosis or reactive depression may be a recognisable psychiatric illness, with or without psychosomatic symptoms. So the first hurdle which a plaintiff claiming damages of the kind in question must surmount is to establish that he is suffering, not merely grief, distress or any other normal emotions, but a positive psychiatric illness. [Lord Bridge: McLoughlin v. O'Brian 1983.]

The court clearly requires from the psychiatric expert witness answers to certain specific questions: Firstly does the plaintiff suffer from a recognised psychiatric illness or may his difficulties be understood in terms of "normal" suffering? As the above judgement by Lord Bridge illustrates, the courts are only too aware that much psychiatric illness lies on a continuum with the normal range of human emotions and suffering. The psychiatrist is no stranger to making difficult diagnostic decisions. The usual concepts of defining disorder apply: are symptoms present to such a degree that they disrupt normal social and occupational functioning or cause significant personal suffering? Do they follow a recognised clinical pattern? Is there an "autonomous" quality to affective symptoms, and does the patient suffer biological symptoms of depression or anxiety? Inevitably, a clinical judgement is required and, as always, a diagnosis should incorporate a collateral history obtained from as many sources as possible.

It is recommended that the psychiatrist should provide a diagnosis in terms of one of the major classifications of diseases, namely the International Classification of Diseases of the WHO (ninth or tenth edition) or the Diagnostic and Statistical Manual (DSM-111-R, 1983) of the American Psychiatric Association. Although in an evolving field of knowledge no classification can be perfect, these more recent systems outline the criteria necessary to achieve a diagnosis and describe the symptoms in considerable detail. As both of these classifications have been produced following extensive international consultation it may be argued that they fairly represent a consensus of views among leading clinicians and researchers in the profession. They may therefore assist a court in evaluating the views of any single practitioner offering "expert" evidence. This may be especially important in hysteria and somatoform disorders (see below) where an expert witness may deny that such conditions exist at all.

Secondly, in what sense does the plaintiff suffer a psychiatric disorder? In other words, the psychiatrist must assist the court in understanding the implications of the diagnosis in terms of the experience of the patient and the pain and suffering involved. The implications for the social and occupational functioning of the patient should be explored, together with relevant treatment options. If possible, the psychiatrist should demonstrate how biological vulnerability, early experience and recent trauma have interacted to produce the symptom pattern which has been described.

Lack of Objective Validation and Malingering

Because the psychiatrist is so dependent upon what the patient tells him about his condition, he must be especially aware of the temptation on the part of the patient to exaggerate his symptoms. Collie [5], a physician retained as medical examiner for an insurance company, documentated the phenomenal rise of industrial accidents over the first few months after the Workman's Compensation Act in 1906. He estimated that, of 3667 accident cases examined by himself, about 8% were malingering. However, he pointed to another sizable group of claimants who, he believed, straddle the borderline between the genuine and the fraudulent. He suggested that the compensation issue created a climate which encouraged the thoughts of claimants to "run along the line of least resistance". In other words, the claimant would be inclined to blame all of his symptoms and difficulties upon the accident or, when faced with returning to unrewarding and laborious work, choose to continue as disabled rather than make the mental and physical effort required to overcome his symptoms. The longer he or she is off work, the more difficult it is to embark upon active rehabilitation.

Henry Miller, a neurologist writing several decades later described a similar process. Miller [21] reported that claims for compensation were often more frequent among the lower social classes, and most often sought from large employers and especially nationalised industries. Miller's work has often been quoted in litigation and deserves some attention. The study was based upon a review of 47 out of 200 consecutive cases of head injury with post-traumatic neurotic symptoms, mostly referred by insurance companies. He concluded that the "cardinal feature" of such patients was the unshakeable conviction of unfitness to work and a resolute refusal to admit to any symptomatic improvement whatsoever. He characterised the patients' attitude as one of "martyred gloom". His follow-up of patients suggested that the vast majority of cases resolved rapidly following settlement of the claim.

Few of Miller's findings have been replicated and his work may be subject to considerable methodological criticism on account of biased sampling, non-blind assessments and unwarranted generalisations. In particular, more recent follow-up studies have suggested that the majority of such patients do not improve after settlement of their claim [1,29,30]. These studies also have methodological problems, but the weight of recent evidence regarding long-term outcome is set firmly against the findings of Miller.

It should be noted that Miller himself avoided a simple conscious/unconscious division of causality: "accident neurosis is not an entirely homogeneous syndrome, but represents a spectrum ranging from gross conversion hysteria at one end of the scale to frank malingering at the other". As we shall see in assessing so-called "functional disorders", the task of differentiating these factors is far from easy.

The first task in establishing the genuineness of a patient's complaint is to take a thorough and complete history. The history given by the patient should be carefully cross-checked with that obtained from a key informant. It is advisable to interview informants separately and, in difficult cases, to gather information from more than one source. A competent defence lawyer will be looking for discrepancies in the plaintiff's history as well as for other adverse factors in the patient's life which may have contributed to the onset of the complaint. A competent psychiatrist will therefore have enquired about these before him. To be "caught out" in the witness box over simple matters of fact undermines the credibility of the expert witness and seriously prejudices the patient's case.

It should be noted that exposure to pre-existing vulnerability factors does not necessarily weaken the patient's case. Indeed, a court may be inclined to view a case more favourably where symptoms precipitated by an accident can be explained at least partly in terms of vulnerability, rather than presenting as a catastrophic and disproportionate reaction occurring "out of the blue". Hoffman and Spiegel [13] correctly argue that "it is not the history of previous events or pre-existing conditions that seriously prejudices the plaintiff's claim but, rather, the plaintiff's attempt to conceal them".

If the psychiatrist believes that he has been deliberately misled by the patient then the credibility of the patient must be called seriously into question. Even if the matters of fact are not central to the diagnosis, the specialist cannot be certain that, having been misled in one area by the patient, he has not also been misled in another and perhaps more crucial aspect of the case. Suspicion should be raised where plaintiffs claim that they had absolutely no previous symptoms or difficulties of any kind before the accident and by those who give colourful or embellished accounts of their symptoms. In such circumstances, the psychiatrist should have no hesitation in conveying his uncertainties to the plaintiff's solicitor. Although a plaintiff's legal advisors will always wish to pursue their client's case as vigorously as possible, counsel would not wish to plead a case which is fundamentally flawed.

Unfortunately, we have little information on the effectiveness of psychiatric opinions in discriminating those who are simulating symptoms from those who are "genuine". Some believe that psychiatrists are not very skilled at doing so [4]. Nevertheless, long-term outcome studies suggesting that compensation does not reverse disability in the majority of cases suggest that frank malingering is much less common than those acting for defendants would wish to believe.

"Functional" Disorders and "Hysteria"

The term "functional" is usually, but not always, used by orthopaedic surgeons or other trauma specialists. The notion of "functional overlay" refers to those conditions where complaints of pain or the reported degree of disability seem out of proportion to the extent or severity of any underlying organic lesion. At best the implication is that the patient has symptoms which are being caused or accentuated by "sub-conscious" factors or, at worst, the patient is malingering.

The history of the term "functional" is one of imprecision and confused usage. Trimble [31] suggests that the word was first used in the late 19th century by an Edinburgh Physician, Andrew Coombe. Gowers [10] (quoted by Trimble [31]) in his textbook *A manual of diseases of the nervous system*, divided neurological disorders into organic and "functional" disease. The latter included those diseases that consisted only "in a disturbance of function... are transient and not permanent, and that are not known to be dependent on organic changes". Similarly, Hughlings Jackson, another prominent neurologist, also wrote "I have ... used the terms 'functional' to describe the *morbid alteration of the normal function* of nervous tissue". These physicians, writing at the turn of the century, therefore delineated abnormalities of *function* from those of *structure*, but understood both in terms of organic disturbance.

A shift in usage of the word occurred in the early part of the 20th century, influenced by a dualism in which the organisation of mind was split off from that of body. With the development of psychological theories in the late Freudian era, theorists came to describe as "functional" those disorders thought to have an emotional or "maladaptive" basis as distinct from those with a physical or organic cause. Hence, Gore [9] wrote "functional disorders are the expressions of abnormally controlled emotional reactions, determined and adjusted by environmental factors and not by any gross or demonstrable pathological lesion".

The use of the word functional must now be considered unsatisfactory and out of date. Firstly, with regard to the nervous system at least, a division into disorders of structure and function is increasingly arbitrary as methods of investigation become more sophisticated. A disorder associated with "no structural change" on yesterday's imaging techniques may show a quite different picture using the most up to date investigations. For example, changes seen on a positron-emission tomography (PET) scan clearly illustrate the *functioning* of the brain, but must also reflect changes in *structure* at the cellular and neuro-transmitter level. The distinction between structure and function in this sense becomes increasingly blurred. Secondly, the wedge driven between psycho-logical and organic factors fails to recognise the essential integration of these factors in the patient's perception and presentation of his disorder. A modern clinical approach to the "whole person" must assess the role of psychological factors and incorporate these into the diagnostic process at all levels. In addition, modern understanding of the role of psychological factors in the perception of pain further militates against an over-simplified mind-body split. The perception of pain is profoundly affected by the emotional condition of the patient, and more specifically by processes of attention, cognition and arousal [7]. Once again, the question can rarely be reduced to the "either/or" issue of whether the pain is functional or organic.

The word "hysteria" is equally problematic, having its origins in notions of the floating womb and because of its close association with psychoanalytic theory. The DSM-111-R of the American Psychiatric Association [6] avoids the use of the word, but retains the concepts of conversion disorder, somatoform disorder and somatoform pain disorder, to describe commonly occurring conditions in which psychological processes play a prominent part in the causation of physical symptoms. Counsel for a defendant may occasionally obtain a medical expert who appears to question whether such conditions exist at all. There may be vague references to the "social role of the plaintiff" or generalisations about the "social phenomenon of illness behaviour in the context of litigation". As suggested above, to avoid presenting the court with a choice between the individual views of two expert witnesses a diagnosis should be offered in terms of one of the major classifications of diseases. In doing so, the expert witness illustrates that his use of diagnoses is broadly in line with an international consensus of experts within his field and ensures that the debate centres upon whether the patient has one of these conditions, rather than whether such conditions exist at all.

In assessing a patient where an orthopaedic surgeon or traumatologist has indentified a "functional component" it is suggested that the following points are noted in assessment:

1. A full history is required as outlined above, with a careful reading over all the available medical reports prepared to date. It is inadvisable to accept

instructions where previous reports are being withheld or presented in an edited version.

2. The psychiatrist should enquire carefully into the ways in which the patient has been disabled as a result of his or her symptoms. He should determine any changes in social as well as occupational functioning and obtain a detailed list of disabilities in areas such as decorating, gardening etc. The history given by the patient should be carefully cross-checked with as many informants as possible, interviewed independently from the patient.

3. It is important to inquire for a history of depression, anxiety or symptoms of post-traumatic stress disorder. Many patients arrive at the psychiatrist's office after undergoing multiple assessments and often bitterly resenting the implication that they are not genuine or have been labelled as "neurotics". They may therefore attempt to play down emotional factors and stress their physical symptoms in order to emphasis the genuineness of their condition. Almost without exception, patients believe that any implication of "psychological factors" means that they are not genuinely experiencing their pain or disability, and the doctor should not be misled by an initial denial of psychological symptoms. Some patients play down present or past emotional problems because of a sense of shame or stigma. In others, symptoms of post-traumatic depression may have recovered, but made a significant earlier contribution to establishing a chronic pain syndrome.

4. It is important to remain impartial. We have already noted that if the psychiatrist has suspicions that the patient is malingering then he must say so. It is preferable for the doubts and uncertainties of the expert witness to be made clear at the time of preparing a report than their being extracted under cross-questioning. In particularly difficult cases, the defendant's solicitor may use surveillance by a private detective to establish the credibility of the patient's history.

5. As noted above it is important to make a diagnosis. Malingering is as much a diagnosis as any other and cannot simply be inferred from an absence of organic change. The doctor offering such a diagnosis must be prepared to defend his judgement in terms of the supporting evidence.

Common Psychiatric Disorders in a Medico-legal Setting

Post-traumatic Stress Disorder

We have seen that in awarding damages the courts accept that "nervous shock" should be considered separately from general pain and suffering. A significant development in the British legal system occurred with the "Zeebrugge arbitrations" on the claims of passengers who survived the capsize of the cross-channel ferry *Herald of Free Enterprise*. Because parties were unable to agree levels of damages for "nervous shock" it was agreed that a selection of cases should be dealt with by arbitration before a panel of three Queen's Counsel. In their decision, the arbitrators said "while the respondents conceded that all the claimants suffered from nervous shock, it was necessary for us to consider the nature of the illness from which each claimant suffered, mainly because identification of the nature of the illness enables conclusions to be drawn about prognosis in most cases". The arbitrators concluded that:

1. Psychiatric diagnosis is necessary to give more information about the nature and prognosis of nervous shock.
2. The DSM-111-R of the American Psychiatric Association provides a useful guide to diagnosis because of its detailed diagnostic criteria.
3. The concept of post-traumatic stress disorder (PTSD) is a recent concept and will almost certainly be subject to revision as knowledge increases. Hence, the arbitrators suggested that diagnostic systems such as DSM-111-R should be used as a guide to diagnosis rather than a statute [25].

It should be noted that the findings of the arbitrators do not constitute a precedent binding on courts; the damages awarded in this case will nevertheless be considered as "lead awards", serving as a template upon which litigators may base their arguments in future. It is therefore important that a psychiatrist advising a court should be thoroughly familiar with the notion of PTSD and its usage in modern diagnostic classifications.

Historical Background of PTSD

It has been long recognised that disturbed emotional reactions may follow exposure to sudden trauma. Most of the early research took place on military populations and tended to focus upon organic factors in causation. For example, in 1786 Benjamin Rush [27] described unexplained "fevers" in previously healthy militia officers returning from the American Revolutionary wars and attributed these symptoms to changes in sleeping position and a return to feather mattresses. A number of World War I combatants suffered reactions which came to be known as "shell shock". Again, organic explanations were sought in terms of carbon dioxide poisoning or changes in atmospheric pressure, and discovery of blood in the spinal fluid of some victims led to a theory of brain damage resulting from proximity to an exploding shell [3].

With the advent of mechanical forms of travel in Victorian times, nervous reactions began to be described in civilians exposed to accidental injury. Charles Dickens gives a detailed account of his own "nervous shock" following a railway accident at Staplehurst in Kent in 1865:

> I was in the carriage that did not go over the bridge, but which caught on one side and hung suspended over the ruined parapet... two or three hours work afterwards among the dead and dying surrounded by terrific sights, render my head unsteady... I am curiously weak – weak as if I am recovering from a long illness... yesterday I felt more shaken than I have since the accident. I cannot bear railway travel yet. A perfect conviction, against the senses, that the carriage is down on one side... comes over me with anything like speed, and is inexpressibly distressing [8].

Much was written during World War II on soldiers displaying "war neurosis" and psychological explanations gained ascendancy over organic causes as investigators focused upon pre-existing vulnerability and neurotic pre-disposition.

The modern concept of Post-Traumatic Stress Disorder has been developed mainly in the USA, largely as a result of research into psychiatric disorders among Vietnam war veterans. The first detailed study by Wilson [32] suggested that chronic stress reactions among these ex-servicemen were far more common than had been previously recognised. Despite the publicity attracted by the suffering of Vietnam veterans, a careful study of the literature shows that similar reactions had been documented and classified throughout this century, in a variety of non-combat situations, including all types of natural and man-made disasters (for example see Kingston and Rosser [17]) .

The Syndrome of PTSD

Nervous reactions caused by stressful events have been described by a colourful array of labels including "accident victim syndrome", "syndrome of dispropor- tionate disability", "entitlement neurosis", "aftermath neurosis", "compensation hysteria" etc. Some terms reflect the important and central role of the trauma in aetiology whilst others underline the putative role of secondary gain or that of the compensation process itself.

The central feature of the modern concept of PTSD is the development of symptoms after an event that is "outside the range of usual human experience". Whilst this clearly applies to natural or man-made disasters, the range of stressful incidents also includes road traffic accidents or other events which the victim may perceive as life-threatening or potentially disabling. The most characteristic symptoms are those associated with *re-living* or re-experiencing the stressful incident. This may take the form of repetitive, intrusive memories, vivid visual imagery or "flashback" experiences in which the victim goes through the full range of anxiety symptoms which occurred at the time of the accident.

The diagnosis of PTSD was incorporated into the third edition of the DSM-111-R of the American Psychiatric Association in 1980 [6]. For the first time, diagnostic criteria were specified for trauma-related stress (see Table.14.1). The DSM-111-R gives symptoms in a detailed and operationalised format in order to increase the reliability of diagnosis between different clinicians. Symptoms are clearly defined and minimum duration criteria are introduced as a measure of clinical significance. This introduces a somewhat arbitrary and rigid component to the diagnostic system, but is an inevitable. cost of greater reliability of diagnosis. The following case illustrates some of the typical features of PTSD:

> *Case History.* A 30 year old secretary was driving home from work when an oncoming sports car spun out of control and crossed the central reservation. In the ensuing collision she did not sustain a head injury, but suffered a whiplash injury to her neck and a dislocated shoulder. Over the following weeks she experienced vivid mental imagery for the car spinning out of control and into her path, especially as she was falling asleep or resting. On these occasions she would jump up startled, with autonomic symptoms of anxiety such as "butterflies", palpitations and sweating. She also began to suffer a repetitive nightmare in which she saw her shoulder being torn off by a large piece of metal flying into her car. She was generally tense, apprehensive and tended to startle more easily. She was tense and apprehensive when driving and took unnecessary avoiding action whenever she saw a car of a similar make and type to that involved in the collision. About 12 months after the accident these symptoms began to decrease in frequency, but she did not recover fully until 3 years after the accident.

Table 14.1. Diagnostic criteria for 309.89 post-traumatic stress disorder

A. The person has experienced an event that is outside the range of usual human experience and that would be markedly distressing to almost anyone, e.g. serious threat to one's life or physical integrity; serious threat or harm to one's children, spouse, or other close relatives and friends; sudden destruction of one's home or community; or seeing another person who has recently been or is being, seriously injured or killed as the result of an accident or physical violence.

B. The traumatic event is persistently re-experienced in at least one of the following ways:
   1. Recurrent and intrusive distressing recollections of the event (in young children, repetitive play in which themes or aspects of the trauma are expressed)
   2. Recurrent distressing dreams of the event
   3. Sudden acting or feeling as if the traumatic event were recurring (includes a sense of re-living the experience, illusions, hallucinations, and dissociative [flashback] episodes, even those that occur upon awakening or when intoxicated)
   4. Intense psychological distress at exposure to events that symbolise or resemble an aspect of the traumatic event, including anniversaries of the trauma.

C. Persistent avoidance of stimuli associated with the trauma or numbing of general responsiveness (not present before the trauma), as indicated by at least three of the following:
   1. Efforts to avoid thoughts or feelings associated with the trauma
   2. Efforts to avoid activities or situations that arouse recollections of the trauma
   3. Inability to recall an important aspect of the trauma (psychogenic amnesia)
   4. Markedly diminished interest in significant activities (in young children, loss of recently acquired developmental skills such as toilet training or language skills)
   5. Feeling of detachment or estrangement from others
   6. Restricted range of affect, e.g. unable to have loving feelings
   7. Sense of a foreshortened future, e.g. does not expect to have a career, marriage, or children, or a long life

D. Persistent symptoms of increased arousal (not present before the trauma), as indicated by at least two of the following:
   1. Difficulty falling or staying asleep
   2. Irritability or outbursts of anger
   3. Difficulty concentrating
   4. Hypervigilance
   5. Exaggerated startle response
   6. Physiologic reactivity upon exposure to events that symbolize or resemble an aspect of the traumatic event (e.g. a woman who was raped in an elevator breaks out in a sweat when entering any elevator)

E. Duration of the disturbance (symptoms in B, C, and D) of at least one month.

Specify delayed onset if the onset of symptoms was at least 6 months after the trauma.

(From: Diagnostic and Statistical Manual [6])

Prognosis of PTSD

The course and prognosis of symptoms has not been well established. In the majority of cases, symptoms usually settle down over a 2-year period, although in a substantial minority they may become chronic and persist indefinitely. There are relatively few data on the course of symptoms because of the difficulty in securing a large, representative sample of accident victims with a follow up sufficiently complete to allow reasonable generalisations. However, in general terms, the longer symptoms persist, the less optimistic the prognosis. Certainly, after 2 or 3 years there is a substantial risk of chronicity.

Practical points

1. Solicitors and doctors should be alert to symptoms of PTSD in accident victims. It should be noted that there is a substantial stigma attached to emotional problems and victims may conceal their difficulties on account of shame or guilt. A brief enquiry concerning emotional difficulties should form part of every medical and legal assessment of an accident victim. Suggested screening questions are: "have you had any nervous problems since the accident?", "Does the accident play on your mind?", "Have you had any difficulties with sleeping or any unusual dream experiences?".

2. It is important that the concept of PTSD is not devalued by widening its use to include all non-specific emotional problems after accidents. If symptoms do not meet the specific criteria, make an alternative diagnosis such as an adjustment disorder or anxiety disorder. If the patient does not reach a level of "caseness", do not make a diagnosis but describe the symptoms in terms of general pain and suffering.

3. Besides making a diagnosis, indicate the severity of the condition. Terms such as mild, moderate or severe are of little value unless described in terms of personal suffering, and social and occupational functioning. Attempt to convey something of the suffering and pain caused by the symptoms whilst remaining factual and accurate.

4. Although the central feature of PTSD is the extent to which the stressor lies outside the range of usual human experience, a previous history of neurotic symptoms is an important predisposing factor [20]. Certain personality types, especially those with "obsessional" or perfectionist traits may be especially vulnerable to the effects of sudden, unpredictable trauma which leaves them feeling "out of control". Assist the court in understanding why the victim has reacted adversely by describing vulnerability factors or predisposing traits in his personality.

5. The court expects a patient/victim to make every effort to mitigate his losses. This involves seeking and accepting whatever treatment is available. An expert witness should therefore indicate what treatment is available and the likelihood of response. It should be noted that the availability of a full range of psychiatric services varies considerably from country to country, and in different parts of the country. This is especially so where more sophisticated behavioural psychotherapy may be indicated. Anti-depressants may stabilise and ameliorate symptoms of autonomic over-arousal, hypnotics may provide short-term relief of insomnia and various anxiety management and behavioural techniques may prove effective in avoidance behaviour; but there are no proven and reliable treatments in PTSD and in every patient a large degree of clinical judgement is involved. In chronic patients especially, symptoms may prove extremely refractory to treatment. The court should therefore be advised accordingly. In considering treatment, the Zeebrugge arbitrators said:

Counsel for the claimants has urged us to bear in mind that, quite apart from the guarded nature of the prognosis, very understandably, some claimants are reluctant to undergo treatment, which involves recollecting the distressing circumstances of the disaster, and may baulk at undergoing such treatment. We have no hesitation in accepting this argument.

Post-concussional Syndrome

The neurological sequelae of head injury are dealt with more fully in Chapter 8. Only those aspects of particular relevance to the psychiatrist assessing such cases will be dealt with here. The reader is directed to comprehensive reviews by Trimble [31], Newcombe [23] and Lishman [19].

Although studies suggest that some 50% of patients with head injury develop post-concussional symptoms, the majority gradually resolve over the year following trauma. Many of the psychiatric symptoms following head injury are similar to those of Post-Traumatic Stress Disorder. However, whereas the central symptoms of PTSD are the repetitive intrusive recollections for the incident, studies show that the most commonly presenting symptoms of the post-concussional syndrome are those of headache, dizziness and fatigue [16, 18, 28]. The remaining symptoms, mainly of a non-specific neurotic nature are detailed in Table 14.2.

Course and Prognosis

Lidvall and co-workers' study in particular provides detailed data on the course and outcome of post-concussional symptoms [18]. Eighty-three patients who had been admitted to hospital with relatively minor injuries were prospectively identified and followed up over a 3-month period. Over this time, all of the symptoms gradually declined, but at different rates and tending to cluster into different syndromes over variable time points. For example, immediately after the injury the most prominent cluster was headache, dizziness, impaired concentration and fatigue. By about 2 weeks, a second cluster had appeared, consisting of anxiety and concentration difficulties. In general terms, headache tended to dominate the picture in the early period whilst anxiety became more prominent later. Patients will therefore show differing symptoms depending upon the point at which they are assessed and it is therefore important to inquire about symptoms over the entire time course since the trauma.

Although the majority of symptoms resolve over a 12–24 month period, in a minority they may persist for longer periods and perhaps indefinitely. Unfortunately, it is difficult to make general statements because studies differ in their sampling of patients, the period of assessment and length of follow-up. It

Table 14.2. Post-concussional Symptoms

Headache	Noise sensitivity
Dizziness	Concentration impairment
Fatigue	Irritability
Anxiety	Depression
Insomnia	Subjective memory impairment

also follows that any enquiry into etiology will be complicated by the nature of the sample of patients studied and the time point in the course of the illness selected for study.

The nature of injury to the brain after less severe head injury has been the subject of considerable debate [19]. The similarity of post-concussional symptoms to those of post-traumatic stress disorder raises the question of the extent to which organic or psychological factors play a role in etiology. A major problem has always been the lack of adequate post-mortem material in these less severe injuries, and the relatively crude technology available for investigating changes in brain mechanisms. An examination of the cranial nerves, motor and co-ordinating functions of the nervous system with an ensuing declaration of "no neurological abnormality" can hardly constitute an exhaustive assessment of the subtle brain mechanisms which mediate motivation, attention, drive and personality. A similar note of caution must be sounded in relation to the findings of psychometric testing. Such tests are useful measures of changes in those parts of the brain subserving motor, sensory and cognitive abilities but have little validity with regard to changes in mood, behaviour, and more subtle aspects of human behaviour such as the ability to persevere with tasks, concentrate on several problems at once and tolerance for frustration and repeated setbacks. These aspects of behaviour and experience, some of which may be regarded as uniquely human, are no less dependent upon the integrity of complex brain mechanisms than more easily measured activities such as adding up numbers and walking in a straight line. The psychiatrist should therefore treat with great caution the opinions of those who maintain that because crude clinical testing has not revealed any abnormality, the question of underlying brain injury has effectively been settled.

With regard to less severe head injuries, Groat and Simmons [11] carried out a series of experiments involving the post-mortem examination of brains of concussed animals. They concluded that "it is evident that some cell loss will occur in all concussions, even in extremely light ones, and in some sub-concussions". Similarly, Oppenheimer [24] carried out post-mortem studies of brains following head injury and found microscopic destructive lesions even after relatively minor head injuries.

Modern in vivo techniques have produced findings consistent with these earlier post-mortem studies. For example, Jenkins and colleagues [14] scanned 50 patients with magnetic resonance imaging and demonstrated twice the number of lesions which could have been detected by computerised axial tomography (CT scanning). More important for the present issue, cortical contusions could sometimes be identified even where there had been *no loss of consciousness*. Deep lesions of white matter could also be demonstrated in some patients where loss of consciousness had lasted less than five minutes. These and other findings underline the need to consider subtle injury to the brain even following relatively "minor" head trauma.

Despite our increasing understanding of impaired brain activity following head injury, psychological factors nevertheless play an important role in the development and maintenance of symptoms. "Psychological factors" range from subtle maladaptive responses to impaired mental function through to the effects of over-protective families and the compensation process itself. Gronwall and Wrightson [12] demonstrated how subtle changes of intellectual function, involving the *rate* at which information is processed, may affect the victim:

A patient who has made a good physical recovery after concussion may feel well enough to return to work. His intelligence appears to be unaffected and he will indeed score normally on standard psychometric tests. However, jobs which he could previously have done easily now require simultaneous attention to a number of factors and are quite beyond his capacity; this he interprets by saying he cannot concentrate. Stress mounts, and with it a headache and irritability.

Increasing tensions with colleagues and irritability at home with the family may follow. These, in turn, may act as a further source of anxiety, setting in motion a process which becomes self-perpetuating. In some patients, the knowledge that they have had a head injury may itself produce anxiety and a degree of hypochondriasis. Amnesia for the accident may serve as a continuing reminder that the victim has suffered an injury at the very centre of his personality. Sudden, unpredictable vertigo or lightheadedness may further consolidate a sense of being "out of control" and increase uncertainties about the future. Medical investigations, chance remarks by doctors, poor explanation of symptoms or over-anxious and smothering responses by his family may all set in motion social and psychological processes that cannot easily be reversed. Lishman [19] has commented upon the role of the litigation process in accentuating symptoms:

> Litigation is not an easy path to follow; hopes are aroused, doubts engendered and conflicting advice is received from doctors and lawyers. The whole process conspires towards a state of chronic conflict and often long drawn out frustration. The repeated rehearsal of symptoms before a variety of audiences, some encouraging, some sceptical, does not help the patient to be clear about what he is truly experiencing.

Table 14.3. Factors relevant to post-concussional syndromes

The nature of the victim

Age
Previous psychiatric illness, including alcoholism
Personality
Pre-existing social and domestic difficulties
Recent adverse life events
Pre-existing cerebral pathology

Traumatic nature, localisation and extent of brain damage

Transient factors (contusion, oedema, intra-cranial pressure, hypoxia, changes in circulation)
Penetrating injury
Length of post-traumatic amnesia

Psychological factors

Gross intellectual impairment
Subtle intellectual impairment (e.g. attention, concentration and information processing)
Physical injuries (deformity, scars, etc.)
Post-traumatic epilepsy
Emotional "shock" of the accident, its impact and meaning to the patient
Work impairment and financial problems
Social and relationship difficulties
Process of litigation

It is well established that those with a previous history of psychiatric disorder and neurotic personality traits are at increased risk for developing post-concussional symptoms. The psychiatrist must therefore explain symptoms in terms of an interaction between the nature of the trauma, pre-existing vulnerability and the role of social and family factors discussed above. All of the possible etiological factors which have been recognised in post-concussional syndrome are summarised in Table 14.3, and should be considered systematically for each patient.

Other Psychiatric Sequelae of Head Injury

Personality Change

"Personality" is a term usually applied to those enduring aspects of temperament, attitudes and behaviour which mark us out as "individuals". Diffuse brain damage may commonly affect personality, especially where the frontal and temporal lobes are affected. Difficulties in assessing personality change have already been touched upon, and the crucial role played by informants in building up a picture of the patient is self-evident. In particular, information about previous personality should be sought from school reports, work reports and any other useful sources of information.

Dementia

We have already noted the work of Groat and Simmons [11] showing neuronal loss after blows to the head. In considering the possibility of developing a full-blown dementia, the work of Blessed et al. [2] has been influential, suggesting that dementia is likely to develop when about 10% of the cortex has been destroyed. This is probably an unreliable and misleading figure, even as a broad rule of thumb, because the age of the victim and pre-existing cerebral disorder may substantially alter vulnerability. For a full review of this subject see Roberts [26] who concluded that "it is possible that a single severe head injury may precipitate, or accelerate, the changes of Alzheimer's Disease, while repeated injury is very likely to do so".

Other Psychiatric Symptoms

Any of the commonly occuring psychiatric symptoms may be precipitated by a head injury. Major depressive illness in particular may often be missed because of a tendency to submerge complaints of depression within the general post-concussional syndrome. Obsessive/compulsive disorders and rarely schizophrenic psychosis have been precipitated by head injury, although it may prove difficult to establish a precise causal relationship.

Practical Points

Courts may readily appreciate the manifestation of gross structural brain damage, for example where a steel bar has penetrated the skull and destroyed a part of the brain. There may be less sympathy however for psychological symptoms which cannot simply be related to the crude destruction of brain tissue. The psychiatrist should attempt to convey the limitations of clinical neurological examination and psychometric testing, and indicate the ways in which head injury may result in subtle trauma to the frontal and temporal lobes and brain stem. The psychiatrist should explain the nature of the suffering associated with anxiety and depressive symptoms, and their repercussions for the patients in terms of his or her social and family life. If the psychiatrist suspects that a chronic syndrome has become established, he should specify the serious long- term implications for the patient and his family.

Psychometric testing may be invaluable in giving an objective measure of intellectual and cognitive functioning. Such tests, for example the Wechsler Intelligence Test, are composed of a number of sub-tests, and the "scatter" of results may give an indication of the site of the damage. The results of psycho-metric testing always require interpretation, especially taking into account the possible confounding effects of depression. In addition, although some tests give an indication of whether a deficit is likely to have been acquired, there is no absolutely reliable measure of pre-morbid functioning, and this must be estimated from informants and the patients occupational achievements.

Preparing a Medical Report

A psychiatrist will be instructed by solicitors representing either the plaintiff or the defendant. He or she will be asked to prepare a medical report outlining what, if any, injuries have been sustained by the plaintiff as a result of an accident, the role of other pre-existing or co-incidental factors and some form of prognosis. Unfortunately, letters of instruction from solicitors are similar to referrals from general practitioners: some give detailed questions with full supporting documentation whilst others amount to little more than a "please see and advise". It is always advisable to seek clarification of the precise questions being asked, and to seek copies of previous reports or statements made by the plaintiff. The following ground rules should be observed.

Be Impartial

The experienced expert witness will soon become aware of the adversarial atmosphere into which he has been drawn. Apparently deeply hostile and combative posturing on the part of his instructing solicitors will often be thrown to the wind after settlement of a case as old opponents share a friendly drink in the bar. The expert witness may be repelled or excited by this atmosphere but he must remain firmly outside of it. His role, as defined by the court, is to give objective, impartial advice based upon his clinical and professional experience. It is regrettable when some expert witnesses give the impression of being "hired guns"; fortunately their predictable views and repetitive track record will become increasingly familiar to judges and duly taken into account in the assessment of their opinions.

Treat Every Case as if it is Going to Court

Over 90% of cases are settled out of court, but an expert witness writing a medical report for a solicitor must be prepared to defend his views in court once they have been committed to paper. Every report should therefore be written in a form which the writer would be able to defend under cross-examination. If the psychiatrist does not wish to appear in court he should decline the opportunity to prepare a report.

The medical report should be factual, detailed and carefully worded. It is important to be aware of how easily psychiatric evidence and jargon can be challenged and the psychiatrist should avoid making assertions that cannot be defended. Evidence of carelessness and imprecision undermine his or her credibility as an expert witness.

Obtain a Corroborative History

The importance of an informant's history has already been emphasised. The general practitioner's notes are also crucial, as many plaintiffs are unable to recall, or prefer not to remember, previous symptoms. It is advisable to obtain a photocopy wherever possible to avoid originals being sent through the post and the GP may be requested to invoice the solicitor accordingly. If the GP refuses to release notes, these may be obtained by the court under Section 37 of the Criminal Proceedings Act. It is unsatisfactory to allow a GP to offer a report of his own as the psychiatrist's opinion would then be based upon his assessment of the general practitioner's version of the medical records. Most general practitioners are likely to release their notes with the written informed consent of their patient, but they are more likely to do so following a politely worded request indicating the nature of the litigation, confirmation that no legal action is being taken by the patient against the doctor or members of his practice, and the name and address of the solicitor involved. It is also advisable to indicate whether the expert witness is acting for the plaintiff or the defendant.

In eliciting symptoms and their relationship to an accident, the psychiatrist should follow sound interviewing techniques. He or she should begin with wide-ranging questions and gradually concentrate upon suspected areas of psychopathology. Where the patient states that a symptom is present following a specific question, he or she should always be asked to describe their experiences in their own words and to give a concrete example. Note whether the patient appears to be susceptible to leading questions and cross-check the history carefully.

Present Findings in an Organised Format

All too frequently medical reports are presented in a disorganised manner with pages of closely spaced, and sometimes inaccurate, typing. A medical report should be presented in a structured and carefully organised format with extensive use of sub-headings. In particular, organise material under headings such as recent history, limitations resulting from symptoms, personal history, previous medical history, mental state, corroborative history and opinion.

The opinion should logically be derived from the preceding history and should ideally anticipate all of the salient points in the mind of counsel. It is advisable therefore to organise the opinion under numbered headings and in response to the questions being asked of the expert witness:

1. What if any symptoms does the patient complain of and what is your diagnosis based upon examination?. Give the diagnosis in terms of one of the main classifications
2. What is the precise relationship of the symptoms to the accident in question?
3. If other factors appear causally related to the diagnosed condition, what relative weight may be apportioned to the accident?
4. What is the relationship of any pre-existing conditions or vulnerability to the development of symptoms in this patient?
5. What is the prognosis? In particular, consider future impairment of social and occupational functioning and the need for any special care and treatment.

Because prognosis can be extremely difficult, a recent ruling allows in certain cases for a judgement before complete recovery, keeping open the possibility of returning to court for further consideration.

Appearing in Court as an Expert Witness

A psychiatrist who goes into court after watching too many television courtroom dramas will be surprised by the slow and laboured proceedings of real life. He may be disappointed by questioning which appears to be based on a hurried and incomplete grasp of the facts of the case and which misses out important material. Just occasionally however, to keep him on his toes, he will find himself on the receiving end of a harrowing cross-questioning which exposes the weakness of his position and penetrates to the central issues of the case.

As in preparing a medical report, the role of the expert witness is to state his views impartially. Witnesses are usually asked to speak slowly to allow the judge to record their replies in long hand. An experienced expert witness learns to turn to the barrister to receive a question and turn back to the judge to deliver his answer. It is not the barrister that he must convince of the merits of his argument, but the judge who presides over the case. By turning and addressing the judge, he can then turn back to the barrister when he is ready for his next question, and so to some extent exert control over the length and structure of his reply. Occasionally counsel may interrupt before the witness has time to finish his sentence: if he feels it is important that he should do so, it is possible to say something like: "I would like to be permitted to complete my answer as there is a danger I may mislead the court".

The expert witness should stick to the facts but be prepared to stand by his opinions. Do not be afraid to ask counsel to repeat a question or to break a rather complicated question into smaller units. A cardinal rule for counsel is never to ask a witness a question to which counsel does not already know the answer. He will, therefore, seek to lead the expert witness by a process of reasoned arguments. The psychiatrist is practised in listening to what people say and in attempting to understand their point of view. He may therefore find himself wishing to acknowledge that a point being put to him has some validity, even though it conflicts with his own view. It is important in these circumstances that he does not appear to be uncertain or prevaricating in his opinion. He could say something like: "there is some validity in what you are saying, but having considered all aspects of this case and having reviewed the evidence in considerable detail, my overall clinical judgement remains the same as that given in my report".

Whilst the occasional "point scoring" can lighten otherwise lengthy and tedious proceedings, it is generally inadvisable. The principle task of the expert witness is to give the court the benefit of his opinion in a straightforward matter-of-fact way and using simple language. His credibility will also be assessed on the basis of his appearance and general demeanour. It is advisable therefore to dress professionally and to be ready to give one's name and professional qualifications.

In conclusion, the most competent expert witnesses are those able to communicate in simple and authoritative terms, using language that is relatively jargon free and arguments that sound convincing to the judge.

References and Further Reading

1. Balla JI, Moraitis SL (1970) Knights in Armour - a follow-up study of injuries after legal settlement. Med Aus 2:355-361
2. Blessed G, Tomlinson BE, Roth M (1968) The association between quantitative measures of dementia and degenerative changes in the cerebral grey matter of elderly subjects. Br J Psychiatr 114:797-812
3. Bourne P (1970) Men, stress and Vietnam. Academic Press, New York, pp10-22
4. Bursten B (1984) Malingering. In: Bursten B. Beyond psychiatric expertise. C Thomas, Springfield Illinois
5. Collie J (1917) Malingering and feigned sickness. Edward Arnold, London
6. Diagnostic and statistical manual. 3rd Ed (revised) (1983). The American Psychiatric Association, Washington, DC
7. Elton D, Stanley G, Burrows G (1983) Psychological control of pain. Grune and Stratton, New York
8. Forster J (1969) The life of Charles Dickens. vol 2. Dent, London
9. Gore DE (1922) Functional nervous disorders: Their classification and treatment. Wright, Bristol.
10. Gowers WR (1893) A manual of diseases of the nervous system, reprinted 1970. Hafner Darient, Connecticut
11. Groat RA, Simmons J0 (1950) Loss of nerve cells in experimental cerebral concussion. J Neuropathol Exp Neurol 9:150.
12. Gronwall D, Wrightson P (1974) Delayed recovery of intellectual function after minor head injury. Lancet ii:605
13. Hoffman BF, Spiegel H (1989) Legal principles in the psychiatric assessment of personal injury litigants. Am J Psychiatr, 146:3
14. Jenkins A, Teasdale G, Hadley MDM, MacPherson P, Rowan JO (1986) Brain lesions detected by magnetic resonance imaging. Lancet ii: 445-446
15. Jolowicz JA, Lewis TE, Harris DM (1971) Winfield and Jolowicz on tort, 9th ed. Sweet and Maxwell, London
16. Keshevan MS, Channabasavanna SM, Reddy GN (1981) Post-traumatic psychiatric disturbances: patterns and predictors of outcome. Br J Psychiatr 138:157-160
17. Kingston W, Rosser R (1974) Disaster: effects on mental and physical state. J Psychosom Res 18: 437

18. Lidvall HF, Linderoth B, Norlin B (1974) Causes of the post-concussional syndrome. Acta Neurol Scand [Suppl] 56:1-144.
19. Lishman WA (1988) Physiogenesis and psychogenesis in the post-concussional syndrome. Br J Psychiatr 153:460–469
20. McFarlane A (1989) The aetiology of post-traumatic morbidity: Predisposing, precipitating and perpetuating factors. Br J Psychiatr 154: 221–228
21. Miller H (1961) Accident neurosis. Br Med J i:919–925, 992–998
22. Modin HC (1975) The trauma in "traumatic neurosis" In: Allen RC, Fernster EZ, Rubin JG (eds) Readings in law and psychiatry. Johns Hopkins University Press, Baltimore
23. Newcombe F (1983) The psychological consequences of closed head injury: assessment and rehabilitation. Injury 14: 111–136
24. Oppenheimer DR (1968) Microscopic lesions in the brain following head injury. J Neurol Neurosurg Psychiatr 31: 299
25. The Personal and Medical Injuries Law Letter (1989) Post-traumatic stress disorder: The Zeebrugge arbitration. Legal Studies and Services Ltd., London.
26. Roberts AH (1979) Severe accidental head injury: an assessment of long-term follow-up prognosis. Macmillan, London, pp 129–139
27. Rush B (1786) Results of observations, 7. London Medical Journal 77: 79
28. Rutherford WH, Merret JD, McDonald (1977) Sequelae of concussion caused by minor head injuries. Lancet i: 1–4
29. Sprehe DJ (1984) Workers' compensation – a psychiatric follow-up study. Int J Law Psychiatr 7: 165–178
30. Tarsh MJ, Royston C (1985) A follow-up study of accident neurosis. Br J Psychiatr 146: 18–25
31. Trimble M (1981) Post-traumatic neurosis. Wiley, Chichester
32. Wilson J (1978) The Forgotten Warrior Project. Cleveland State University Press, Cleveland, Ohio

PART 3:

**Legal Advice for Doctors
Involved with Medico-legal
Problems**

CHAPTER 15

The Solicitor's Problems

G.C. Reed

The object of this chapter is to assist both solicitors and doctors In understanding each other's role in medico-legal cases and how they can best assist one another to deal with the case in hand. The observations are directed to the consideration of ordinary medico-legal cases. The particular problems that apply to medical negligence cases are dealt with in Chap. 17.

Instructing the Doctor

It should be obvious that the more useful information the solicitor can provide to the doctor the easier it will be for the doctor to carry out his enquiries and to provide the solicitor with a helpful report. It is therefore essential that the solicitor obtains as much useful information as he can and passes that on to the doctor when instructing him.

If the solicitor is acting for the plaintiff he should obtain the following information and pass it on to the doctor when sending instructions to him:

1. The plaintiff's name, address and date of birth
2. A brief description of the injuries that the plaintiff claims to have suffered without necessarily going into any technical detail and a general account of the symptoms the client says he still has
3. Where the client received treatment for those injuries and the name and address of his general practitioner
4. Details of any relevant pre-accident medical condition
5. An account of how the injury or illness was alleged to have been caused. The solicitor will need to obtain details of the circumstances of the accident in order to consider the questions of liability. In addition the doctor will need to know what happened to the plaintiff so that he can consider the mechanics of any injury suffered and give full consideration to the questions of causation that may arise.
6. The plaintiff's occupation, prospects of promotion and any other activity that has been adversely affected by the injury

7. Any material features of his social circumstances such as, for instance, whether he is single and has to look after himself, whether he lives at the top of a block of flats with an unreliable lift

8. His National Insurance number. There may be material Department of Social Security (DSS) records. In any event this will be required to enable the solicitor to obtain particulars of the state benefits that have been paid and which have to be taken into account pursuant to the Social Security Act 1988.

Solicitors acting for defendants are largely dependent on the information provided by their opponent when gathering the material details they require before instructing their doctor. They may be reluctant to ask their opponent for too much information, particularly at an early stage, for fear of provoking a head of claim that the claimant had not considered or intended to raise. It is the defendant's solicitor's job to test the claim put to him and not to assist his opponent in preparing the plaintiff's claim. Prior to the commencement of proceedings the defendant's solicitor will need to rely on the information given by the plaintiff's solicitors of their client's claim. If the action has begun, the defendant's solicitors will have the Statement of Claim and any Further and Better Particulars of that pleading that deal with questions of injury, loss and damage and pursuant to the new rules, a report from the plaintiff's medical expert.

Copies of those documents should be sent to the doctor instructed by the defendant's solicitors for him to check the accuracy of their contents against the information he is able to obtain from the plaintiff, his findings on examination and the contents of any available medical records. Solicitors acting for defendants may also be able to obtain some useful information from their client, particularly in employer's liability cases. If the employer has questioned the bona fides of the plaintiff there is often some substance to his comments. There may also be some material information in Police reports of road accident cases and in the work's accident records and in particular the report to the DSS (Form B176) which the claimant must submit before he is entitled to industrial injury benefit.

In many cases the plaintiff's solicitor will have disclosed copies of his medical reports to the defendant's solicitor before the defendant's solicitor commissions his own medical evidence. He must do so in any event when serving the Statement of Claim or Particulars of Claim pursuant to the recent Rule changes. In general it is not desirable for a defendant's solicitor to send a copy of the other side's reports before the doctor he is instructing has carried out an examination of the plaintiff. The defendant's doctor must reach his own conclusions before considering the reports of the plaintiff's doctor. He should not assume that the findings of his opposite number are accurate or reliable. Following recent changes in the Court Rules pursuant to The Rules of the Supreme Court (Amendment No.4) 1989 and The County Court (Amendment No.4) Rules 1989, a plaintiff's solicitor is not able to serve the Statement of Claim or Particulars of Claim in the County Court in personal injury cases unless that pleading is accompanied by a medical report or reports describing the injuries sustained. It is normally desirable to get proceedings under way at an early stage and so the plaintiff's solicitor must obtain medical evidence before he can take any step beyond issuing and serving the Writ. To comply with that obligation he should therefore ensure that he has commissioned a medical report as soon as he reasonably can, even though he knows that a final prognosis is not going to be available for some considerable time. In those cases where there is going to be delay before a definite prognosis can be given it will probably be sufficient, to comply with the new Rules, for the solicitor to simply ask the doctor to compile a preliminary report for disclosure from the general practitioner's or hospital notes. This report will be adequate if it describes the injuries suffered and their consequences in sufficient detail to enable the defendant to know, at least in general terms, what claim he has to face.

Reports from the Treating Doctor

Should a plaintiff's solicitor commission a report from the consultant who has been responsible for the plaintiff's medical treatment? In straightforward cases this may be sensible. The doctor who dealt with the treatment will have first-hand knowledge of the plaintiff's history, ready access to the notes and ability to interpret them. Indeed a preliminary report, produced from the notes alone, will be more expeditious.

There are, however, disadvantages in consulting the doctor who was responsible for the plaintiff's treatment even in cases where no question of medical negligence arises. The doctor who has been responsible for carrying out any surgical procedure may be unrealistically optimistic about the likely end result and not take a wholly objective view of the plaintiff's prognosis. Difficulties may arise in making a detached assessment of a patient, known and treated over a prolonged period. Any assessment may be coloured by sympathy or the lack of it depending on whether or not the patient has been co-operative. If in doubt the plaintiff's solicitor should seek independent advice.

Under no circumstances should the solicitor acting for the defendant seek a report from a doctor who has been involved in the plaintiff's treatment. The defendant's solicitor will not be able to ascertain whether there are any features which render that consultant unsuitable. More particularly the plaintiff's solicitor should not permit the defendant's solicitor to commission a report from any doctor who has been involved in the treatment. In the event there would be no control of the information available to the defendant's doctor on which any opinion may be founded.

When Should the Doctor Be Instructed?

Until the plaintiff's condition has stabilised and he has largely if not wholly recovered from the injuries sustained insofar as he is going to, it is likely to be very difficult for any doctor to give a final prognosis. In straightforward cases a plaintiff's solicitor will normally only want to obtain one medical report and will not, therefore, want to seek that report too soon in case a stable condition has not been reached by the time the doctor examines. He must ensure, however, that his report is ready for service on the defendant of the Statement or Particulars of Claim.

However, it must be remembered that most doctors who have established reputations in medico-legal work will have substantial waiting lists. In some fields of specialty, particularly orthopaedic surgery, a solicitor can expect to wait an average of 6 months before he can obtain a date for the doctor to examine the plaintiff. There may be some further delay after the examination before the report is produced if the doctor does not have immediate access to all the notes and other medical records he needs to see. The solicitor should try to take into account the progress the plaintiff will make during that period of delay and hope that the plaintiff will have reached a stable condition by the time the doctor is able to examine, even though the plaintiff may not be fully recovered at the time the doctor is first instructed.

The Doctor's Role

It must be remembered that whilst doctors, like solicitors, are instructed to act on behalf of one particular party, in medico-legal cases their roles and obligations are not identical. The doctor is instructed as an independent expert who will be called upon to give to the court his honest professional opinion on the injuries suffered by the plaintiff and the consequence of those injuries without favour. The solicitor is instructed to represent his client's best interests and, subject to his obligation not to mislead the court, will only be concerned to present to his opponent and to the court such evidence as will assist him in advancing his client's case.

It follows, therefore, that the solicitor is under no obligation to inform the doctor he has instructed of any facts that he knows of which are adverse to his client's case. The doctor must not assume that the solicitor has related all the material facts. For instance, the solicitor may be fully aware that his client has had a bad back for years or that he has had several convictions for dishonesty but he is under no obligation to tell the doctor he is instructing about such matters. The onus is upon the doctor to discover and report upon any material features which he considers may be adverse to the case of the party instructing him. The solicitor does, of course, run the risk of his expert medical witness having no credibility at all at the trial if that expert has not taken into account material features relating to the plaintiff's history. These facts, which might be adduced from other sources, could affect the assessment of the plaintiff and cause the doctor to change the opinion.

Choosing the Doctor

A plaintiff's solicitor can arrange to have his client examined by as many different doctors as he wishes until he and his client obtain a medical report that supports the case they wish to advance. The solicitor is under no obligation to disclose every report he obtains, only those he intends to rely upon. He need not even disclose the fact that he has obtained other reports that he does not wish to rely upon. The only sanction limiting the number of medical reports a plaintiff's solicitor can obtain is one of cost. A successful plaintiff will not be able to recover from his opponent the cost of obtaining a medical report on which he does not wish to rely. The cost, however, has to be borne by the plaintiff. The Legal Aid Board will limit the number of expert opinions a plaintiff may obtain if supported by public funds.

A defendant's solicitor is in an entirely different position. Only medical evidence necessary to consider and test the claim may be obtained. There is no automatic entitlement to have the plaintiff examined by whoever the defendant's solicitor wishes. Investigations are limited to those that can be justified as necessary.

The defendant's solicitor must, therefore, decide in the light of the allegations contained in the particulars of injury set out in pleadings or in correspondence, what medical evidence he needs to investigate those allegations. He must obtain facilities from his opponent for the plaintiff to be examined by a particular doctor in the particular field or specialty that is appropriate for consideration of the injuries complained of.

It may be necessary for the defendant to obtain opinions from more than one specialist medical adviser. If the plaintiff's injuries cover more than one specialty then it would be appropriate for the defendant to arrange for an examination by one consultant from each of the specialities that is necessary to cover the range of injuries involved. Ordinarily a defendant would not be entitled to an examination by another doctor in the same specialty as a doctor who has already examined the plaintiff unless he can demonstrate a specific need to do so. Defendant's solicitors must therefore choose their expert witnesses with care.

There is one qualification to this limitation. In High Court cases the automatic Directions provided by Order 25 Rule 8 permit each party to call two medical witnesses at the trial provided that reports containing the substance of their evidence have previously been disclosed. There is nothing in this rule which says that those two experts must be of different specialties and so a defendant's solicitor may be able to obtain a second opinion as of right from another specialist in the same field as the one from whom he has already obtained a report. He must appreciate that by doing so, however, he may be limiting his entitlement to obtain a report from a specialist in another field of medicine if it subsequently transpires that he ought to do so.

The plaintiff is not entitled to stipulate which doctor his opponent may consult but he is entitled to refuse facilities for medical examinations on his opponent's behalf from doctors who have been involved in his treatment and from doctors that his legal advisors have retained for the purposes of his claim. He may only object to being examined by the doctor nominated by the defendant's solicitor if there are good reasons for doing so. Such a reason is, for instance, the fact that the doctor nominated by the defendants is likely to conduct his examination or make his report unkindly or unfavourably (*Star* v. *National Coal Board* [1977] 1 A11 ER 243). The onus is firmly upon the plaintiff to establish that he would be prejudiced by an examination by the particular doctor concerned, if he wishes to object to the specialist nominated by the defendants.

It is incumbent on a plaintiff who claims damages for personal injuries to afford the defendant a reasonable opportunity to have him medically examined. The court has power to stay the proceedings unless and until he does so if he should decline. The court will only make such an Order, however, if it is in the interests of justice to do so. The onus of establishing the need lies on the party applying for such a stay to show that he cannot properly prepare his case without the medical examination he is seeking (*Lane* v. *Willis* [1972] 1 A11 ER 430).

Normally the plaintiff may not impose conditions on a medical examination on the defendant's behalf that has been demonstrated to have been necessary, other than reimbursement of his expenses and losses in attending that examination. He is not normally entitled to insist that a particular relative or his own medical or legal adviser be present when the examination takes place. It may, however, be possible for a plaintiff's solicitor to stipulate that the plaintiff be accompanied during the examination by a friend or third party if the plaintiff is nervous or if the defendant's doctor has a reputation for roughness or hostility (*Hall* v. *Avon Area Health Authority* (Teaching) [1980] 1 A11 ER 516).

What Investigations May the Doctor Undertake?

In making himself available for a medical examination the plaintiff is consenting to the medical advisor carrying out a physical examination of him. That examination would not constitute an assault unless it goes beyond the normal investigation that would ordinarily be required for the preparation of a medico-legal report. The plaintiff would be entitled to refuse to undergo an examination that is unpleasant, painful or risky unless the party seeking to undertake that investigation can demonstrate that the interests of justice imperatively require the test to be carried out. So for instance the court was not prepared to require the plaintiff to submit to patch testing in a case of industrial dermatitis because there was a real risk of the dermatitis breaking out again if that test was undertaken (*Aspinall* v. *Sterling Mansell Ltd.* [1981] 3 A11 ER 866). The test is whether the objection or the request for the investigation sought is reasonable in the light of the information or advice which the respective parties receive from their advisors. A real but minimal risk of some short-term injury to the plaintiff's health from the investigation proposed can be justified if the defendant genuinely believes that he cannot defend the case without that investigation. The defendant must agree to compensate the plaintiff for any injury that does arise from the investigation (*Prescott* v. *Bulldog Tools Ltd.* [1981] 3 A11 ER 869).

In general, solicitors will not be able to anticipate what tests a doctor will wish to carry out. The doctor must not, therefore, assume that by being asked to examine the plaintiff he automatically has authority to carry out such investigations as he considers to be necessary to prepare his report. If he wishes to carry out any investigation beyond the normal tests that are carried out on examination, he must obtain express authority from those instructing him. Strictly speaking, permission to commission radiographs should be sought before arrangements are made although normally it is in order to put these in hand if the plaintiff agrees. Most doctors would consider it unwise to perform any invasive investigation for medico-legal purposes regardless of whether they have been granted permission to do so and certainly should not carry out such tests in the absence of express permission.

In addition to carrying out an examination of the plaintiff an examining doctor will of course also obtain particulars of the plaintiff's history and complaints by questioning him on these matters. He should confine his questions and his subsequent report to those matters that are necessary for him to express an opinion as a doctor and to deal with the specific points raised by those instructing him.

Consequently, questions about how the accident occurred must be limited to establishing such facts as the doctor needs to have to be able to understand the mechanics of the injury suffered so that he can better understand what that injury was and whether it was a consequence of the incident complained of. He should not deal with matters that relate purely to the liability aspect of the case such as whether there had been complaints about the amount of lifting the plaintiff was required to undertake or whether the car the plaintiff collided with was displaying lights or not.

The doctor may encounter cases where a plaintiff refuses to answer any questions about the circumstances of the incident complained of and how the injury was caused. There have even been instances where the plaintiffs have been instructed by their solicitors not to answer such questions. If that does occur the doctor must report to the solicitor instructing him that such a refusal to co-operate has occurred and should then list the questions or at least the kind of questions that he asked the plaintiff to answer but to which he received no reply. Such observations are normally best put in a covering letter accompanying the report.

Access to Medical Records

The doctor does not have an automatic right to see any medical records. By making himself available for a medical examination the plaintiff does not consent, by implication or otherwise, to the doctor seeing any notes about him. It must also be remembered that the medical records themselves are unlikely to be in the plaintiff's own custody, power or control.

If the doctor is instructed by the plaintiff's solicitor he is entitled to assume that he will get such co-operation as he considers necessary from the solicitors instructing him and their client to enable him to complete his report. Even so, he ought to seek the authority of the plaintiff, through his solicitors, before applying for any such notes and specify what notes he needs to see and why. If the doctor does not obtain the authority he considers he needs to see records he regards as material, he must at the very least say so in his report. He should make it clear that any opinion he has expressed is provided on the basis of the limited information available to him. If he considers he is unable to express an opinion without seeing records that have been denied to him he should decline to report at all.

No such presumption applies when the doctor is instructed on behalf of the defendant. Before the defendant's doctor is entitled to see any of the plaintiff's records he will have to justify a need to do so. There will be no difficulty in justifying that need where it relates to the hospital notes and radiographs for the treatment the plaintiff has received following the accident in question. However, the defendant's doctor would not be able to justify the need to see the general practitioner's records if the GP has not been involved in the treatment for the injury, unless he can demonstrate why such records are going to be of assistance to him. If he is told that the plaintiff has had a similar or related medical complaint prior to the accident in question then again he should have little difficulty in justifying the need. The plaintiff's advisors may seek to limit any disclosure to those records that are directly related to the injury in question. When such limitations are imposed it can be extremely difficult to distinguish between those notes that are material and those that are not. Very often it is only the doctor who is preparing the report who can say what notes he considers to be material. If the doctor considers he has been denied access to all necessary records then this should be stated.

It must be remembered that there may be a number of sources of material medical records in addition to the hospital and general practitioner's notes. Many employers have a works surgery and the company nurse will keep records of each employee's attendance at the surgery. However, most works nurses consider that company medical records are confidential and will not even make those notes available to the employee's own company unless the employee specifically gives authority for their release. The Department of Social Security may require the plaintiff to undergo medical examinations in connection with his applications for benefit. The plaintiff may have received private medical treatment from a chiropractor or osteopath. If a plaintiff's employment has been terminated on health grounds the employer may have obtained a report from an occupational health physician. The doctor ought to ascertain during examination what material records exist and ask the instructing solicitor to provide an authority for the disclosure of those notes.

When medical records are sought from third parties, an authority in writing and signed by the plaintiff must be obtained, specifying the notes that are to be disclosed and stating to which doctor the notes may be supplied. If the authority is not specific the holder of the records may well refuse to disclose the notes. The holder of the medical records may also seek confirmation that the notes are not required for the purposes of pursuing a claim against whoever holds the records. If such confirmation is sought it needs to be answered very carefully and in such a way that does not prevent a claim from being pursued against the holder of the records in due course if it becomes apparent from subsequent enquiry and perusal of the notes in question, that such a claim is appropriate.

If the plaintiff refuses to provide the defendant's medical advisor with authority for disclosure of the medical records, the remedy is for the defendant's solicitor to make application for third party discovery against the holder of the records pursuant to Section 33(2) of the Supreme Court Act 1981 and Order 24 Rule 7A of the Rules of the Supreme Court. It must be remembered that that application can only be pursued against the holder of the records and not the plaintiff himself even though the only reason why the records have not been released may be the plaintiff's refusal to provide an authority for their disclosure. If that is the case the appropriate remedy may be for the costs of the application for third party discovery to be paid by the plaintiff in any event.

Disclosure of Medical Evidence

Order 38 Rule 37 of the Supreme Court provides that the substance of a medical witness's evidence shall be disclosed in the form of a written report to the other parties to the action unless directions to the contrary are given. The Court will only order that medical evidence can be called, without prior disclosure of the reports, if the expert evidence deals with the manner in which the injuries were sustained or the genuineness of the symptoms of which complaint is made. Even in medical negligence cases, therefore, the doctor must assume that any report he writes is intended for disclosure.

It follows, therefore, that the doctor should confine the contents of his medical reports to these matters described in Chapter 2 which sets out what should be contained in a medical report. The doctor must appreciate that his report will be disclosed to the other side at some stage if the commissioning solicitor intends to rely upon it and probably also to the plaintiff himself. If the case goes to trial the judge will be provided with a copy and the report will form the basis of the medical witness's evidence in chief and he will be cross-examined upon it.

Whilst the vast majority of cases settle before trial the doctor should assume that each report he writes is in respect of one of the few cases that ends up in court.

The doctor must, therefore, be confident of the opinions he expresses in his report. He must be sure of the facts upon which his diagnosis is made and be able to substantiate his opinions from either his own experience of medical practice or the research of others in the field in question. Whilst the burden of proof in civil cases is to the balance of probabilities only, there must nevertheless be grounds for the conclusion that the doctor has reached.

Many doctors adopt the practice of sending with their medical report a covering letter that is not intended for disclosure. This is a useful way for the doctor to communicate to those instructing him information that should not be contained in the medical report. The kind of information included in such a covering letter would relate to questions of liability, such as reporting that the casualty notes at the hospital revealed that the plaintiff was drunk on admission; comments on the other side's medical evidence that has been disclosed or the experience of the other side's medical advisors in dealing with that kind of medical problem, assist in the cross-examination of the other side's medical witnesses. Recommendations as to further investigations the instructing solicitor might undertake, such as the commissioning of a follow-up report, special tests, a report from a medical advisor of another specialty or an enquiry agent should be put in a covering letter as well.

The covering letter should not relate to the facts concerning the medical condition of the plaintiff established on examination of him, on questioning him or from the medical records nor should it contain an opinion from the doctor on those matters, all of which should be in the report itself. Furthermore, if the information the doctor wishes to convey to his instructing solicitor is something upon which he might be required to give evidence it should, in accordance with the provisions of Order 38 Rule 37 mentioned above, be included in the report.

The automatic directions in personal injury actions pursuant to Order 25 Rule 8 of the Rules of the Supreme Court provide that there shall be mutual disclosure; that is, exchange of medical reports within a specified period in the absence of any special circumstances, entitling medical witnesses to be called, without their reports having been previously disclosed. The Order states that reciprocity will be normal but in exceptional circumstances or to save costs, disclosure by one party only may be ordered and the other party may be permitted to defer disclosure. For instance, where a defendant has not had a medical examination and there is no reason to suppose that the plaintiff's report will not be agreed (RSC vol. 2 para. 746.).

The practice of mutual contemporaneous disclosure was, however, questioned in the case of *Turner* v. *Carlisle City Council* (1989) 8CL 259 which provided that if the defendant did not have his own medical evidence when the time for disclosure occurred, the plaintiff remained under an obligation to disclose his report without condition. The plaintiff could not subsequently object to the defendant commissioning his own report if he did not wish to agree the plaintiff's medical evidence and then disclosing any report that he obtained and relying upon the evidence of that medical witness at the trial.

The provisions of Order 25 Rule 8 have been further amended by the recent Rule changes which came into effect on 4 June 1990. The Rules of the Supreme Court (Amendment No. 4) 1989 and The County Court (Amendment No. 4) Rules 1989 provide that a plaintiff must disclose medical reports in support of the substance of his claim for damages for personal injury when serving his Statement of Claim or Particulars of Claim. If the plaintiff needs to obtain further medical evidence dealing with complications or developments to his condition since the reports disclosed with the pleadings were obtained, the new rules allow him to do so. They also provide that those follow-up reports must also be disclosed.

It would appear that, notwithstanding the provision of Order 25 Rule 8 relating to mutual disclosure, a plaintiff must now disclose his medical evidence before there is any obligation upon the defendants to consider what, if any, medical evidence they wish to rely upon, or for them to disclose the appropriate reports. The application of the new Rules is still to be considered by the courts at the time of writing and until this has been decided there can be no certainty as to the manner in which they will be applied.

Once disclosure of medical evidence has taken place the solicitor receiving his opponent's reports should ask his own medical advisor to consider the differences between that doctor's findings and conclusions, and the other medical witnesses involved. He must, therefore, be sent copies of the reports. He should also be sent copies of other material records such as the Department of Social Security notes, occupational health and work surgery notes and enquiry agents reports for comment.

Ordinarily a plaintiff's medical record supplied pursuant to the authority the plaintiff has given will only be available to the doctors to whom the authority refers. If those records contain entries upon which the doctor relies to support the opinion he has given, he must specify to the instructing solicitor the source of the information he considers to be important. By doing so the solicitor will then be able to take the necessary steps to obtain copies of those medical records. Copies can be prepared for use at the trial or, at the very least, steps taken to ensure that the records are produced at the trial, by the issue of subpoenas against whoever holds the records concerned.

In personal injury actions all reports of medical experts should be lodged at court as soon as possible after setting down whether or not they are agreed. Each report should be marked with the name of the party on whose behalf it has been obtained, the date and a statement of whether or not it has been agreed (Practice Direction (QBD: Personal Injuries Action) (1990) 1 WLR 93). The purpose is to enable the judge to form a view of the areas in contention in the expert evidence and thus make the trial more efficient. If the reports are not agreed they do not become evidence in the case. They are merely lodged to give the judge an opportunity of assessing the areas of dispute. It remains necessary for the expert to give oral evidence if the reports are not agreed.

Joint Examinations and Reports

Whilst Order 25 Rule 6.2 of the Rules of the Supreme Court appears to encourage joint medical examinations of a plaintiff this practice is not really compatible with the adversarial English legal system. The usual practice is for each party to obtain his own medical evidence and only disclose to his opponent the evidence upon which he intends to rely at the trial. The opportunity to assess whether or not a party wishes to rely upon a report does not exist if the report is a joint one since his opponent will have a copy of it.

There are, however, a few circumstances in which a joint examination is desirable. If opposing sides' doctors have observed differing objective facts on their examination of the plaintiff, it might resolve the question as to who carried out his tests correctly and obtained the accurate results. If it is considered desirable that the plaintiff should undergo a hazardous or unpleasant test it would be preferable for him to undergo that test once only in the presence of both sides' doctors rather than twice if the tests were to be carried out independently.

If there are issues between the medical witnesses many judges prefer the doctors to have met in an attempt to resolve their differences, thus enabling the judge to avoid having to make a difficult decision in a field in which he has no expert knowledge. If the doctors can resolve their differences by such a meeting in the sense that one is able to convince the other by cogent reasoned argument that he is wrong, then it is as well to know how that issue will be resolved before the trial rather than at the trial. Doctors must appreciate, however, that a meeting between them in an attempt to resolve issues in the medical evidence in this way should not be simply an attempt to thrash out a compromise. If an expert witness genuinely believes that his opposite number is wrong he should be prepared to stand up in court and say so and not simply accept a middle road which neither doctor really believes is correct. If there really is a material issue between the doctors it is the judge's task to resolve it.

On occasions there will appear to be an issue between medical advisors simply because they undertook their examinations at different times or considered different aspects of the injury with the result that certain features will appear to have been omitted. Very often when this occurs there will, in fact, be no issue between the doctors at all and if that is the case, the doctors may well consider it appropriate to produce a combined report setting out the full history for use at court. They should not meet to prepare such a combined report, however, unless expressly authorised by those solicitors instructing them to do so. If, after meeting, they find that there are, in fact, issues between them they should not put their names to a joint report that is not their joint opinion.

Provisional Damages

Since 1st July 1985 courts have been able to make awards of provisional damages pursuant to Section 6 of the Administration of Justice Act 1982. The entitlement to make a provisional award was recently extended to the County Court as well as the High Court by The County Court (Amendment No. 4) Rules 1989 S6. Section 32a of the Amended Supreme Court Act 1981 applies to an action for damages for personal injuries in which there is proved or admitted to be "a chance that at some definite or indefinite time in the future the injured person will, as a result of the act or omission which gave rise to the cause of action, develop some serious disease or suffer some serious deterioration in his physical or mental condition".

If the court is satisfied that a provisional award is appropriate it will make an assessment of damages on the assumption that the injured person will not develop the disease or suffer the deterioration in his condition and order that further damages may be paid at a future date if he actually develops the disease or suffers the deterioration feared.

In order that the solicitor can consider whether an award of provisional damages is appropriate or should be resisted if claimed, he will need to ask some specific questions of the doctor consulted on his client's behalf. These questions are:

1. Is there a real chance of a deterioration occurring or a disease being contracted as a direct consequence of the original injury or incident?
2. Would that deterioration or disease be serious and what would be the consequence of it upon the plaintiff's lifestyle and occupation?
3. During what period is the deterioration or disease likely to occur if it is going to occur at all?

These questions should be specifically raised by the solicitor who wishes to consider the possibility of a provisional award being made in the case in question. If they are raised, the doctor must answer each question in turn if the requirements of the Section are to be fulfilled. He should do so in a separate letter to his report as it may well be that the solicitor or his client will not wish to deal with the case on a provisional damage basis but, nevertheless, rely upon the doctor's general findings on examination of the plaintiff.

The principal difficulty that arises when considering whether a case is appropriate for an award of provisional damages, is ascertaining whether there is merely a "chance" of the deterioration or disease occurring, as opposed to the doctors being able to "forecast" that it will occur. Thus where the plaintiff has suffered a head injury he may have apparently made a complete recovery but there could be a chance that he will subsequently develop post-traumatic epilepsy. If he does not, then it would be wrong to compensate him for the risk that he might do so. If he does actually develop epilepsy as a result of the accident he may well be entitled to a very substantial award. Alternatively, where a plaintiff has suffered a fracture involving the articular surface of a joint the doctor will probably be able to forecast that he will develop osteo-arthritis in that joint at some stage in the future. As the prospects of this occurring and its consequences can be assessed with reasonable accuracy well before the degeneration arises, it is possible to quantify that deterioration. The plaintiff can be compensated for it at the same time as dealing with the quantification of his injuries and losses to date. So an award of provisional damages in that case would not be necessary.

If an award of provisional damages is made the court will specify in its Order the deterioration or disease from which it considers the plaintiff may suffer. The period during which it would be prepared to re-open the case and consider making a further award in the event of that complication arising will also be stated. The court will retain various documents relating to the case for the period it has specified including any medical reports that have been disclosed and relied upon. The doctor may well have made notes of his examination or perusal of the records to assist him in preparing the reports that he has produced. He may well wish to refer to those notes if he has asked to see the plaintiff again at some stage in the future to consider the deterioration or disease that is alleged to have occurred. He should, therefore, be notified by the solicitor of the terms of the order that has been made and should be asked to ensure that he retains his papers relating to the case for the duration of the period during which the case could be re-opened.

An award of provisional damages is not appropriate merely because there will be a delay before the doctors can give a final prognosis. If that is the case the correct procedure would be for there to be split trials dealing with liability first and the assessment of quantum later when a final prognosis is available. A plaintiff who successfully establishes liability on the part of the defendant can obtain an interim payment until the final award is made. If, of course, there is going to be delay before a final prognosis can be given it will greatly assist the lawyers if the doctor can give an estimate as to when he should be able to make a final assessment.

Arrangements for Attending Court

The vast majority of cases are settled before trial and if settlement is reached then, of course, the doctor will not have to give evidence. There will, however, always be some cases that go to trial and the doctor must be prepared to attend the trial to give evidence in accordance with his report if called upon to do so. If he is not willing to attend court in those few cases that go to trial the doctor should not accept instructions to undertake medico-legal work.

When a case is set down for trial the procedure for listing the action for trial will vary depending upon which court the case is set down in. The procedures are as follows:

1. *High Court action set down in the Royal Courts of Justice in London.* If, after setting down, the parties do nothing further, the case will simply come into the list, often at very short notice, and the parties and their witnesses, including any experts, will be expected to attend when it does. This is clearly an undesirable procedure in cases where doctors have to give evidence, because very few medical witnesses can make themselves available at short notice without prior warning. Consequently the parties should apply for a fixture. They must ascertain the availability of their witnesses for

the period when the court is likely to be able to deal with the case and then appear before the Clerk of the List with details of that availability so that he can fix a date. Once a fixture is given the court will only be prepared to vary the arrangement it has made for the trial if there is a very good reason why that fixture is no longer a convenient date. When the fixture is given it may not appear to be a priority listing and, indeed, there may be several cases listed for the same day ahead of it. However, there is so much flexibility in arranging trials in London because of the large number of courts sitting at any time, that it is usually possible for a case to be brought on for trial on the appointed date once a fixture has been given.

Once a trial begins in the High Court either in London or in a provincial Crown Court it will normally continue into the next and subsequent days until it is concluded. If this is likely to occur the solicitor should warn his witnesses, especially the doctors that they may be needed on more than one day. In very lengthy trials the solicitor should try to agree a timetable with his opponent so that the doctor only attends court when necessary.

2. *Crown Courts in the Provinces.* After the case has been set down for trial it will appear in a warned list in which the court publishes a schedule of all the cases it hopes to deal with during a specific period. The listing officer of the Court concerned will require the parties' solicitors to inform him of their, and their witnesses availability during the period in question. The court will then publish a cause list in which it appoints dates for trials to commence, hopefully (although not necessarily) in accordance with the availability the solicitors have given. As with fixtures in London the case will only be removed from the list once a date has been appointed if there is a very good reason for it to be removed. Unlike trials in London there is no certainty that the case will actually be dealt with on the date appointed. The Court of its own volition will take it out of the list at short notice if the judge at the trial centre in question is required to do urgent criminal work which takes priority over civil cases. In addition, because there are only likely to be one or two judges sitting to deal with civil work in any provincial trial centre at one time, there is no flexibility to move cases from one court to another if a case earlier in the list runs over and occupies the date appointed for a subsequent trial.

In some cases, even in provincial centres, it may be desirable for the parties to apply for a fixture if they have a case that is going to take a long time to try and which involves a large number of expert witnesses who are unlikely to be available at the same time and at short notice. In those cases the parties should apply to the Crown Court Listing Office for a fixture to be given explaining why this is necessary. If the court agrees, the parties should then ascertain when their witnesses are available to attend court and a date will then be fixed that is convenient to the parties. Crown Courts are, however, reluctant to grant fixtures because they probably will not know the itineraries of the judges they will be getting far enough in advance to do so with confidence. In addition, they will not know how much criminal work they are going to have to deal with so far in advance. This must take priority over civil cases even when a fixture has been given.

3. *County Court.* Once a case has been set down for trial in the County Court or transferred to the County Court for trial pursuant to the Practice Direction

enabling the more straightforward High Court cases to be tried by a County Court judge (*Practice Direction* [1983] 3 All ER 95.) the court will simply fix a date for trial without prior consultation with the parties to ascertain the availability of their witnesses. The parties must then ascertain whether their witnesses can, in fact, attend a trial on the date appointed and ordinarily the court will only remove the case from the list if it has been notified that a material witness is not available within 7 days of it having appointed a date. The cases are only likely to be taken out of the list after that 7-day period if there is a good reason why the Court had not been told sooner that the date fixed was not convenient. Normally the trial will take place on the date fixed by the court but very often the court will have to deal with urgent matrimonial work listed at short notice before starting a civil trial. As a consequence it is rare for County Court trials to make a prompt start on the date that is fixed. If the case is not concluded on the date that has been appointed it will be adjourned part-heard until another convenient date can be fixed that is suitable to the parties, that is, the witnesses who have still to give evidence, the judge and the advocates.

It will be apparent that it is often extremely difficult to make arrangements for a trial of those County Court cases that involve several expert witnesses who have many other commitments and those cases that are likely to last more than one day. As a consequence many County Courts in the larger trial centres operate a running list for these more substantial trials from their and the surrounding County Courts to be dealt with in a similar way to Crown Court cases.

It must be remembered that arrangements for listing cases for trial are all based upon the principle that the judge is ensured of having sufficient work to do. Allowance is made for the fact that many cases settle at a late stage often on the morning of the trial and that some will have to be taken out of the list at short notice. In addition solicitors find it difficult to forecast how long a trial will take. As a result, listing officers will put more cases in the list than the court is able to hear if all those cases remain effective. Whilst this system remains there will continue to be a significant number of cases that simply do not get reached on the date fixed for trial or at least have to be taken out of the list at short notice when it may be too late for expert witnesses, such as doctors who have to plan operating lists and clinics, to make alternative arrangements during the short period of notice they are given. The consequence of this is an inevitable increase in expense to the litigant.

In recent years there has been considerable public concern at the length of litigation. Personal injury actions in particular have been criticised for delay. The Lord Chancellor's Department is determined to ensure that the courts are no longer responsible for any significant periods of delay. There is consequently pressure from the court to list cases for trial notwithstanding any difficulties the witnesses may have in making themselves available because of other commitments. There is a growing lack of sympathy for other commitments doctors may have, which probably arises as a result of the considerable delays that occur between the doctor being instructed and his being able to examine and report. Courts are even frequently unsympathetic where the doctor has been asked to attend a court in another trial centre to give evidence in some other case.

One of the consequences of this problem has been that many solicitors have found it necessary to serve subpoenas upon all the witnesses they require at a trial, including the doctors they wish to call, to establish a priority over cases that other trial centres are attempting to list and over other commitments the doctors in question may have. Doctors must appreciate that when this happens it is usually because the solicitor in question has no alternative but to serve a subpoena to protect his client's position at trial.

CHAPTER 16

Counsel's Advice to the Medical Expert

R. Maxwell QC

This chapter is intended to comment upon the role of the medical expert who produces medical reports and plays a forensic role if called upon to testify at trial. The relevant questions are looked at specifically in the context of civil proceedings where typically (but certainly not invariably) a doctor's evidence is concerned with the issue of compensation.

At the outset it is important to remember that the medical expert plays a function in litigation under English law which is, by its nature, adversarial. According to the adversarial system of litigation, one party, the plaintiff, sues the other, the defendant, and seeks to prove a case for damages; the two *parties* are regarded as adversaries.

The medical expert is involved in the adversarial procedure because he* is able to provide evidence and is, therefore, a witness, whose evidence is liable to be used at a trial, i.e. in court. The vast majority of claims for damages never see the light of day in a court but are settled, or otherwise disposed of, at some earlier stage. Whether the claim is resolved by agreement prior to a trial or by a judgement at a trial, the evidence of the medical witness will have played an important part either in the form of a written report or, possibly, at trial, by way of oral testimony.

It is in the nature of the adversarial system that a party relying upon the evidence of a medical expert will seek to use that evidence to further his case or to detract from his opponent's case. However, even though such are the tactics of the protagonists in the litigation, they do not reflect the proper function which the medical expert undertakes, which is simply to provide expert evidence. Generally that evidence will concern the nature and extent of pain, suffering and loss of amenity (including disability and incapacity for work and other purposes) both past, present and future, which affect an individual so far as that expert is able to judge matters based upon his independent (and expert) opinion. If the matter goes before a court at a trial, then the expert's medical evidence, if relevant, will be put before the judge (either in written form, if the evidence is agreed, or by way of oral testimony if the doctor is called as a witness). It is, though, only evidence, including evidence of opinion, which the

---

* The author fully recognises the fact that experts, doctors, plaintiffs, etc., are just as likely to be female and hopes female readers will forgive him for using the male case; this is for convenience only and without prejudice.

expert provides. Such a witness does not decide the issue, because he may not usurp the judicial function. His function is to provide the judge with both expert opinion and, in addition, the necessary scientific criteria for testing the accuracy of that opinion, so that the judge can then form his own independent judgement on the issue by applying such criteria to the facts of the case. Though justice is said to be blind, the judge must not blindly follow an expert but must see, and understand and then adjudicate upon the medical issue.

Preliminary Considerations

Keep Within Your Expertise

It is important to remember that a doctor, asked to provide a medical report about a claimant, is presupposed to have the appropriate expertise to be able to provide a relevant opinion and report. That does not always follow. The doctor should always consider whether he has the right expertise to be able to provide any report. Those who are medically inexpert do not always realise where the boundaries of a field of expertise enjoyed by a particular doctor lie. The medically inexpert ought, though, to be able to rely upon the medically expert to say whether or not a particular injury or problem affecting a plaintiff is outside that expert's province.

Are You Adequately Instructed?

There are two factors in particular to bear in mind. The first is that you ought to have been given written instructions which set out clearly your terms of reference and which, therefore, establish exactly what those instructing you want to know. Proper instructions will set out generally the subject headings which are to be covered (as to which see further below) and also particular areas of concern. Examples of the latter might be where the expert has to consider whether a plaintiff is acting reasonably in declining some recommended form of treatment; whether a plaintiff reasonably needs some specific appliance or equipment or nursing care or the like; whether a plaintiff has recovered some degree of working capacity and, if so, to what extent. The list of particular subjects that may need consideration is infinite. Look out for instructions to provide comment on some such particular factor that is of concern.

It is a fact of life in litigation that sometimes the instructions given to a medical expert are less than adequate and may amount to no more than "provide a medical report". Sometimes it may be necessary for the medical expert to enquire first as to what the terms of reference for such a report are, for example, where a plaintiff may have had more than one accident giving rise to discrete problems. Although it will often be possible for the expert to provide a medical report (taking into account the general considerations set out below) even if instructions have been inadequate, nevertheless in such circumstances the sensible medical expert will ask whether any further matters call for additional comment.

Are You Sufficiently Informed?

It sometimes happens that the only information available to the medical expert is what the plaintiff has to say. In a simple case this might not cause any major problem. The fact that the plaintiff is able to tell the doctor that he had a broken leg, coupled with the doctor's own clinical examination and assessment based upon experience, may produce what is for all practical purposes a sensible opinion. There is, though, always a risk that the doctor may have been left without information that would materially affect his opinion; for example, that a fracture involved the articular surface of a joint, that there was an episode of deep vein thrombosis, or even that there was a head injury which has left the plaintiff with a lack of insight into the true nature of his problems.

It is dangerous to provide a report without adequate information and no sensible doctor would take the risk of proceeding on the mere *ipse dixit* of the plaintiff. The sensible doctor will require, at the very least, hospital and medical notes relating to the plaintiff, a sight of radiographs or other such medical investigations that have been carried out. Where relevant the general practitioner's records and, perhaps, a further and better description of the accident or other traumatic event which is said to have been the cause of the plaintiff's ills may be needed.

The Golden Rules

Be Independent

The important factor to bear in mind is that the vehicle which carries the expert's evidence to Court - or if appropriate to a settlement out of Court without the need for any hearing - is a claim for damages. One party will be seeking to maximise the claim for damages and the other to avoid or reduce that claim. The use made by lawyers of expert medical evidence reflects those cardinal features of litigation. The medical expert must avoid becoming enlisted on behalf of a party. The medical expert must always be objective and independent. The medical expert is not a mercenary who merely follows the cheque. He tells the truth as he genuinely believes it to be and not trimmed or coloured so as to favour those who instruct him.

The doctor in this context faces two dangers. The first is that there is a temptation to regard the party on whose behalf the doctor is acting as a person whose interests have to be not merely protected but promoted by the doctor. Such a partisan approach has to be avoided.

The other danger is that the doctor may perceive that the doctor's interests are better served by providing evidence of a kind that he supposes will persuade those instructing him to retain him again in future cases. This commercial approach of, in effect, creating goodwill must equally be avoided.

If the advice in this context causes offence, then none is intended. However, it is surprising and sad to find doctors who, far from remaining detached and independent, become on the contrary over-zealously combative in their enthusiasm for what they regard as "their side".

Moreover, the best reputation that a doctor can have is to be independent. Any doctor marked out as a plaintiff's doctor or a defendant's doctor may enjoy, in the short term, a measure of one-sided popularity but, like any fashion, that is liable to fade. The doctor who is independent and objective and fair will find his services called upon equally by both sides for as long as the doctor wishes to be involved in such work, and even more importantly will enjoy the trust of the Court.

By way of a cautionary note, it has to be added that those who lack independence and objectivity are usually exposed as such eventually, with a resulting and seriously detrimental effect upon their reputation as an expert witness.

Always Have in Mind the Trial

The recommendation here is that the medical expert witness should, whenever called upon to express his view, test and assess the validity of that view by considering whether it represents what he would say if called upon to testify as a witness. Although only a very small proportion of cases get as far as a trial before a judge, most other cases are settled on the basis that the result reached by compromise is one which the parties feel was likely to reflect the result which a judge would come to. In those cases, the parties will have relied upon what the doctor has to say. It is important, therefore, that in the large number of cases which are settled without recourse to a trial, the medical expert has set out accurately and authoritatively what his views are. He must avoid inaccuracy and carelessness, because views vitiated in that way may lead the parties to a false evaluation of the claim.

From time to time, the medical expert will find that cases, where he has provided a report, do go to court. In that situation it is just as important, and in one respect even more so, that the medical expert should have expressed his views with regard to the possibility of a trial. If the expert has had such a possibility in prospect, then he will have expressed himself in the report(s) in the same way as he would if called upon to do so orally in the witness box. It is, therefore, vital that the expert should look carefully at his words. Firstly, it is no more than humane to do so: the report concerns a living (usually) claimant who would understandably be distressed if told, for example, that expectation of life has inevitably or probably been reduced, or that amputation might be required, or the like, whereas in fact the doctor meant only to say that there was a possibility of some marginal reduction of life or an outside chance of an amputation. Secondly, accuracy and care in the formulation of the views that the doctor wants to express will allow a correspondingly accurate and reliable quantification of the claim. Thirdly, the doctor can avoid the embarrassment of having to concede in the witness box that he had not noticed what he said, did not mean it, and now wishes materially to alter the effect of the written medical report. Thus, the medical report should reflect neither more nor less than the evidence which the expert would give to the judge by way of oral testimony.

The Medical Report: Achieving Clarity of Communication

The subject headings of the relevant areas of information in respect of which the lawyers seek the doctor's views are commonplace. The purpose for which that information is sought is sometimes not understood by the doctor, or may not be made clear by the lawyers. From the doctor's point of view, there is a risk that the doctor may treat the creation of a medical report as being no more than a repetition of the documentation that results when some injured person is admitted to a hospital ward and a medical history is taken, a diagnosis formed and treatment recommended. The reference is not far-fetched. If the first few sheets of typical ward clinical notes are examined, it will be seen how similar the subject-matter of a medico-legal report often is: history of present condition; past medical history; details of treatment so far; diagnosis; recommendations.

The fact that there is a similarity is not a criticism. The information under these headings is clearly relevant, but for different purposes in each case. In the ward, such information is relevant for the purposes of treatment. In litigation, the purpose is quite different. In medico-legal work, the doctor's expert views translate not into treatment (although coincidentally on occasions this may happen) but into an assessment of the difference between, on the one hand, the plaintiff as he would have been without the accident as against, on the other hand, the plaintiff as he has been, is and will be as a result of the accident. The purpose of adducing and evaluating evidence on the issue of quantum is to see what difference some traumatic event has effected upon the plaintiff, so that he may be compensated by an award of damages. The theoretical basis for the award is to make up to the plaintiff for the devaluation in the various aspects of his life that flow from the traumatic event.

Although the purpose of the exercise is to produce compensation by way of damages, that does not mean that the doctor should involve himself in the exercise of contriving or maximising a claim or in seeking to defeat such a claim. The function of the medical expert evidence, namely to assist in quantifying the claim, simply emphasises the commercial and economic reality of litigation. The doctor, though, must still remember the need to be independent and to have as his priority the purpose of being helpful to the Court rather than to the cause.

The medical report provides an invaluable window through which the plaintiff can be viewed. Sometimes it is the only window and this may be the case, for example, where a defendant or the defendant's insurers have information about the effect of an accident on a plaintiff only by virtue of what a medical report says.

Of course, if a case goes to court, a judge will have more viewpoints on the plaintiff than simply a medical report or series of medical reports because the judge will see for himself (probably) the plaintiff and hear his and others' evidence about the effect of the accident on the plaintiff. In cases settled out of court, though, the medical report will be the sole or main means of providing an assessment of the effects of some accident upon a plaintiff. It is important then that the medical report should set out in a convincing and authoritative manner the doctor's views. For guidance in the technique of writing a report the reader is referred to chapter 2. Some further comment is now offered on those matters of interest to the legal mind.

Layout

Certain basic rules are best followed if a visually impressive and readable document is to be produced:

Size

It is best to avoid a variety of different paper sizes and preferable to have one uniform size. Ultimately, a bundle of medical reports will be produced for the trial judge on A4 size paper and, on the whole, it is preferable if the doctor produces his original report on A4.

Identification

The report ought to be clearly dated, together with some clear indication as to which party has requested it and whether the report is a first report or second and so on. Thus, on the first page the report may be instantly identifiable if set out with a heading:

> First Medical Report on [name] of [address], at the request of [name of solicitors], Solicitors for [party].

Numbering

Each and every page must be numbered.

Sections

It is important that the report should be broken up into different sections of relevant information and that each such section, which may comprise one or more paragraphs, be given a separate subject heading. Suggestions as to appropriate subject headings are set out below. Since, from time to time, more than one report on a particular plaintiff will be provided by a doctor, it is very important that in subsequent reports the doctor should, for the sake of continuity, maintain uniformity in the subject headings.

Subject Headings

The following is a representative rather than an exhaustive list of relevant subject headings that are commonly of interest in actions for claims for damages for personal injuries:

Plaintiff: background information

History of accident (or other traumatic event)

Subsequent history

Plaintiff's current complaints

Relevant past or other medical history

Findings on examination

Diagnosis

Assessment and grading of present and future disability

Special needs

Recommendations (including, if appropriate, treatment or further investigations and review).

It is necessary to consider each of these in turn in order to explain why those involved in litigation have an interest in such matters:

Plaintiff: Background Information

Since the object of compensation is to make up to a plaintiff, as far as money can, the difference between the plaintiff as he would have been without the accident and the plaintiff as he is in fact, having suffered the accident, background information about the plaintiff will provide a necessary datum point. Here, the window first opens to allow a view of the plaintiff and typically, in order to envisage the plaintiff properly, information will be needed under the following subheadings.

Age. The plaintiff's date of birth should be noted, together with his age at the date of the report and the length of time in years and months since the accident occurred. If the plaintiff's age is worthy of comment, then make it, as for example that he is a sprightly octogenarian or that his appearance is of a man much older than his age, or whatever.

Sex. Usually the sex of the claimant is apparent but not always. Better to indicate, for example, by the use of Mr/Mrs/Ms.

Apparent State of Health. Some general description of the plaintiff is helpful so as to indicate the plaintiff's general state of health and demeanour. It is useful to have information about a person's weight, height and apparent level of physical fitness.

Work. Since loss of earnings is so important a part of a claim for damages, it is vital to investigate the plaintiff's pre-accident and post-accident working capacity in some detail. The starting point is to find out what work the plaintiff used to do. That will involve obtaining information from the plaintiff as to what his job involved, what physical or mental efforts were required of him, how well he coped with it, what hours he worked, whether he was settled in the job or likely to move or be promoted, how much he enjoyed the work or otherwise. If the job involved any special skills, or expertise, then they need to be identified. Similarly, the plaintiff's post-accident working history needs to be described and details given of work which the plaintiff has done.

Hobbies, Sports and Leisure Pursuits. Again, with the aim in mind of establishing a picture of the plaintiff as he was before by way of comparison with the
plaintiff as he is after the accident, details need to be found from the plaintiff
about his hobbies, sports and leisure pursuits in those two different situations. If
the plaintiff had any particular success in any field of endeavour, then it should
be stated.

Social Status and Circumstances. Some detail needs to be given about the
plaintiff's social status and circumstances and this will involve enquiry as to
where he lives and with whom. It may well be necessary (see below) to make a
domiciliary visit as, for example, in the case of a plaintiff seriously injured and
complaining that his present accommodation is unsatisfactory or that inadequate arrangements for care and attendance exist. The doctor will want to know
whether there are supportive relatives or friends, caring for the plaintiff, how
much the plaintiff is independent and able to look after himself and whether
more needs to be done to provide a suitable quality of life for the plaintiff.

History of Accident (or Other Traumatic Event)

"History of present condition" is a concept already well known to a doctor, but
it takes on a different shape in legal proceedings, where it is necessary for a
plaintiff, in order to succeed in his claim for damages, to show that some
specific injury or resulting financial damage was caused by the relevant event. In
this context, the relevant event is usually to be regarded as the occasion of
trauma which it is alleged was caused by some negligence or breach of duty on
the part of the defendant, or perhaps some further consequence of that original
trauma such as an operation or form of medical treatment. Thus, the lawyers –
on both sides – have a legitimate interest in seeking an explanation as to how a
person came to be injured or ill and when this happened and, possibly, where it
happened. To some extent, the doctor may seem to be acting as a detective at
this point but appearance belies the reality. There are clear limitations on what
the doctor is or should be expected to do. Essentially the question for the
doctor is whether or not the doctor is of the expert opinion that if the account
as to how, when and where some traumatic event occurred is accepted, then in
his opinion it is credible to conclude that the injury or damage has been caused
as a result. The doctor, in this context, is not required to make up *his* mind, as a
judge would, as to whether such explanation should be believed, although
occasions do arise when the doctor can and should offer useful comment on
this issue of credibility. This might happen, for example, where the doctor
doubts that some direct impact with the lumbar spine could have caused as a
consequence a slipped disc such as appears to be the cause of the plaintiff's
problems.

The doctor, too, has a legitimate interest in investigating the cause of some
injury or the etiology of some condition. His evidence is to help explain to a
court how some relevant state of affairs came about. The explanation is
incomplete if the doctor fails to enquire into the initiating circumstances.

Often this part of the investigation is without controversy and relates to what
is common ground between the parties. It should never be assumed that this is
so, however. Even if a letter of instruction to the doctor indicates some history

of the injury, the astute medical witness will, nevertheless, make his own enquiries unless instructed not to do so.

Subsequent History

Because a plaintiff will doubtless be claiming damages for pain, suffering and loss of amenity, and probably for resulting loss of earnings as well, it is important to know what has happened from the time of the original injury or the onset of the original condition up to the date of the report or, in the case of a subsequent report, from the date of the previous report to the date of the present one. From time to time up to the date of the trial, the doctor will be asked to update his first report by the provision of subsequent reports. Thus what is described here as "subsequent history" gradually becomes longer.

The subsequent history will, to some extent, be derived from the hospital notes and certainly they will be the main source of information as to the medical treatment of the plaintiff, both whilst he was an inpatient and subsequently as an outpatient.

In addition, though, information may well be provided by the instructing solicitor, or by way of access to the general practitioner's records, as well as what the claimant has to say; it is a significant aspect of the evidence. The lawyers' interest in what the doctor has to say is partly that of reading the factual account that emerges from what the doctor discovers, but is also to a significant extent that of seeing what assessment the doctor makes of the amount of pain, suffering and loss of amenity affecting the plaintiff during the period prior to the date of the report and how far the doctor credits that the pain and suffering has been as great (or as little) as asserted by the plaintiff or, possibly, as asserted by a medical expert on the other side. Again, the lawyers will want to know how far their medical expert credits that the plaintiff has been, say, incapacitated for work or some particular social or leisure pursuit during this period.

Plaintiff's Current Complaints

It is appreciated that the current state of the plaintiff does not necessarily reflect the plaintiff's final state when he reaches whatever plateau of improvement may be available to him. It is though, very important that the doctor should provide a detailed account of what the plaintiff is complaining at the date of the relevant medical report, preferably noting the plaintiff's words. That obviously is necessary where the plaintiff has reached maximal recovery. In a case where further medical reports will be required, a detailed account provides a valuable basis for comparison when some subsequent report is obtained.

At this stage of the report, the doctor is concerned with the plaintiff's assertions as to what is wrong and this is essentially a subjective area. The area of investigation, of course, is divided into two. Quite apart from the subjective element, there is the further vital question - the objective area - where the doctor states the extent to which he credits that the subjective complaints are valid.

A useful distinction can be drawn between complaints volunteered by a plaintiff compared with those which result only from some leading question from the doctor. It should be remembered that some plaintiffs are not particularly articulate and may need prompting and encouragement in order to reveal what troubles them.

At this point the medical expert needs to remind himself that the ultimate purpose of the exercise is for the lawyers, by agreement or by adjudication of the Court, to establish what the consequences of the relevant trauma or illness have been. The consequences as complained of by the plaintiff may relate to details of the plaintiff's life of a seemingly trivial or otherwise uninteresting nature. However, the fact that the doctor may have but a passing interest in a plaintiff's complaints of difficulties in working on the coal face, in having sexual intercourse, or in looking after his budgerigars, is neither here nor there. The doctor needs to establish what the complaints are because what the lawyers or the court, where appropriate, need to know is the extent to which the doctor credits the problems as complained of. Without establishing what the complaints are and recording what may otherwise seem to be hum-drum detail, the doctor cannot begin to make a proper assessment and say to what extent he thinks that the plaintiff has the alleged disabilities or continuing difficulties or whether they are related to the relevant event said to have been caused by some negligence or breach of duty on the part of the defendant.

There would seem to be no reason why the doctor should not obtain a full and detailed history of what the plaintiff feels to be the problem. Unfortunately, what is sometimes reported back to the lawyers, and sometimes to the court is along the lines "I was only in there for ten minutes – he just didn't want to know – he never said a word and he didn't even look at me," and so on. This is not a complaint that some doctors are rude or that some deal with medico-legal appointments as though they are process workers on some production line. It is not a plea that doctors should be more friendly, sympathetic towards or supportive of plaintiffs. It is simply a reminder that the medical expert witness needs to have an extensive interest in the plaintiff's current state as complained of subjectively because eventually the doctor will consider those subjective complaints in the light of his objective findings and expert opinion. He must form some appreciation of what he credits that the plaintiff can or cannot do, the extent to which any such disability is related to the relevant traumatic event. He must assess and grade the alleged disability. If effective and proper enquiry into this aspect of a claim demands more of a doctor's time, then he will, doubtless, charge accordingly. Since the claim will be quantifiable to a more accurate extent, the time taken is cost-effective.

Relevant Past or Other Medical History

Because compensation is paid only in respect of the consequences of some relevant traumatic event, it is necessary to identify and isolate those consequences from any other disabling condition that may affect a plaintiff. Therefore, it is important to enquire into relevant past medical history. Bearing in mind that the purpose of the exercise is to compensate the plaintiff for the difference between the plaintiff as he is and will be as a result of the accident compared with the plaintiff as he would have been without the accident, it is vital to consider what has happened to the plaintiff already and what would have happened in the future without the accident.

Thus, if a steel erector, for example, falls to the ground and breaks his legs so that the resulting disability prevents him from working again as a steel erector, he would no doubt claim for resulting loss of earnings past, present and future. However, enquiry into his past medical history might, for example, throw up a significant spinal condition which on a balance of probabilities may be thought to be likely to have caused him to leave work as a steel erector within 5 years. That would then limit the claim for loss of earnings accordingly.

Past medical history is a wide category and includes not only other traumatic accidents but also mental illness, disease, constitutional conditions and defects, etc.

The existence of a past medical history does not necessarily enure to a defendant's advantage. Sometimes the relevant traumatic event may have exacerbated some otherwise unrelated condition, for example, where the stress of an accident and its consequences adversely affect some underlying hypertension. Sometimes an otherwise unrelated condition by its mere presence makes the effects of the accident that much worse as, for example, where a one-eyed man suffers injury to his remaining good eye.

The relevance or otherwise of a past medical history may give rise to considerable problems so far as the application of legal principle is concerned. However, the doctor's responsibility is to provide the basic data to enable the lawyers to apply the relevant legal principles. This is an aspect of a claim where the doctor should anticipate further correspondence with the instructing solicitors to enable the application of such legal principles to be properly made.

In an appropriate case enquiry into past medical history is best dealt with by seeking access to the general practitioner's records and such other medical records, including occupational health histories where available, as may exist.

Findings on Examination

It would be presumptuous for a lay person (in medical terms) to indicate how any medical examination should be conducted. In making a report about the medical examination, the doctor can fairly assume that the reader will have some, albeit limited, knowledge of medical terminology and access to a medical dictionary. He ought not to assume a level of understanding such as might be expected from another doctor. Some simplification and, where necessary, clarification is called for. This does not mean that the medical information upon which the doctor's diagnosis and other views may be established should be excised from the report. It does mean that the doctor should pause to think whether the information will, without more explanation, be readily comprehended by non-medically qualified personnel. If there is any doubt on that score, then further comment and explanation should be offered as necessary.

The following suggestions are made:

1. Diagrams and photographs to show the effect of a lesion, the restriction of movement and so on can provide visually impressive explanations.
2. Some idea of the comparative loss of any range of movement in a joint ought to be given, with an assessment of what would have been the range of movement without the accident.
3. Scarring is best explained not only by a written description but by at the very least a diagram and better still a photograph. Photographs are best taken by an appropriate professional photographer. If the solicitor has not already

arranged for this to be done, then the doctor may have access to a medical photographic service where it can be arranged. Photographs should show fairly the state of scarring, not only as isolated lesions but also in relation to the plaintiff as a whole so that an overall assessment can better be made. Ultimately, the written description and photographs will not be the only evidence of scarring and almost always before any damages are agreed upon or ordered, there will have been an inspection by the lawyers or judge.

4. Injuries giving rise to loss of vision or loss of hearing will necessarily be reported upon by doctors whose medical terminology will probably require careful explanation so that the practical effect of the relevant injury can be understood. It is important that the medical findings be recorded so as to indicate how many decibels hearing loss there may be, but it is just as important to give as far as possible some grading of that hearing loss in terms of overall disability and by way of comparison against normal hearing. The same comment may be made with regard to an injury giving rise to interference with vision.

5. It is sensible to make written notes of the examination and then to keep those notes until the claim is finally disposed of. A note of a relevant finding or of some comment made by a plaintiff is potent evidence if any challenge is made against the accuracy of the doctor's report. It should be remembered that a written note may not only refute an unwarranted challenge but also confirm the validity of a challenge where the doctor may have inaccurately remembered or misinterpreted his findings. Of course, if the doctor has followed the golden rules, he has nothing to fear. He will wish to be independent and objective and fair and thus will not be troubled if the note confirms the challenge. If he has written the report with care so as to represent what he would say if the matter went to court, he will have taken care to avoid the situation arising where he has misinterpreted the findings on examination.

Diagnosis

Diagnosis should as far as possible be firm and clear. Except in the most obvious cases, some indication should be given of the reasoning that leads to the diagnosis, including an explanation as to the mechanics of injury in the context of the relevant accident or other traumatic event. If, exceptionally, the doctor does not know what diagnosis to reach, then this must be stated, but with a detailed explanation as to what prevents a diagnosis.

The matter of diagnosis is important for two reasons. Firstly, it will enable the parties to see whether they are in agreement about the nature of the underlying injury or condition. Secondly though, the parties will be enabled to categorise the injury and to quantify the injury by having regard to previous decided awards for such injury.

Assessment and Grading of Present and Future Disability

In an appropriate case the lawyers are concerned to assess and grade the nature and extent of a present and future disability. This is a crucial part of the process.

The doctor has to give practical effect to his findings by offering an opinion as to the nature and extent of real disability that affects or is likely to affect this plaintiff in his day-to-day life, both in terms of work and socially. This exercise is appropriate whether reporting for plaintiff or defendant.

The doctor needs to consider also not only the present, but the future, and to give a prognosis. The prognosis is essentially a medical matter where the doctor explains what will happen in terms of a particular injury or condition, but from a lawyer's point of view the prognosis has to be looked at in a wider context so as to see what difference deterioration makes to the quality of the plaintiff's life in all respects. Thus, whilst medically it may be sufficient for a doctor to say with regard to an injured ankle joint that osteo-arthritis may set in within 10 years, the lawyer and ultimately the judge would need to know what that means in practical terms. How much more pain and restriction of movement will there be? How far will locomotion be affected? Will further treatment be required? How much more of a problem, in other words, will osteo-arthritis be?

Again, the doctor needs to remember that the object of the exercise is compensation to represent the difference between the plaintiff as he was and would have been without the accident, compared with the plaintiff as he is and will be as a result of the accident. Of course, this involves some degree of crystal ball gazing, but nobody is better qualified than a doctor to give a forecast and courts appreciate that often the matter cannot be stated in terms of certainties, but only by way of finely balanced estimations of odds that may approach guesswork.

So far as incapacity for work is concerned, this is a vital part of the claim. It may well carry the major portion of the damages with it, if a plaintiff cannot do any work or is reduced to some lesser and lighter job than he previously carried out. It is an aspect that affects not only the past up to the date that the doctor is seeing the plaintiff, but also the current state and the future.

The lawyers want to know how far the plaintiff is disadvantaged as a result of the relevant event as far as his work is concerned. Can he do his old job? If not, why not? What job could he do? Will there be improvement so that in due course he can do some increased work? All this may translate into hard cash by way of damages. It is, of course, an aspect of the case where a greedy plaintiff may try to pull the wool over the eyes of the expert.

In order to carry out a sensible and meaningful investigation, the doctor needs to find out what the plaintiff used to do as a job and why he says he cannot do that job any longer. He then needs to assess whether he, the doctor, credits that there is this alleged disability and, finally if the plaintiff is handicapped then what alternative work the doctor thinks the plaintiff to be capable of. The lawyers are dependent to a great extent upon what the doctor says here. The doctor needs to be careful in his assertions. He begins, though, by forming some sensible view of what the plaintiff did in his old work. That may require the doctor making further enquiry to satisfy himself that he knows what the work involved. In coal-mining areas, for example, it is doubtful whether a doctor could sensibly express a view as to whether or not a plaintiff could work, say, "in the pit bottom" but not "on the face" without having some detailed information on which to base his judgement. That might be obtained from the plaintiff by question and answer. It might involve asking the solicitor for assistance in order to help understand the problem. It may even involve visiting the work place to view the job.

It must equally follow that the doctor here may *not* credit the alleged problem with work and may come to the conclusion that it is over-stated by the plaintiff to the extent of being unreasonable. The doctor should say so. If he thinks a plaintiff should be back at work, then it would be misleading to give any other impression. Of course, in the majority of cases the plaintiff's bona fides is beyond question but it would be naive to think that this is universally true.

Therefore, if the doctor does regard the plaintiff's alleged incapacity for work as well founded, he should say so. He ought not though, except in the most obvious case, to rely merely upon what the plaintiff says. Given that a plaintiff is saying that he cannot do this or that, then, as far as can be achieved within the consulting room, the doctor should see for himself how real the problem is. The astute doctor will in cases of any doubt be alive to the possibility of looking at the plaintiff outside the consulting room.

Special Needs

The growth area in claims for damages nowadays lies in a claim for the provision of some medical treatment, perhaps even para-medical treatment, claims for aids, appliances and so on, and claims for nursing or quasi-nursing or other care and assistance. The question is always whether or not such expenditure is being or is to be reasonably incurred for a plaintiff. A doctor will often be approached to express a view about this.

It is often better that the doctor should make some domiciliary visit in order to see the plaintiff in his own environment and find out exactly why he needs such care and assistance. The danger in the context of such claims is that medical expert witnesses may be either too dismissive of the claim or too uncritical of such a claim. Such claims merit careful attention because they can sound heavily in damages. Therefore, the claims need to be assessed objectively. The lawyers need to know to what extent the doctor credits the claim and that question for the doctor is whether or not in the doctor's view such expenditure would be *reasonably* incurred. That is not to be answered by comparing the lot of the plaintiff, who in that respect at least may be fortunate enough to have the chance of suing for damages, with the lot of some patient without that opportunity. The test is not whether the plaintiff can get along without the expenditure but whether or not it is reasonable to incur such expenditure.

Recommendations for Treatment and Further Investigations/Review

It may be that the doctor feels that some further specific treatment should be considered. The doctor is not advising the plaintiff but is making such comment to the solicitors who have requested the report. The doctor's comments may then be brought to the attention of the doctor who has charge of the plaintiff. If any further treatment is suggested, then the plaintiff may want to recover the cost of that on a private patient basis and the doctor will probably be asked for details of such likely expenditure.

Quite apart from medical treatment, the doctor may feel that some form of rehabilitation either by way of training for work or physiotherapy or the like is appropriate. Again, details of the recommendations would have to be given.

It may though, be that the doctor feels that further medical investigations are necessary, or that some further time must elapse before any definitive medical opinion can be given. He should indicate what further medical investigations are required or when would be an appropriate date for him to provide a further medical review.

For the most part, English law contemplates that damages will be provided on a once and for all basis. There are occasions where "provisional" damages may be awarded. Unless the doctor is instructed otherwise, he should assume in the first place that the claim involves an award of final damages, that is to say where damages are assessed once and for all. If a solicitor wants to find out whether a claim is appropriate for provisional damages (that is, an award for some damages now with a later award if there is some serious deterioration or disease that supervenes), then the solicitor will give appropriate instructions and formulate the question that is relevant in the particular case for the doctor to answer. If the doctor finds that he is presented with a question that he does not regard as a sensible question that allows some appropriate answer, then he should tell the solicitor.

In the event of a doctor reporting that the effect of some accident or condition is that there is a risk of some serious deterioration or disease supervening, then he will probably find that the solicitor follows this up in correspondence by enquiry with regard to the possibility of provisional damages.

In dealing with the prognosis both in general terms and specifically in the context of such a risk of serious disease or deterioration ensuing, the doctor is not expected to do more than express an opinion. He is not guaranteeing what will happen. The prognosis that the doctor gives is needed to explain to what extent in that doctor's opinion the pain and suffering will continue, improve or deteriorate; the extent to which the plaintiff will remain incapacitated for work or the stage at which he will become incapacitated for work; how far social and leisure pursuits will be affected; how far care and assistance will be required and what sort and degree of care and assistance, and so on. The lawyers will use the prognosis to help work out the claim for damages.

The prognosis may vary from time to time and in particular from report to report. There is nothing embarrassing about the doctor changing his formulation of the prognosis, provided that at each stage the prognosis has been worked out and assessed objectively and with as much care as is reasonable. If at the end of the exercise, the medical expert opinion is the next best thing to guesswork in this context, then it is still better than any guess which a lawyer might make.

The Medical Expert as Witness

Sometimes, in a small proportion of cases, the medical issue proceeds to trial and the medical expert is called as a witness.

If the litigation is properly conducted, then the medical expert should avoid what regrettably happens too often, namely, that he finds himself suddenly and without warning required to attend a trial. Perhaps he may be subject to a subpoena, in a case where he may have provided a report or reports over a period of years but not recently, and where he has no knowledge of what, if any, current medical issue is involved. That scenario, which occurs with depressing regularity, means that the doctor's evidence is almost *in vacuo.* What ought to happen is that well before any trial date, a sensible solicitor will find out from his doctor what the doctor's views are of the medical evidence on the other side, whether any further medical examination of the plaintiff and, therefore, any further report is needed, and whether the doctor needs access to any other documentation or material. The doctor may be invited to have access to such material, as for example the general practitioner's records. He might even be asked to have access to other material, such as a video recording of the plaintiff, perhaps showing what the plaintiff can do when viewed unawares.

The careful medical witness will want to consider the medical issues in some depth. It may be one where he feels additional comment is required. Perhaps further research in medical text books and articles is needed and relevant references noted. A bibliography may be needed. What was previously *in vacuo* may now expand when the medical issue is subjected to the forensic experience.

It is therefore vital that well before trial, the final and definitive version of the medical expert's views should be sought. Such version will not necessarily be the same as that expressed after the last medical examination of the plaintiff. In order to find out the final and definitive version, the medical expert needs to be given the opportunity to take stock so that he can say in the first place whether there is, indeed, a medical issue at all and, if so, then to comment upon that medical controversy in a particular case and to modify and qualify or confirm and corroborate what he may already have said.

Any medical expert apparently called upon to speak to his report or reports by way of evidence ought to respond by asking to know the context in which that evidence is to be given: what other medical evidence is available? Can there be the opportunity for a further medical examination, if necessary? Can there be a conference with counsel?

The facility is now available for a "without prejudice" meeting of experts, and the court has the power to order this in an appropriate case. The purpose of such a meeting is to identify the parts of the expert evidence which are in issue. If there is such a meeting, then the experts may prepare a joint statement indicating those parts of their evidence on which they are and those on which they are not in agreement. If doctors are asked to attend such a meeting, they should establish exactly what the terms of reference are. They should beware the temptation to regard the meeting as inviting them to arbitrate upon a case or as an invitation to strive to reach the middle ground. Such a meeting does not have as its purpose that of splitting the difference, only of establishing the areas of agreement or disagreement in the evidence.

Where, though, a doctor on taking stock of his views as expressed in previous reports, concludes that some modification or shift in his opinion is appropriate, then this really should be done sooner rather than later. It ought not to be the case that the doctor reveals what he now believes only at trial.

Often the conflict of medical opinion is shown to be more apparent than real, or at all events much narrower than had been thought, if the opportunity is given to the doctor to refresh his memory about what has been said by him, to scrutinise what he has said, and to view it in the context of other medical evidence available in the case. In that situation, the division of medical opinion may be revealed to be no more than a matter of semantics. Sometimes the division can be bridged. Better that this should be done before the expense of a trial is incurred.

The Trial

Suppose, in spite of all, a claim is going to trial. What are now offered are some practical tips intended to ease the doctor's task and delay anxiety that may be felt by the novice medical expert giving evidence for the first time.

The Subpoena

It may be that the solicitors who have instructed you serve you with a writ of subpoena which is a daunting document whereby the Monarch commands you to attend the trial and the solicitors may well offer conduct money ("a reasonable and sufficient sum of money to defray the expenses of coming and attending to give evidence and of returning from giving evidence"). Do not be alarmed. Equally do not be offended. You are not being treated in a manner unbecoming to your station. This is a standard method of securing the attendance of a witness. It may well be your salvation if it is necessary for you to show a reason why on some particular date(s) you are not available but required to attend a court sitting. That might be the case, for example, where two different actions in which you may be involved as a witness come on for trial in different courts on the same day.

However, the law will, so far as is reasonable, have regard to your convenience. If it is difficult for you to attend as required then make your difficulties known to your solicitors and ask for help. In appropriate cases it may be possible to alter the date of a trial.

Arrangements for Attendance

You are entitled to know when, where and for how long your attendance is required. It is important to establish what arrangements are made for meeting the solicitors who have required you to attend the trial. A typical court centre is a large building. You will need to know exactly where to go and where you will be met. Equally you will need to know at what time you should be there. These details are really no more than matters of common courtesy. They should be dealt with by the solicitor, but if they are not, then demand to be told.

It is also important to establish for how long your attendance will be required. This is very much a matter for the solicitor and counsel to decide upon. Do not expect that your involvement will be limited to the time when you are in the witness box giving evidence. Remembering that a case is typically made up of opening address by plaintiff's legal representative - evidence from plaintiff and witnesses including expert witnesses - defendant's evidence and defendant's witnesses including expert witnesses - closing addresses by legal representatives - judgement. You are unlikely to be released until after all relevant expert evidence has been heard. That does not mean that you will be required to be in constant attendance until that point but you will need to be there, if called upon to do so, for the purposes of hearing relevant material until that time. In the typical sequence just set out that may well mean that you have to hear the opening address, the plaintiff's evidence and evidence of other relevant witnesses both for the plaintiff and the defendant. The extent to which you need to attend is a matter for the lawyers to consider and then to inform you.

Pre-trial Conference

If there is a medical issue then almost certainly the lawyers will want to see you in conference (or, if a silk (QC) is involved, in consultation) and this will be arranged prior to the trial starting. It may be on the day or a few days before trial or on the first day of trial (typically at about 9.00 am to 9.30 am prior to trial commencing at 10.30 am). This is an important meeting since by this stage the relevant issues for the court to decide will have become crystallised. It is by way of an informal discussion. It serves various purposes. You may be called upon to develop views that you have expressed and to consider views expressed by other experts. You may be asked to identify the essential points that support one view and tend to refute another.

Probably you will be told how in practice your evidence will be dealt with when you are called to the witness box. So, for example, you may be told that your reports will be put in and taken as read so as to represent your evidence generally but that you will be asked to develop particular points. Your attention may be drawn to what the lawyers think might be weaknesses or strengths in your or others' reports and you may be asked to comment.

If you have any questions (and all the more so if you have any problems or doubts) about the medical issues then this really is the last time to express them.

Preparation

Before coming to the court you should have prepared your evidence with some care. That does not mean that your evidence should be contrived. You should though, have reviewed all the relevant papers, including all available medical records and reports. You should avoid a situation where in the witness box you seem to be taking a trip down Memory Lane and to be dealing with matters which until that very moment you had entirely forgotten. In short make sure you are familiar with the available material.

Patience and Discretion

Being at court involves a certain amount of waiting. Be patient. Do not assume that time is being wasted. Relax and enjoy the respite from the typically hectic day of a doctor. Let the lawyers get on with their business and while you are waiting, almost certainly issues are being resolved which may lead possibly to settlement of the claim or to agreement of the medical evidence.

Do not take it upon yourself to seek out the medical expert on the other side with a view to resolving the medical issue yourself. Apart from pleasantries it is better to avoid such contact. If the lawyers want the doctors to put their heads together they will arrange for this to be done and state the terms of reference.

Giving Evidence

The good expert is one who tells the truth so far as matters of fact are concerned and is honest and objective so far as matters of opinion go. He is independent and seeks to assist the court rather than trying to be partisan. There are no tricks. It is not a matter of dress, demeanour or delivery. The expert, however, is not the conductor of the performance. He is in the hands of the legal representative who decides what questions to ask. Of course, in response to those questions the expert may give a virtuoso performance.

The key to giving evidence is to listen to and answer the questions. Usually the terms of the question show the nature of the answer that is appropriate, whether it is to be limited to a short "yes" or "no" or to give the opportunity for some lengthier and perhaps reasoned reply.

The answers are given to the questions put by the lawyer and to that extent it is a dialogue, but those answers are intended to be for the assistance of the judge who decides the case. It is important then to make sure that the answer is given in a manner that allows the judge to understand and to note the words used. The dialogue then does not proceed at normal conversation pace. The judge needs to make a note of what is being said. The expert will need to speak more slowly than normal. He is not, though, dictating the answer to the judge, who may note only such parts as are considered relevant. The expert should give the judge the opportunity of doing precisely that.

Since the answers are intended for the judge it is usually better physically to turn to the judge when giving the answer. Some judges require that to be done. It produces an unusual aspect to the dialogue in that the doctor faces the lawyer to hear the question but replies to the question facing the judge. If in doubt how to address the judge, ask the solicitor or counsel whether he is "my lord" or "your honour". If still in doubt address him as "sir".

When called to give evidence the expert will have moved from a seat in the court to the witness box. He should take with him his medical reports, other relevant medical reports from other experts in the case and any other documents that he thinks may well be required, for example, his own original notes, possibly his references in medical text books and the like. Such material will amount to an *aide mémoire*. However, the doctor should not refer to such material without either being expressly invited to do so (e.g. "Look at your report dated April 1st, Doctor...") or without asking permission to do so (e.g. "May I just look at my original notes on that point?").

However, care must be taken as to what is transported into the witness box. The doctor may have documents which, for whatever reason, are confidential and have not been disclosed. Better then to establish with the lawyers who have instructed him what documents and material he may take into the witness box. In that particular context the doctor should have been told exactly which of his reports or letters have been disclosed to the other side and, sensibly, such disclosed reports and letters will have been marked as such, so that material which has not been disclosed will not be referred to.

The occasion of giving evidence is not the time for the doctor to attempt some brilliant coup by a reference to medical literature or some feature in the case that he has never previously commented upon. We do not have trial by ambush. There should already have been made full disclosure by each side of relevant medical evidence. If medical text books or works are to be cited in support of an opinion then that should already have been disclosed prior to trial in some relevant medical report. If in doing his homework prior to trial the doctor does come upon some further relevant feature that he thinks should be mentioned he should reveal that as soon as possible to the lawyers who instruct him so that they can arrange for further disclosure to be made to the other side.

Although lawyers may have some image in mind of the ideal medical witness, experience in the court shows that persuasive expert witnesses who carry the day on a particular issue display widely differing characteristics. By and large, they do not show themselves as argumentative or resenting challenge to their opinion. Generally, they are aware of the need to make the judge understand their view and this is usually to be achieved by answering the questions put and doing so in a calm and helpful manner. There are though exceptions, as all lawyers are aware, where for example the court has to endure a theatrical, antagonistic and wordy performance from an expert but, nevertheless, remains willing to be persuaded that there is some essential truth to be heeded in that expert's evidence.

Other Evidence

You will probably have to hear other evidence in the case. You may have to listen to the plaintiff to hear what he has to say in the witness box. If it helps you then make notes of what he says. If you have any relevant comment to make then make notes of your comments and ensure that they are given to the solicitor who instructed you.

Equally you will probably have to hear the evidence of other medical witnesses perhaps for both sides. Where opinions differ there is a temptation for feelings to run high. That must not happen. Again, in paying attention to what is said you may want to make notes. If you have relevant comments make a note of your point and pass it to the solicitor.

In order that you can hear the evidence that is relevant make sure you are seated in a position where you can hear and see what is going on. If you have a problem in that respect then make sure you tell the solicitor.

Your role is concluded at the trial when you reach the point where your lawyers indicate as much. They may have to ask the judge for his leave to release you from further attendance as a witness. Do not depart from the trial without making sure that it is appropriate for you to do so.

Of course having left the trial you probably will not at that stage have found out how the medical issue was resolved by the judge. If the result of that issue is of interest then arrange with the solicitor to be informed later of what happened, but remember that sometimes it may be more comfortable not to know.

CHAPTER 17

The Legal Basis of Medical Negligence

B. Knight

In virtually all systems of law, there is a presumption that every inhabitant must take reasonable care not to injure his neighbour. If he fails to do this, he may fall foul of the State by committing an offence under the criminal law – or be liable to the injured neighbour in a civil action. In countries with an Anglo-Saxon system of law, such as the UK, North America and most of the Commonwealth, such a civil action will lie within the law of "tort". A "tort" may be simplistically defined as a "civil wrong", a dispute between two parties, one of whom claims that the other has caused him damage.

Negligence is a limitless field, the essence being that there has been a breach of a duty to take care, resulting in damage. Medical negligence is in no way different to any other type, except that that it occurs in the context of diagnosis and treatment. The legal aspects are identical whether it be a crane-driver allowing a sack of flour to drop upon a stevedore or a surgeon carelessly ligating a ureter.

Applying the general legal definitions, one can identify four essential components of negligence, medical or otherwise. It must be emphasised that all four must be present and proven before the patient-plaintiff can succeed in his action against the doctor-defendant:

1. The doctor must have had a duty of care to the plaintiff
2. There must have been a breach of that duty
3. The plaintiff must have suffered damage
4. The damage must be a consequence of the breach of the duty of care.

As these elements are central to the whole concept of medical negligence, each must be looked at in depth.

The Duty of Care

A doctor has a duty of care to his patient, but the definition of *who* is his patient needs exploration. Certainly in law, the whole general public are not a given doctor's patients, even though there may be strong ethical reasons why a doctor should always render medical help to anyone in urgent need – and, of course, an

NHS general practitioner has a *contractual* duty to treat any emergency within his practice area. Naturally, any person on a formal medical list or in an institution such as a hospital or clinic to which the doctor has a contract of employment, or his private patients are the people to whom the doctor owes a direct duty of care.

Much more informally, the doctor also owes a full duty of care to anyone he *intends* to diagnose and treat, irrespective of any contractual obligation, receipt of a fee, etc. Immediately the doctor decides to give medical care to a person, a full doctor-patient relationship is established, with which goes a duty of care and the responsibility to exercise prudent medical behaviour. Not only need there be no formality or fee, but the "patient" may not even be aware of the doctor's existence. For example, at the scene of an accident, a passing doctor may find that the victim is deeply unconscious, but once he bends down to assist that victim, he assumes a duty of care and is fully liable for the result of any negligent act, unless some statutory provision exists to indemnify him.

The establishment of a duty of care tends to shade off into a grey zone where the doctor's ministrations blend into what might be called purely social relationships. If a doctor at a dinner party or a golf club casually answers a friend's request on how best to treat a headache, then whether or not that person can sue the doctor if they suffer a violent idiosyncratic reaction to the recommended aspirin, would have to be tested in each individual case. *Prima facie*, it would seem that he does have a duty of care.

Every person seen by a doctor does not necessarily remain as his patient indefinitely. If a doctor has an individual on a practice list or sees a private patient regularly or on a number of occasions, the last not too remote, then that patient can legitimately claim that the doctor had a continuing duty of care; but if a person was seen only once and/or a considerable time previously, so that it could not be said that the same disease process was under supervision, the doctor may well have no duty of care remaining. He could not be held liable for an act of omission in declining to attend that patient on a later occasion. Even where one person is undoubtedly a doctor's patient, there can be occasions where the doctor's refusal or inability to attend when required need not be negligent; for example, if another patient had a greater medical need at the same time.

Apart from certain contractual obligations in the National Health Service, a doctor has no obligation to accept any new person as his patient and therefore need not set up a duty of care at the person's demand. Apart from the ethical aspects mentioned earlier, a doctor can ignore the needs of any sick person on the road, in an aircraft or even one calling at his private surgery. Indeed, the medico-legal risks of emergency treatment, especially in road accidents, were formerly so great in the United States that many State Legislatures had to bring in "Good Samaritan" laws to indemnify physicians, so that they would no longer refuse to stop to render assistance at the roadside.

A duty of care may not be set up in certain situations where the doctor is not acting in his capacity as a "healer", but for other reasons, usually at the behest of a third party. Medical examination for acceptance for life insurance is a common example, as would be a "medical" for employment or the armed forces. Port health and immigration examinations, admission to prison and several other situations are similar. The police surgeon examines both victims and accused persons on behalf of law enforcement agencies; medical experts examine for injury or disability assessment and community physicians, research workers and occupational health physicians make examinations during various surveys.

The common factor is that the examining doctor is not acting in the immediate and personal interest of the person examined, who can thus not truly be called a "patient". The nature of these examinations should always be explained, so that the person is under no misapprehension as to the purpose of the procedure. Though no "healing" duty of care is set up, the doctor still has a duty not to harm the patient, such as breaking off a needle in the arm during a venepuncture. He cannot be sued in tort for misdiagnosis etc., though the commissioning third party could bring an action for breach of contract if, for example, an insurance doctor recommended a poor risk person for a large life insurance, or a medical expert gave a totally erroneous prognosis in a personal injury case, so that the quantum of damages was wrongly calculated.

However it may be established, the duty of care owed by a doctor to his patient is not of a fixed level. There is certainly a minimum standard, which is set by the final examinations of the medical school which accredits new doctors and which is monitored by the supervisory registration or licensing authority, such as the General Medical Council in Great Britain.

A house officer or intern must display a standard of care and proficiency which can reasonably be expected of such a junior doctor, working under the supervision of his seniors. He obviously cannot be expected to have the knowledge and experience of a professor or consultant. Should something go wrong, it will be matter of fact, judged by peer review, as to whether he could have been expected to avoid or deal with that situation at his level of expertise. At the same time, no junior doctor must hold himself out to his patients as possessing the attributes of a more senior doctor. If he does, and something goes wrong, he will then be judged at the level of what he professed himself to be capable of, rather than at his true station in the hierarchy.

Thus a doctor must be competent and also diligent, which are two different qualities. In a notorious (and thankfully rare) instance of criminal medical negligence in 1925, where Dr. Bateman was accused of causing the death of a woman in labour by performing a grossly traumatic forceps delivery when he was drunk, the judge stated that:

> If a person holds himself out as possessing special skill and knowledge, he owes a duty to the patient to use diligence, care, knowledge, skill and caution in administering treatment. No contractual relationship is necessary nor is is it necessary that the service be rendered for reward. The law requires a fair and reasonable standard of care and competence. If the patient's death has been caused by the defendant's indolence or carelessness, it will not avail to show that he had sufficient knowledge; nor will it avail to prove that he was diligent in attendance if the patient has been killed by his gross ignorance and unskilfullness". (*Rex* v. *Bateman* [1925] 94 LJKB 791.)

No doctor is expected to possess the available knowledge of his specialty, nor be able to apply all known diagnostic and therapeutic techniques. However, a doctor of a particular grade is expected to have a standard of knowledge and proficiency commensurate with his status. He should be aware of all major advances in his branch of medicine, but need not be familiar with all the recent literature, such as the contents of last week's *British Medical Journal*. For example, a patient being transfused during an operation had his arm extended and abducted for several hours, developing a brachial palsy as a result. The patient sued the anaesthetist, pointing out that the dangers of this technique had been published a few months earlier in *The Lancet*. The anaesthetist admitted that he had not read the article, and the patient won his case. However, it was reversed by the Appeal Court, where it was said that doctors did not have to read and follow every article in the medical press, but should adopt proven techniques when they became standard practice. (*Crawford* v. *Board of Governors of Charing Cross Hospital* [1953] CYL 2518 CA; *The Times*, 8 December 1953.)

The Breach of the Duty of Care

Over 150 years ago, the proper standard for a doctor's work was addressed by Chief Justice Tyndall, who said:

> Every person who enters into a learned profession, undertakes to bring to it a reasonable degree of care and skill. He does not undertake, if he is an attorney, that at all events, you shall gain your case. Nor does a surgeon undertake that he will perform a cure – nor does he undertake to use the highest degree of skill. There may be persons who have a higher education and greater advantages than he has, but he undertakes to bring a fair, reasonable and competent degree of skill. (*Lamphier* v. *Phipps* [1838] 8 C&P 475.)

A medical practitioner breaches his duty of care to his patient when he fails to reach the standard of skill which is required of him. This may be either because he is ignorant or incompetent (though he should not then have passed his finals and become registered) or because from carelessness, indifference, fatigue or even illness or intoxication, he does not apply his skill. An exceptionally talented doctor may be negligent if be does not apply sufficient of that talent, but conversely, an inadequately trained or inexperienced doctor may be negligent even if he strains his insufficient skills to the utmost. The decision as to whether the doctor was in breach of his duty of care is determined by peer review. Other doctors with knowledge of the same field of practice give their opinion as to whether the actions of the doctor, in the particular circumstances applying at the time, were consistent with the practice of a responsible body of doctors. This is the well-known "Bolam test", named after a negligence case in 1957. Here the judge, Mr Justice McNair, said that

> A doctor is not guilty of negligence if he has acted in accordance with a practice accepted as proper, by a responsible body of medical men skilled in that particular art. (*Bolam* v. *Friern Hospital Management Committee* [1957] 2 All ER 118; 1 WLR 582.)

It should be noted that there need not be universal (nor indeed even a majority) approval of the doctor's actions, only that "a responsible body" of opinion agrees with him. In a Scottish case, it was said that

> In the realm of diagnosis and treatment, there is ample scope for genuine differences of opinion and one man clearly is not negligent merely because his conclusion differs from that of other professional men, nor because he has displayed less skill or knowledge that others would have shown. The true test for establishing negligence is whether he has been proved to be guilty of such failure, as no doctor of ordinary skill would be guilty if acting with ordinary care. (*Hunter* v. *Hanley* [1955] SLT 213; 1955 SC 200.)

The Bolam principle is crucially important to the medical profession, as it lays down the vital fact that a doctor's professional behaviour is to be judged by other doctors, not lawyers, politicians or administrators. There is increasing criticism and indeed, antagonism to this right to peer review, especially in the United States, where the courts wish to accrete more power to themselves in this respect. Thankfully in Great Britain, the principle has been upheld time and time again, yet a judgement of the House of Lords in 1985 (in the Sidaway case, which concerned informed consent), the first signs of hardening of judicial attitudes was apparent when the word "rightly" was slipped into the Bolam principle. This indicated that in the future, the courts would reserve the power to over-rule peer review, if they felt that even the opinions of a responsible body of doctors were untenable in the eyes of the law. (*Sidaway* [1985], *The Times*, 22 February 1985; Annual Report, Medical Protection Society, London, 1985, p.17.)

Almost any diagnostic or therapeutic procedure in medicine is a potential source of negligence. One is reminded of the apochryphal "Murphy's Law", which says that "Anything than can go wrong, eventually will go wrong!". The same law was propounded in a more legalistic fashion by an eminent English judge, who made the now famous observation that "The categories of negligence are never closed". This indicated that one can never compile a complete catalogue of negligent acts, in medicine or any other sphere of activity, because as medical techniques increase in number and develop in complexity, so further opportunities for mishaps arise. It is therefore futile in this chapter to even begin to enumerate the possible breaches of the duty of care, but experts in other chapters have discussed the potential hazards of their particular fields of medicine.

In general terms, a breach of the duty of a doctor to exercise reasonable care may be either an act of *commission* or of *omission*. Leaving an artery forceps in the abdomen or giving two incompatible drugs is a positive act, whereas failing to visit a genuinely sick child or omitting to have a radiograph taken where clinically indicated is an act of omission. If harm is a consequence, both types of behaviour may equally well constitute grounds for an action in negligence. Because such actions often come to notice a very long period following the actual mishap, care must be taken to assess the circumstances as they were at that time, and not at the time of trial, which may be many years later. With the rapid advances in medical techniques, the peer review system must be operated in retrospect and the disputed event evaluated by medical knowledge and attitudes of the time.

Negligence Versus Error of Clinical Judgement

By no means all medical mishaps are negligent. Indeed, taking overall the things that go wrong in hospitals, clinics and general practice every day of the year, only the tip of the proverbial iceberg ever surfaces as grounds for patient's complaints. Of these, only a small minority ever turn into legal actions, and of these, only 4%-5% ever reach a court of law, the rest being either abandoned or settled.

A large proportion of medical errors are never recognised as such by patients or their bereaved relatives and we have the anomalous situation where many marginal and indeed, trivial or mischievous allegations are pursued with vigour, yet many undoubted acts of incompetence and error are met with sincere thanks and gratitude by uncomprehending patients and their relatives.

On the other side of the coin, much that is presumed to be negligent by patients, their families and the community at large (especially the popular media) is non-negligent mishap, which is no one's fault whatsoever. Medicine is a biological science combined with a therapeutic art and can never have the exactness of mechanical engineering, architecture or other more precise fields of activity. As yet another senior judge said in a famous dictum "doctors cannot be insurers", guaranteeing a perfect cure or result. As long as a doctor meets the requisite standard of care commensurate with his station in the medical hierarchy, by showing sufficient skill, knowledge and application, he cannot be guilty of negligence, however disastrous the result.

Medical treatment is not yet a contractual obligation, such as a builder enters into when he agrees to construct a house to certain specifications. If he falls short of the desired and agreed result, the client can sue him, but a doctor can never offer a warranty of a perfect, even acceptable result. So many extraneous and untoward factors enter the process of diagnosis and treatment; even the plastic surgeon who agrees to a mammoplasty can never exclude the occurrence of a fatal pulmonary embolism from silent deep vein thrombosis following the operation, however rare it might be.

Thus the common misapprehension amongst the public that most undesirable complications must somehow be the fault of the doctor, is quite unfounded. Even if the doctor makes what in retrospect, was an error of judgement, that is not necessarily negligent. If he was diligent, employed the correct diagnostic procedures, but in good faith drew the wrong conclusion from a set of alternatives or did not employ the optimum treatment, he may still have made only an error of clinical judgement, rather than been negligent. It is not sufficient for the plaintiff to claim that some other doctor, especially one of greater professional status, would have done it differently and achieved a better result. If peer review is of the opinion that a substantial body of similar doctors would have acted in that way under those particular circumstances, then the patient cannot succeed in his action.

The Patient Must Suffer Damage

The third element of medical negligence is that some injury, disadvantage or damage must befall the patient. Even if there is a clear duty of care and the facts prove that a breach of that duty occurred, the patient-plaintiff still cannot recover any compensation unless he can show that damage was suffered.

As an extreme, rather facetious example, a patient might attend a doctor complaining of a wart on the back of her hand. After examination, the doctor hands her a bottle of concentrated sulphuric acid and advises swabbing the wart with this twice a day. Outside the surgery, the patient decides that the doctor is an idiot and declines to apply the treatment. Thus she has suffered no damage and by rejecting his advice, cannot sue the doctor for negligence; except perhaps on the flimsy grounds of mental anguish or perhaps having suffered a delay in obtaining proper treatment.

The Damage Must Flow from the Breach of the Duty of Care

It is not sufficient for the patient to claim that damage followed the alleged negligent act – it must be proved that the damage was a *consequence* of that act. This is the thorny problem of "causation", so dear to the hearts of civil lawyers. It has arisen in many major medical negligence cases, especially those involving drugs and vaccines, where a direct link between the administration of those substances and some congenital or neurological disaster may be vehemently in dispute.

As will be discussed below, in civil cases causation must be proved "on the balance of probabilities", meaning that the damage was more likely than not to have flowed from the breach of duty of care. This can be very difficult in some instances, though the burden of proof is far lighter than that in the rare criminal medical negligence cases, where the causative link must be proved "beyond reasonable doubt". As with the fact of breach of duty of care, causation can only be settled by peer review by medical experts, with the court (if the dispute reaches that stage) acting as umpires.

Often the causative link is obvious to everyone: if a doctor performing a pituitary function test mistakenly injects 20 times the intended dose of insulin and the patient dies in hypoglycaemia within hours, the issue of causation will not detain the lawyers for long; neither would it if a patient requiring amputation of the left leg, emerges from hospital with the right leg missing.

On the other hand, if the connection between the doctor's act of commission or omission is too remote, or if the damage would have been inevitable, irrespective of the doctor's actions, then the patient cannot succeed at law. An example of the last was where an Accident and Emergency doctor declined to see three nightwatchmen complaining of stomach-ache and sickness, telling a nurse to refer them to their GPs. All three were suffering from acute arsenical poisoning, but the widow of one who died failed when she sued the doctor, as her husband would have died whether he had been seen by the doctor or not. (*Barnett* v. *Chelsea and Kensington Hospital Management Committee* [1969] 1 QBD 428; [1968] A11

Novus Actus Interveniens

No classical education is required to translate this legal term, which sometimes has a marked bearing upon either the culpability of a doctor or the compensation awarded to a patient. It is sometimes hard to differentiate from the next issue, that of contributory negligence, but really means that some extraneous factor intervened. For example, a surgical registrar, attempting to suture a cut tendon at the wrist, made such a poor job of it that later, a consultant hand surgeon was required to undertake a corrective operation. Due to his own error, the consultant transected the radial artery and caused severe damage to the hand. The potentially actionable negligence of the junior doctor was swamped by the later disaster and any disability the patient might have had from the poor tendon repair would have been overtaken by the gross loss of function caused by the new intervening act.

In another leading case, a man fell from a ladder and cut his leg, due to the negligence of his employers. He went to his doctor, who gave him anti-tetanus serum without a test dose. The man developed severe encephalopathy 9 days later, which left him severely disabled. He sued both employer and doctor, but the courts (including an Appeal) dismissed the doctor from the suit, even though the employer claimed that his actions were a "novus actus" which removed their responsibility. The judges indicated that as the encephalopathy did not appear for 9 days, a test dose, even if it had been given, would not have contraindicated the giving of ATS. (*Robinson* v. *The Post Office* [1974] 2 A11 ER 574; [1974] 1 WLR 1176 CA.)

Contributory Negligence

If a doctor acts negligently and the patient suffers harm, the legal remedy may be markedly modified if the patient commits his own act of commission or omission which worsens the medical situation. This may be voluntary or involuntary, wilful or innocent. There have been examples of patients tampering with surgical wounds or dressings to delay healing or cause infection, in order to worsen the damage and increase the compensation. However, most contributory negligence arises from misunderstanding. A common one is the omission to return to the doctor, outpatients or a GP's surgery when directed to by the first doctor.

For example, a casualty officer may put on too tight a plaster, which leads to peripheral ischaemic damage, but had told the patient to return next day or go to see his GP. If they omit to do so, and the toes become gangrenous in a week, then all the damage consequent on the incorrect application of the plaster cannot be laid at the door of the first doctor.

Contributory negligence – in any field of tort, not just medicine – is governed by statute, the Law Reform (Contributory Negligence) Act of 1945.

This provides that:

> Where any person suffers damage, partly as his own fault and partly as the fault of others, a claim in respect of that damage shall not be defeated by reason of the fault of the person suffering the damage; but the damages recoverable in respect thereof shall be reduced to such an extent as the Court thinks just and equitable having regard to the claimant's share in the responsibility for the damage.

Though generally, the onus of proof of negligence is on the plaintiff, if contributory negligence is alleged by the defendant, it is up to him to prove its existence, not for the plaintiff to have to deny it. He must show that the patient failed to take such care for his own well-being as a reasonable man would reasonably have been expected to take in those particular circumstances. Though this may not defeat the claim altogether, it may well appreciably reduce the damages, if it can be shown that the subsequent actions of the patient contributed to his eventual disability.

"Res ipsa loquitor", the Facts Speak for Themselves

The general principle in any civil action for negligence is that the patient-plaintiff must prove the facts alleged against the doctor-defendant, but one legal situation exists where the reverse is true, the defendant having to refute the allegation if he can. This is the "res ipsa loquitor" doctrine, where the facts appear so flagrant that no proof is required from the complainant. For example, where the wrong patient, side or digit is operated upon or where instruments or swabs are left in the abdomen, this doctrine may be invoked, though not necessarily so, as there may he some good medical reason, such as an untoward complication, which made a rapid wound closure urgently necessary.

The doctrine may be especially useful to the plaintiff where he cannot identify any individual doctors or other staff as being the person(s) responsible. The whole team or their employing hospital, has to try to explain how the undesirable event came about, rather than sit back and let the plaintiff attempt to prove his case against each individual.

Lord Justice Denning put the matter clearly in a case where a patient went into hospital to have treatment for a Dupuytren's contracture and was discharged in a worse state. The judge said:

> The plaintiff would have been unable to prove that some particular doctor or nurse was negligent, but he was not put to that impossible task. He said "I went into the hospital to be cured of two stiff fingers and came out with four stiff fingers, my hand being useless. That should not have happened if due care had been used – explain it if you can." (*Cassidy* v. *Ministry of Health* [1951] I A11 574; [1951] 2KB 343 CA.)

Damages

"Damages" are financial compensation and must, of course, be distinguished from "damage" which has been discussed above. The object of a civil action in tort is to obtain financial compensation which will, as far as is possible, restore the injured party to the condition in which he was before the tort occurred. Money cannot replace a wrongly amputated arm or revive brain function after anaesthetic hypoxia, but it can help to restore the quality of life or in the event of fatal negligence, support the family of the lost bread-winner.

Damages fall into two main categories, "general" and "special". General damages are those awarded for what might be called the subjective effects of the injury. These consist of pain and suffering, loss of enjoyment and quality of life, loss of the function of the damaged part of the body, loss of expectation of longevity, secondary effects on the remaining physical and mental health, etc. These less tangible and measurable factors are often the subject of legal wrangling, compared with the more calculable items in special damages. All kinds of losses may be claimed, many legitimately. A former music lover may have been rendered deaf by a surgical mishap and thus has lost the enjoyment of that particular pleasure. An attractive spinster may have been facially or bodily disfigured and thus her expectations of a favourable marriage may have been reduced. A keen sportsman may not be able to follow his favourite pastime, and many other deprivations consequent on medical negligence may be pleaded.

Special Damages

Special damages are usually larger than general damages, as here the process is an actuarial exercise to quantify the financial consequences of the injury. They include medical expenses, the costs of remedial treatment, costs of modifying the life style (such as a disabled person having to move from a house to a bungalow), but may be overshadowed by the costs of 24-hour nursing attendance for the rest of life.

Even more commonly, the largest element may be for loss of both past and expected earnings, where death or severe disability has occurred and there are dependent relatives. This exposes the fallacy of believing that there is a fixed tariff for any anatomical part, even though in general damages there may well be a relatively modest compensation for loss or damage to various organs or limbs. An eye is not just worth X thousand pounds and a hand Y thousand. It is to whom the eye or hand is attached, that constitutes the major consideration. The eye of an expert diamond cutter is worth far more than one belonging to a jobbing gardener, and cutting the finger tendons of a professional concert pianist is very much more costly than the same injury in an auctioneer.

The projected salary or private earnings until retirement is a major factor in calculating special damages, so it is far less expensive to iatrogenically damage a postman of 62, rather than a 30-year old merchant banker. Past pecuniary loss will be paid with interest, though complex calculations are necessary for the computation of anticipated income, perhaps over 40 years, with allowance being made for salary increments, inflation and other factors. The length of time for which he or she will have dependent spouse, children and others, will also enter the equation. These days, the estimation of the quantum of a claim for both special and general damages is a profession in itself, with loss assessors expert in gathering up every compensatable item, from estimating the expense of maintaining a garden where the householder has been rendered incapable, to the cost of enlarging doorways for a wheelchair. The claim will then be either the subject of negotiation between the lawyers for each party - or, in the few cases that go to trial, be awarded by the judge after he has considered all the circumstances.

Trial by jury in negligence cases is now virtually unknown in the British Isles. It survived until very recently in Northern Ireland and the Irish Republic, but even there has been largely abandoned, much to the relief of organisations such as the Medical Protection Society, who indemnify doctors against damages and legal costs. A jury was almost always far more sympathetic to the plaintiff than a judge sitting alone.

In the UK, the damages are paid as a lump sum, no satisfactory system of phased payments having yet been accepted. This not infrequently leads to unintended consequences, when a huge sum, perhaps approaching a million pounds sterling, is paid to the victim of a neurological catastrophe - yet within a short period the patient dies, leaving money intended for many years' nursing care and other support in the hands of the relatives, with no mechanism for restoration to the defendant.

Who Is Sued?

Anyone can serve a writ on another, but the matter will not get very far unless the case has substance. A patient-plaintiff can choose who to sue, though sometimes, the problem is in choosing the right target, especially where a large medical team have participated in treatment and the alleged culprit(s) may be hard to identify. It is here that the doctrine of "res ipsa loquitor" may be useful, as explained earlier.

Otherwise, the patient can sue a single doctor, or more than one or a partnership or the employer of the doctor(s). If the doctor is a private practitioner or, in the UK, a general practitioner contracted to the Health Service, the target is obvious, as the doctor is personally liable, together with any partners. In a private hospital, the hospital owners are liable, but depending on the contractual relationship of their medical staff, this may or may not extend to those doctors. Some may be full employees, especially more junior staff, but others may be consultants or contractors, where there is no "master-servant relationship". However, both hospital and doctors can be sued severally or jointly by the plaintiff.

If a defendant feels that he is either not liable at all or jointly liable with another doctor or a hospital, clinic, etc. he can pull them into the action by means of "third party proceedings". Alternatively, if he loses the case, he can bring his own action against them to try to obtain a financial contribution from them.

The time limit for bringing a legal action for personal damages, which includes medical negligence cases, is theoretically 3 years from the time of the event. However, especially in medical suits, the 3 years does not begin running until the patient discovers the damage, which might not become apparent until years after the "limitation period" has expired.

In the cases of "infants" under 18 years of age, the time does not begin running until they reach the age of majority, so damage to a newborn may still be open for litigation almost 21 years later.

In addition to these statutory limitation periods, the courts have a wide discretion, which they often exercise, to allow actions that are "out of time" to be brought. These facts make it all the more imperative for doctors to keep good clinical notes on all their patients and for both they and hospitals and clinics to retain records for a considerable number of years.

Medical Liability and Indemnity

Doctors may be servants, contractors or independent entities. Where a doctor is a salaried employee of a hospital, Health Authority, commercial firm or public corporation, he is a servant of that employer. This is important, because the concept of "master-servant relationship" then operates, under which the employer is liable for the torts of his employees. In the British National Health Service (NHS) hospitals, doctors have a contract of service with the Health Authority, Health Board or whatever administrative structure operates the hospital. The doctrine of "master and servant" then ensures that the employer is responsible for the negligent acts of its servants, which includes porters, nurses, technicians and doctors of all grades.

Until 1 January 1990, the NHS had an agreement with the doctor's protection and defence societies that the medical staff would hold personal insurance to indemnify themselves and the hospital for that part of any negligence that was due to the doctors, whilst the hospitals would carry the risk for all other staff. The object of doctors preferring to carry their own risks was originally due to their intense desire to preserve clinical freedom, as they felt that if the employer paid their damages, he could also dictate the way they worked. In 1990, this agreement ceased, mainly because both employer and employee found the costs of indemnity had escalated so much. Now the "master-servant" relationship has returned under so-called "Crown Indemnity", but this applies *only* for NHS hospital and community health staff carrying out their contractual duties. General practitioners are not included, as they are independent contractors, providing their services on a capitation basis to Family Practitioner Committees, so they are not servants and have to arrange their own indemnity.

Under the law on partnership, two or more partners are considered to be one legal "person", much as a limited company or "plc" is regarded as a single entity. Thus all the members of a partnership are equally liable for the negligence of one of them, even if they were at the other ends of the earth when the trouble occurred. It is common, when establishing a partnership in general practice or private clinic, for the members to include an indemnity agreement, whereby a "guilty" partner will recompense the others if he causes them to suffer damages for negligence.

Any private practitioner must carry his own risks, which includes any NHS doctor working outside his contract, such as locum appointments, Category Two (i.e. medico-legal) work and any voluntary or emergency aid, including "Good Samaritan" acts at the roadside. Crown Indemnity is strictly limited to legal aid and payment of damages from negligence arising from contractual obligations; it does not cover any other type of medico-legal problem, such as coroner's inquests, disciplinary enquiries, General Medical Council matters, criminal negligence, other forms of malpractice, courts martial, etc., so all doctors should still ensure that they have obtained medical protection of sufficient degree from one of the mutual societies.

Subject Index